PRINCIPLES OF GERIATRIC NEUROLOGY

CONTEMPORARY NEUROLOGY SERIES AVAILABLE:

Fred Plum, M.D., *Editor-in-Chief*
Series Editors: Sid Gilman, M.D.
Joseph B. Martin, M.D., Ph.D.
Robert B. Daroff, M.D.
Stephen G. Waxman, M.D., Ph.D.
M-Marsel Mesulam, M.D.

PRINCIPLES OF GERIATRIC NEUROLOGY

ROBERT KATZMAN, M.D.
Professor
Department of Neurosciences
University of California, San Diego
La Jolla, California

JOHN W. ROWE, M.D.
President
Mount Sinai School of Medicine
The Mount Sinai Hospital
New York, New York

 F. A. DAVIS COMPANY • Philadelphia

Printed in the United States of America

Last digit indicates print number: 10 9 8 7 6 5 4 3 2 1

NOTE: As new scientific information becomes available through basic and clinical research, recommended treatments and drug therapies undergo changes. The author(s) and publisher have done everything possible to make this book accurate, up to date, and in accord with accepted standards at the time of publication. The authors, editors, and publisher are not responsible for errors or omissions or for consequences from application of the book, and make no warranty, expressed or implied, in regard to the contents of the book. Any practice described in this book should be applied by the reader in accordance with professional standards of care used in regard to the unique circumstances that may apply in each situation. The reader is advised always to check product information (package inserts) for changes and new information regarding dose and contraindications before administering any drug. Caution is especially urged when using new or infrequently ordered drugs.

Library of Congress Cataloging-in-Publication Data

Katzman, Robert.
    Principles of geriatric neurology / Robert Katzman, John W. Rowe.
       p. cm. — (Contemporary neurology series ; 38)
    Includes bibliographical references and index.
    ISBN 0-8036-5232-1 (hardbound : alk. paper)
    1. Geriatric neurology. 2. Nervous system—Aging. I. Rowe, John W. (John Wallis),
  1944– . II. Title. III. Series.
    [DNLM: 1. Nervous System Diseases—in old age. W1 CO769N v. 38 / WL 100 K194p]
RC346.K373 1991
618.97′68—dc20
DNLM/DLC
for Library of Congress   91-28286
                                                 CIP

PREFACE

During the twentieth century, the number of people over 65 years of age in the United States will increase tenfold. This is a measure of the success of today's medicine in treating and preventing acute diseases, especially infections, cardiovascular disease, and strokes. This very success, however, has created new problems. With the increase in the number of the very elderly (over 75), there has been a resultant increase in the occurrence of age-related chronic diseases. The consequent problems range from accelerating social and economic costs to the frustration of physicians caring for patients whose disease and disability progress despite the physician's best efforts. As doctors who care for the elderly—whether our training has been in neurology, psychiatry, internal medicine, family practice, or geriatrics—we can no longer pass off these diseases as inevitable consequences of aging; we need to begin to apply the same analytical clinical and experimental approaches to these diseases that have been successful in other aspects of medicine. The need for similar attention to understanding the diseases of aging also exists for other health professionals who care for the elderly, such as nurses and nurse-clinicians, physician associates, psychologists, gerontologists, and even nursing home administrators.

Geriatric neurology as a body of knowledge and as a discipline needs input from both neurologists and geriatricians. We have attempted to incorporate both disciplines in this book. Chapters 2, 4, 7, 8, 10, and 13 are revisions and extensions of chapters in *The Neurology of Aging*, edited by Drs. Katzman and Terry.* Chapters on neuroimaging by Dr. Duara and on neuropsychologic assessment by Drs. Butters and Salmon are wholly new additions to this neurologic point of view. Drs. Salzman, Besdine, Dicks, Lipsitz, Johnson, Resnick, and Rowe have added important insights from geriatricians working with neurologic problems. Thus we hope to combine the efforts of these two points of view in this new monograph.

Throughout this book there has been particular emphasis on Alzheimer disease. We recognize that more than half (perhaps two thirds) of those in nursing homes suffer from senile dementia, usually due to Alzheimer disease. Indeed, Alzheimer disease is the third most important

---

*Katzman, R and Terry, RW (eds): *The Neurology of Aging*. FA Davis, Philadelphia, 1983.

chronic disease after cancer and cardiovascular and cerebrovascular disease.

However, many of the other major problems of the very old—difficulty in walking, falls, urinary incontinence, defective temperature regulation, sleep disorders, loss of hearing, and in many instances impaired vision— also result from disease of the central or peripheral nervous system. Our understanding of the processes involved in these disorders is still in the early stages, but a body of knowledge has developed (and is now rapidly expanding) which we believe will be helpful to the physician and health professional. This book is intended to provide both background and practical information in these many regards to all the several kinds of health workers involved in the care and study of the elderly.

We wish to thank Robert Davignon and Linda Weinerman for their skilled assistance in editing the entire volume for the authors.

ROBERT KATZMAN, M.D.
JOHN W. ROWE, M.D.

CONTRIBUTORS

Richard W. Besdine, M.D.
Professor of Medicine
Travelers Professor of Geriatrics and
    Gerontology
Director
Travelers Center on Aging
University of Connecticut Health
    Center School of Medicine
Farmington, Connecticut

Nelson M. Butters, Ph.D.
Chief
Psychology Service
San Diego Veterans Administration
    Medical Center
Professor in Residence
Department of Psychiatry
University of California, San Diego
    School of Medicine
La Jolla, California

Robert S. Dicks, M.D.
Assistant Professor of Medicine
Assistant Director, Geriatric
    Fellowship Program
Travelers Center on Aging
University of Connecticut Health
    Center School of Medicine
Farmington, Connecticut
Director of Geriatrics
Hartford Hospital
Hartford, Connecticut

Ranjan Duara, M.D.
Medical Director
Wien Center for Alzheimer's Disease
    and Memory Disorders

Mount Sinai Medical Center
Miami Beach, Florida
Associate Professor
Radiology and Neurology
University of Miami School of
    Medicine
Miami, Florida

Palmi V. Jonsson, M.D.
Reykjavik City Hospital
Reykjavik, Iceland

Robert Katzman, M.D.
Professor
Department of Neurosciences
University of California, San Diego
    School of Medicine
La Jolla, California

Lewis A. Lipsitz, M.D.
Irving and Edyth S. Usen Director of
    Clinical Research
Hebrew Rehabilitation Center for the
    Aged
Roslindale, Massachusetts
Assistant Professor of Medicine
Harvard Medical School
Boston, Massachusetts

Neil M. Resnick, M.D.
Chief of Geriatrics
Director
Continence Center
Brigham and Women's Center
Harvard Medical School
Boston, Massachusetts

John W. Rowe, M.D.
President and Professor
Departments of Medicine and Geriatric
    Development
Mount Sinai School of Medicine
The Mount Sinai Hospital
New York City, New York

David P. Salmon, Ph.D.
Assistant Professor in Residence
Department of Neurosciences
University of California, San Diego
    School of Medicine
San Diego, California

Carl Salzman, M.D.
Associate Professor of Psychiatry
Harvard Medical School

Director of Psychopharmacology
Massachusetts Mental Health Center
Boston, Massachusetts

Robert Terry, M.D.
Professor
Department of Neurosciences
University of California, San Diego
    School of Medicine
La Jolla, California

Leslie Wolfson, M.D.
Chairman
Department of Neurology
University of Connecticut School of
    Medicine
Farmington, Connecticut

CONTENTS

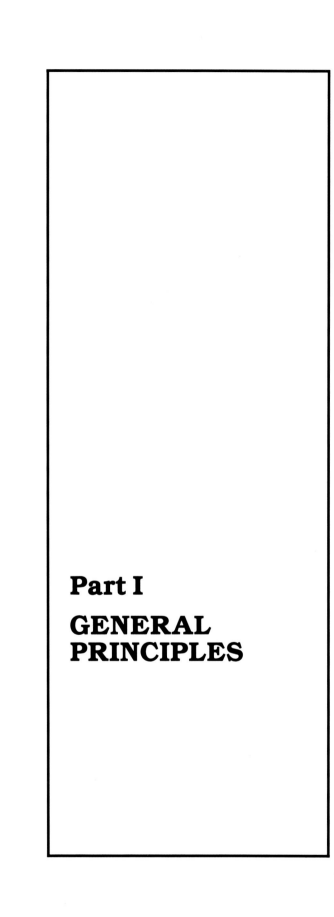

Part I
GENERAL PRINCIPLES

Chapter 1

PRINCIPLES OF GERIATRICS AS APPLIED TO NEUROLOGY

John W. Rowe, M.D., and
Robert Katzman, M.D.

THE CHANGING DEMOGRAPHY OF
  AGING: IMPACT ON THE RELATIVE
  PREVALENCE OF DISEASES OF
  THE NERVOUS SYSTEM
THE PHYSIOLOGY OF AGING
SUCCESSFUL AND USUAL AGING AS
  SUBTYPES OF "NORMAL" AGING
THE INTERACTION BETWEEN
  PHYSIOLOGIC CHANGES AND
  DISEASE IN THE ELDERLY
ILLNESS BEHAVIOR IN THE
  ELDERLY
THE IMPORTANCE OF FUNCTIONAL
  CHANGE WITH ADVANCING AGE
AN APPROACH TO COMPREHENSIVE
  FUNCTIONAL ASSESSMENT OF
  THE ELDERLY
THE ROLE OF THE GERIATRIC
  NEUROLOGIST IN THE 1990s

The recent surge of interest in gerontology and geriatrics parallels the increase in the elderly in the US population. The number of persons over age 65 rose from 3 million in 1900 to 25 million in 1980, an eightfold increase. Census bureau projections indicate that there will be 31 million persons over age 65 by the year 2000. This demographic shift has serious implications for our social security system and has led to the rapid growth of retirement communities for the well elderly and nursing homes for those with chronic disease. An even more striking phenomenon has been the increase in the over-age-75 population—the "old-old" in the new jargon. There were 900,000 individuals over age 75 in the United States in 1900, a number that had grown to 10 million by 1980, an 11-fold increase, and that will exceed 13 million by the year 2000.[24] Brody and Foley[4] project that by the year 2050 "50% of the population will survive to their 85th birthday and in that year the population aged 85 and over will constitute at least 15 million people." Thus, interest in the neurology of aging is understandably a recent development.

A series of articles by Critchley[8] in the *Lancet* in 1931 appears to have been the first attempt to examine the topic in a systematic fashion. Earlier, Clarke[7] authored the Bradshaw Lecture on "The Nervous Affections of the Sixth and Seventh Decades of Life," an article interesting chiefly as a historical curiosity, since the diseases of late middle age of most concern to Dr. Clarke included tuberculous meningitis, neuroses, hysteria, and neurasthenia! Current concepts of neurology have thus evolved in this century. In contrast, Critchley's emphasis on the gross and microscopic changes associated with the "senile brain," the clinical aspects of dementia, and the changes in the neurologic examination in the aged remain pertinent today.

THE CHANGING DEMOGRAPHY OF AGING: IMPACT ON THE RELATIVE PREVALENCE OF DISEASES OF THE NERVOUS SYSTEM

The demography of aging has become important for neurologists and others interested in disease processes associated with aging, because prevalence and clinical presentations reflect both the total number of elderly persons and the age distribution within the over-65 segment of the population.

Anthropologic and historical data suggest that both the life expectancy and total possible life span of humankind were fairly constant for at least 100,000 years, until the 19th century. Cutler[10,11] estimates that 100,000 to 200,000 years ago *Homo sapiens* developed a maximum potential life span of just over 100 years, a span that has since remained constant (the oldest proven life span is said to be 120 years).[26] Despite the evolution of such a life span, actual life expectancy was significantly shorter. In the harsh environment of prehistoric times, life expectancy is estimated to have been about 30 years, varying in different societies from the mid-20s to 40 years.[10,11,27] Surprisingly, there was little increase in life expectancy during eras when civilization flourished, as in the classical Greek and Roman periods.

It was not until the 19th century that a significant change in life expectancy began to occur, one that accelerated at the turn of the century and continued to the mid-1960s. This change reflected the recognition, understanding, and conquest of bacterial and some viral infections. Fatal infections of childhood, adolescence, and adult life have become increasingly rare. In the mid-19th century a newborn child in the United

States could expect to live 40 years; in 1900, 49.2 years; in 1964, 70.2 years[31,36]; in 1978, 74 years[37]; and in 1986, 76 years.[38] The death rate at age 30 was 10 times greater in England in 1820 than it was in the United States in 1975 (Fig. 1–1). As fatal disease of the young was eliminated, a significant difference in male and female life expectancies became apparent; in the United States in 1980, life expectancy of a newborn girl was 77.5 years and a newborn boy 70.0 years. The survival curve of women in the United States is now beginning to approach the ideal limit that would be reached if the only deaths before senium were those attributed to accidents and trauma (Fig. 1–2).

In the mid-1960s a number of writers noted that although life expectancy had greatly increased if measured from birth, only minimum gains in expectancy had been made for persons over age 65. Cardiovascular disease had re-

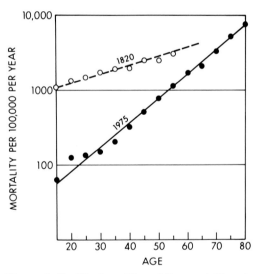

Figure 1–1. The logarithm of the mortality rate is a linear function of age. The data labeled 1820 represent the mortality data in Northhampton used by Gompertz in his first calculations of the mathematical relationship of mortality rate and age.[14a] The data labeled 1975 represent the US mortality figure (entire population) for that year.[36] Note that in persons age 30 the death rate in 1820 was *10 times* that of 1975. Note also that the two lines converge at advanced ages. (From Katzman and Terry,[21] p 5, with permission.)

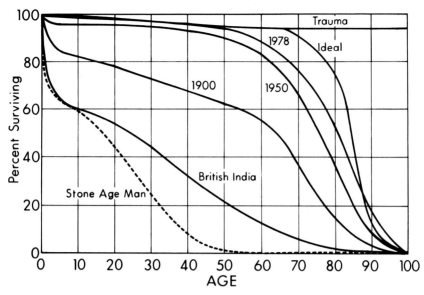

Figure 1–2. The marked shift in survivorship that has occurred during this century. The estimates of Stone Age man and of British India in the early part of this century are from Comfort.[7a] The curves labeled 1900, 1950, and 1978 represent survival curves for women in the United States.[36,37] The ideal curve represents the estimated survival curve if death were due to physiologic aging and trauma.[16] Note how closely survivorship of women in the United States in 1978 approaches the ideal curve. (From Katzman and Terry,[21] p 6, with permission.)

placed infections as the number one cause of death in the elderly, and mortality due to cardiovascular disease had actually increased in the 1950s and early 1960s.[36] Hence, the possibility of significantly increasing life expectancy within the aged population seemed dim.

It has turned out, however, that the pessimism of the 1960s was premature. In the years 1966 to 1979, a rapid and significant fall in the death rate of the elderly became evident and was most pronounced among those over 85, with a drop of more than 2% per year.[33] This decrease was due in part to the continued success in containing the death rate resulting from winter influenza epidemics, but it predominantly reflected a decrease in the incidence and death rate of cardiac and cerebrovascular disorders.[12,13,36,37] During the period from 1980 to 1986, the death rate in the over-85-year-olds appeared to decline at a slower pace[38] using traditional vital statistics tables, but a more complete analysis of recent trends needs to be undertaken.

THE PHYSIOLOGY OF AGING

Over recent decades, increasing interest in aging and the medical problems of older persons has fueled substantial growth in physiologic, psychologic, and sociologic research on aging. Investigators involved in such studies recognize the critical importance of separating pathologic from age-related changes. Thus, for physiologic studies, careful guidelines are developed to exclude individuals whose results might not represent "normal" aging, but rather changes related to specific disease processes. Results on the remaining population are believed to represent "normal" aging, with confidence regarding the age relatedness of the findings resting more on longitudinal studies of age changes than on cross-sectional comparisons of age differences, which are sensitive to cohort and other effects. Numerous studies on carefully screened, well-characterized populations have demonstrated major effects of age on a number of clinically relevant variables, including hearing, vision, renal functions, glucose tolerance, systolic blood pressure, bone density, pulmonary function, immune function, sympathetic nervous system activity, and a variety of cognitive and behavioral measures. Such nonpathologic aging effects are important to understand not only as reflections of the aging process but also because they serve as a physiologic substrate for the influence of age on the presentation of disease, as reflections of response to treatment and the complications that ensue.

The decline in most variables that change with age is linear into the eighth and ninth decade. Although healthy 80-year-olds have accumulated more of the changes secondary to aging than their younger counterparts, they are not losing function at a more rapid rate.

Although many important physiologic variables, including cardiovascular, immune, endocrine, renal, and pulmonary functions show fairly substantial losses with advancing age, an important characteristic of these data sets is their substantial variability. With regard to physiologic factors, the variance often increases with advancing age so that older people are less like each other, not more like each other. In many data sets in which the average change in the aged group is a very substantial decrement from the results seen in youth, one can easily find some older persons with minimal or no physiologic loss when compared with the average younger person.

Age-related changes in one organ or organ system are not necessarily predictive of changes with age in other organs. If an apparently healthy 60-year-old is found on serial prospective measurements to have a glomerular filtration rate that is declining at a certain slope, this information is of no value in predicting the rate at which the individual's pulmonary or immune function or that of any other organ is changing over time. This apparent failure of various organs to be synchronized in their age-related changes is evidence against the presence of a central biologic clock. In other words, currently, one cannot construct a "functional age" variable that is composed of the results of several age-sensitive measures that predicts performance on a separate age-related physiologic or psychologic test better than the individual's chronologic age.

SUCCESSFUL AND USUAL AGING AS SUBTYPES OF "NORMAL" AGING

Although it has served gerontologic research well, the focus on dichotomizing findings into either disease or normal aging categories has important limitations. This approach tends to neglect the previously discussed substantial heterogeneity among older persons with regard to many physiologic and cognitive variables. It tends to imply that the physiologic changes that occur in older individuals in the absence of disease are harmless and do not carry a significant risk, and, finally, the identification of certain physiologic changes as normal suggests that these changes are the natural state of affairs and, thus, cannot or should not be modified.

A growing body of evidence indicates that the physiologic changes of normal aging in the absence of disease, in addition to being quite variable, are in many cases associated with substantial attributable risk for adverse health events and are potentially modifiable. The contribution of the intrinsic aging process to decrements observed in aging populations may be substantially less than previously recognized with factors such as personal habits, diet, exercise, nutrition, environmental exposures, and body composition playing important roles in modifying or aggravating the effect of the aging process per se.

Rather than focusing purely on differentiation of the effects of disease versus normal aging, gerontologic studies should recognize that the normal aging group includes two important subsets. One subset is composed of those individuals who demonstrate minimal age-associated losses in a given physiologic function (e.g., immune function, bone density, carbohydrate tolerance, renal function, and cognitive function). These individuals might be viewed as aging "successfully" with regard to the particular variable under study. Individuals who demonstrate successful aging in a constellation of physiologic functions rather than just one, present a state of minimal physiologic loss and robust physiologic function in advanced age, a pure aging syndrome. This successful aging group currently represents a small but potentially increasing portion of the overall normal aging population, the bulk of which is represented by the group that might be termed "usual" aging. For a given physiologic variable, the usual aging group has significant impairments compared with their younger counterparts, but these impairments are not so severe as to qualify as diseases. Examples of usual aging would include mild increases in systolic blood pressure, postprandial blood glucose, or obesity, or decreases in renal or pulmonary function. As noted previously, the physiologic losses in the usual aging group display large interindividual differences and those individuals with the greatest usual "age effect" are at increased risk for the emergence of a specific disease or disability.

We should also be aware that older persons who display usual aging for a given function may be able to improve their function and thus potentially reduce their risk of adverse outcomes. Thus, the focus of study moves gradually from the evaluation of the emergence of diseases in an aging population to elucidation of those factors that regulate the transition of individuals from a successful to a usual state of aging and vice versa.

With these general considerations in mind, the specific physiologic changes associated with normal aging will be reviewed from the perspective that they can be considered to fall into a number of specific categories regarding the relationship of aging and the emergence of disease.

THE INTERACTION BETWEEN PHYSIOLOGIC CHANGES AND DISEASE IN THE ELDERLY

Physiologic Variables That Do Not Change with Age

From a clinical standpoint, perhaps the most important physiologic change that occurs with age is no change at all. Too frequently, clinicians are apt to ascribe a disability or abnormal physical or laboratory finding to old age, when the actual cause is a specific disease process. An example of this lack of change may be seen in hematocrit. Frequently, elderly individuals will be found to have low hematocrit levels, and the clinician will categorize the patient as having "anemia of old age." The physician may fail to pursue the underlying basis of the anemia, believing that the normal aging process had induced the anemia and that no investigation or treatment is warranted. However, data from several sources, including the Framingham study, indicate that in healthy, community-dwelling elderly people there is no change with age in hematocrit.[15] Thus, a lower hematocrit in an elderly individual cannot be ascribed to "anemia of old age," but deserves a proper investigation and treatment.

Physiologic Changes by Which Specific Diseases Become Less Likely or Less Severe with Age

Although aging is characteristically considered to be associated with a greater prevalence or severity of disease, it is quite possible that the physiologic changes associated with normal aging result in more diseases being less likely or less severe in advanced age. *Disorders based, at least in part, on altered immune system response, such as systemic lupus erythematosus, myasthenia gravis, and multiple sclerosis (MS), are seen more commonly or are clinically more severe in younger individuals than in older individuals.* It is feasible that the changes that occur in the immune system with age might result in a less robust immunologic response to the inciting agent or event in these disorders.[14] In this regard, recent findings of increased auto-anti-idiotypic antibody production with age suggest a basis for lessened autoimmune disease in the elderly.

Another example of a disease that may often run a less virulent clinical course in the elderly than in younger adults is carcinoma of the breast. Many cancer specialists feel that carcinoma of the breast has a more aggressive natural history in premenopausal than in postmenopausal women. In addition, the likelihood of breast carcinoma responding well to hormonal therapy increases with the number of years after menopause.

Physiologic Changes That Alter the Presentation of a Disease

This poorly understood area has long been recognized as having major importance to the practice of geriatric medicine. Many diseases that occur in both young and old adults have manifestly different clinical presentations and natural histories in the two age groups. These disorders should not necessarily be looked on as being less severe or more severe in the elderly, but just *different.*

One example of a common disorder that presents very differently in the elderly compared with the young is uncontrolled diabetes mellitus. In children and young adults, uncontrolled diabetes is generally manifested by diabetic ketoacidosis, with elevations of blood glucose to levels between 300 and 500 mg/dL and coincident severe metabolic acidosis associated with markedly elevated levels of circulating ketones. Conversely, elderly individuals with uncontrolled diabetes will frequently present with hyperosmolar nonketotic coma, altered consciousness, striking elevations of blood glucose (often to levels exceeding 1000 mg/dL), and a relative or absolute lack of circulating ketones or acidosis.

Impaired Homeostasis in the Elderly: Physiologic Changes That Increase the Likelihood or Severity of a Disease (Age-Related and Age-Dependent Disorders)

This category encompasses the previously described age-related reductions in the function of numerous organs that place the elderly person at special risk of increased morbidity from diseases in those organs.

As discussed earlier in this chapter, there is no pleasant plateau of the middle and late years during which physiologic function is stable; instead, there is a progressive age-related reduction in the function of many organs, including major losses in renal, pulmonary, and immune functions. Simultaneous linear reductions in homeostatic capabilities in several organs result in a geometric reduction in the total homeostatic capacity. When coupled with the functional impairments associated with disease states, this constricted homeostasis is responsible for the markedly increased vulnerability of the elderly to morbidity during acute illness or trauma, major surgery, or administration of medications.

One example of the clinical importance of age-related normal physiologic change is the impact of age on the course of bacterial pneumonia. Acute bacterial pneumonia is more likely to induce serious clinical manifestations in the elderly because of the markedly lessened physiologic reserve. Healthy individuals in the ninth decade of life frequently will have lung function equal to only one half of their 30-year-old counterparts. In addition, over the past decades, significant advances have been made in our understanding of marked reductions in immune competence that occur with age. Immunosenescence is likely responsible, in some ways, for the increased severity of infections in the elderly. Thus, an elderly individual with pneumonia not only is more likely to become hypoxic but also is less likely to contain and control that infection in the respiratory tract than a young individual.

In addition to altering the severity of a disease, aging changes may increase disease prevalence. In this regard, the distinction between age-dependent and age-related diseases, highlighted by Brody and Schneider,[5] is useful. As they point out, morbidity and mortality from *age-dependent* diseases and disorders (e.g., coronary artery disease) increase exponentially with advancing age. *Age-related* diseases and disorders, such as MS and amyotrophic lateral sclerosis (ALS), increase in frequency to a "specific age and then decline in frequency or continue at less than an exponential rate of increase." These authors present a model that relates "aging processes to age-dependent diseases and disorders such as Parkinson's and Alzheimer's diseases." According to this model, age-dependent losses occur in either cell number or cell function of specific critical cell populations. With aging, individuals within the population at large reach a threshold for susceptibility to age-dependent diseases such as Parkinson disease (PD) and Alzheimer disease (AD). Subgroups at increased risk may either "lose cell numbers or cell function of specific critical cell populations at a faster rate or are born with either fewer functioning cells or have

been exposed to environmental insults." However, in the case of idiopathic PD there is clear-cut pathologic evidence of an active neuropathologic process leading to the cell death of dopaminergic neurons (as determined by a more than sixfold increase in phagocytosing microglia in the substantia nigra [SN] of PD brains[25]) superimposed on any loss of dopaminergic cells that may occur as part of normal aging.

Postencephalitic parkinsonism may represent an example in which an "environmental" factor interacts with aging processes to increase the prevalence of a disease. It is well established that aging is associated with a significant progressive reduction in basal ganglia dopamine content. During the 1920s, an epidemic of viral encephalitis, which may have begun during the 1918–1919 influenza epidemic but was termed *von Economo's encephalitis*, swept the western world, only to disappear by 1930. This encephalitis often left devastating changes in the form of cell destruction in the SN and neurofibrillary tangles (NFT) in the midbrain. The result was a most severe form of parkinsonism often associated with eye movement disorders and oculogyric crises. These symptoms, however, often occurred or became more intense years after the acute viral infection and in the absence of an ongoing viral infection. The aging process apparently added to the neuronal destruction wrought by the virus, leading to delayed onset and later progression of the extrapyramidal symptoms.

Another example whereby age-related alterations in function increase the prevalence of a disease is accidental hypothermia in frail elderly. This disorder has a high mortality rate and occurs not only in individuals exposed to unheated rooms in the winter, but also in elderly individuals in heated rooms who appear to spontaneously develop marked lowering of body temperature. Essentially absent in healthy young individuals, accidental hypothermia occurs with increasing frequency with advancing old age. Although the underlying mechanisms are poorly understood, alterations in sympathetic nervous system responsiveness seem likely to be a major contributor.

Herpes zoster is an excellent example of a nonfatal age-related neurologic disorder that may occur as a consequence of the aging of the immune system. Herpes zoster, or shingles, is a viral disorder ordinarily affecting a single dorsal root ganglion, which leads to a vesicular eruption in the dermatome supplied by the dorsal root ganglion, with consequent severe pain due to the involvement of the ganglion itself. Occasionally, the infection also involves adjacent spinal cord segments. It is now known that herpes zoster virus is identical to the varicella virus that produces chicken pox during childhood. Present evidence suggests that when we first contract chicken pox, the varicella virus enters our body and may be incorporated within the genome of many cells.[18] However, it does not express itself as herpes zoster until later in life, displaying typical age dependence as shown in Figure 1–3. Factors leading to the activation of herpes zoster are unknown, but are assumed to involve immune mechanisms, because the virus commonly becomes active during immunosuppression. Thus, the substantial decline in immune competence during aging may contribute to the onset of

herpes zoster. One mechanism of immunologic activity change during aging is an actual increase in the activity of suppressor T cells.[2,28] An important recent finding is that lesions in the anterior hypothalamus lead to a reduction in the proliferative response of T cells, independent of any effect of hypothalamic lesions on hormones.[9] It is interesting to speculate whether changes in the anterior hypothalamus that may occur with aging might ultimately be involved in the changes that lead to the expression of herpes zoster in the absence of exogenous immunosuppression.

There are other instances where this model of age-disease interaction pertains. For example, in Chapter 8 we will discuss a subgroup of elderly patients whose brains at autopsy show features such as neuritic plaques (NP) and NFT but who had shown neither clinical nor neuropsychologic features of dementia prior to death. In these patients, the large neurons in association neocortex, a class of cells at particular risk in AD, were much greater in number than in demented AD brains and also somewhat greater than the number in age-matched control brains. However, other mechanisms can lead to an apparent age dependence; an example is 1-methyl-4-phenyl-1,2,5,6-tetrahydropyridine (MPTP) parkinsonism. MPTP, an analogue of meperidine and synthesized as a "designer drug," produced an epidemic of parkinsonism in young drug addicts.[22] Subsequent studies both of individuals exposed to this toxic drug and of experimental animals have shown that, indeed, this molecule produces a disorder that is an excellent model of "idiopathic" PD, both clinically and pathologically, as MPTP specifically destroys dopaminergic neurons in the SN compacta.[23] The molecule is converted by the enzyme monoamine oxidase B (MAO-B), present in glial cells, to MPP+, the toxic metabolite of MPTP[6]; MPP+, in turn, is actively taken up by dopaminergic neurons, leading to cell death.

Brody and Schneider[5] cite MPTP par-

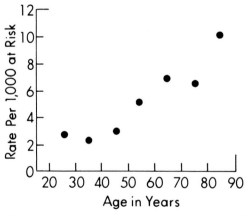

Figure 1–3. Herpes zoster as a function of age[21]. (Adapted from Hope-Simpson.[18])

kinsonism as an example of the potential importance of environment on an age-dependent disease. A more direct relationship to the aging process has been shown by the recent discovery that the amount of MPTP required to produce parkinsonian symptoms is greatly reduced in aging animals.[16,19] One might a priori have assumed that the greater sensitivity to the drug resulted from a decrease in functional reserve in the extrapyramidal system, perhaps due to loss of dopaminergic SN cells in normal aging. However, it has been found that the effect of aging in lowering the threshold to MPTP is due to the increased level of MAO-B in the basal ganglia. MAO-B is an enzyme whose concentration in the brain increases with normal aging.[32,34] The increased level of MAO-B, in turn increases the conversion of MPTP to MPP+. Thus, age-dependent MPTP susceptibility is apparently related primarily to an aging increase in a single critical enzyme rather than to the loss of nigral neurons that may occur during normal aging.[23] This basic research finding has led to the use of an MAO-B inhibitor (deprenyl) to slow the course of PD.[35]

Physiologic Changes That Mimic Specific Diseases

Some changes that occur with aging may be seen to mimic specific clinical entities, thus causing confusion regarding the diagnosis of specific diseases in the elderly. Perhaps the best and most widely recognized instance of this is the decrease in carbohydrate economy, reflected in a decreased performance on oral or intravenous glucose tolerance tests, that occurs with advancing age in the absence of diabetes mellitus. A substantial body of evidence indicates that the defect is in part due to age-related postreceptor decreases in insulin action and in part due to the "usual" aging effects associated with obesity, sedentary life style, improper diet, and use of diabetogenic

medications. If the hyperglycemia of aging is not taken into account, normal older individuals may be incorrectly diagnosed as diabetic.

Physiologic Changes That Have a Direct Clinical Impact

As noted previously, for many decades gerontologists and geriatricians have drawn a clear line between the changes that occur with age and those associated with specific disease states. We have staunchly defended the view that aging is not a disease but a normal process that must be clearly understood to adequately diagnose and treat the increasing burden of illness that will befall a rapidly enlarging aging population. Substantial data in several different areas suggest that this approach is no longer tenable. There is no question that some physiologic changes of aging are not harmless, but rather have adverse clinical sequelae.

Although one can argue about the specific criteria for the definition of a "disease," one generally acceptable definition would include any process that results in adverse clinical sequelae measured as either morbidity or mortality. Under this definition, there are clear changes that occur with advancing age that appear to be normal characteristics of the aging process and that would also qualify as diseases. Of the potentially long list of such processes, three will be briefly reviewed.

More than any other biologic change, menopause seems to be accepted as age-related. Although menopause is thus clearly "normal," it has become abundantly clear that this normal change is associated with an increased risk for certain diseases such as osteoporosis and atherosclerosis as well as for symptomatic clinical manifestations such as hot flashes, which are associated with sleep disturbances and in many individuals are so frequent and severe as to be disabling.[17]

A second change that occurs with normal aging and has direct adverse clinical consequences is cataract formation. Posttranslational modification of central lens proteins with advancing age results in an increasing opacity as well as a decreasing flexibility of the lens, which is manifested as a reduced capacity to accommodate to near vision.[39] The reasons for the development of cataracts in some individuals and not in others are poorly understood. Lens opacification or cataract is a common cause of blindness in older Americans, although new operative procedures and lens implants reduce the disability from this disorder. Thus, this normal age-related change, in its most extreme form, would seem to clearly represent a disease treated by a surgical procedure.

A third characteristic type of change with advancing age that would appear to have direct clinical consequences is arteriosclerosis. This thickening of the walls of major arteries must be distinguished from atherosclerosis, which represents the development of plaques on the vessel intima that encroach on the lumen. Arteriosclerosis appears to be a normal consequence of age-related changes in the extracellular material in arterial walls and is reflected in decreased compliance and increased stiffening of vessels with advancing age.[29] This is manifested in increased systolic blood pressure.

ILLNESS BEHAVIOR IN THE ELDERLY

Underreporting of Illness

An important factor underlying functional impairment in the elderly is the failure of many persons to seek assistance. Studies in several countries with varying health care systems indicate that symptoms of serious and treatable diseases often go unreported. Health problems reported by frail elderly persons are thus frequently only the tip of the iceberg of treatable illness.

This apparently self-destructive behavior springs from the notion on the part of older people that advanced age is necessarily accompanied by illness and functional decline and that many symptoms are thus to be expected rather than treated. Other contributing factors include cognitive impairment; fear of the nature of the underlying illness; and concern about the costs and other negative aspects of hospitalization, diagnostic evaluation, or treatment.

As Besdine[3] has pointed out, nonreporting of symptoms of underlying disease in elderly persons is an especially dangerous phenomenon when coupled with the passive American organizational structure of health care delivery, which lacks prevention-oriented or early detection efforts. He notes that aged persons, burdened by society's and their own ageist views of functional loss with aging, cannot be relied on to initiate appropriate health care for themselves, especially early in the course of an illness.

Multiple Diseases

The coexistence of several diseases has a profoundly negative influence on health and functional independence in the elderly. The number of pathologic conditions in a person is strongly related to age. Elderly persons who live in the community have 3.5 important disabilities per person,[1] and the hospitalized elderly have evidence of six pathologic conditions per person.[40] The entire array of diseases present in an individual patient must be considered as treatment plans are developed.

Atypical or Altered Presentation of Disease

A fundamental principle of geriatric medicine is that many diseases have signs or symptoms in the elderly that differ from those in their younger counterparts. These alterations can take two major forms. First, specific characteristic symptoms of a disease in middle age may be replaced by other symptoms in old age. For instance, in acute myocardial infarction (MI), some studies have suggested that elderly persons are less likely than younger adults to present with chest pain.[30] On the other hand, acute MI is not silent in older persons; instead, they have a variety of other acute signs and symptoms, including syncope and the sudden onset of left ventricular failure. The second difference is that elderly persons may present with nonspecific signs and symptoms, such as confusion, weakness, weight loss, or "failure to thrive," instead of specific symptoms indicating the organ or organ system affected.

THE IMPORTANCE OF FUNCTIONAL CHANGE WITH ADVANCING AGE

The emphasis in the provision of health care to the elderly should be on maintaining functional capability. Although most older Americans living in the community are cognitively intact and fully independent in their activities of daily living, a substantial portion of elderly patients who are not institutionalized report major activity limitations due to chronic conditions. Major functional impairment is clearly age related within the elderly, increasing from approximately 5% of individuals age 65 to 74 requiring assistance in basic activities to nearly 35% to 40% by age 85. Even if one maintains functional independence into old age, the risk of becoming frail for a long period is still high. For independent persons between the ages of 65 and 70 years, "active life expectancy," that portion of the remaining years characterized by independence, represents about 60%, a portion that falls to 40% at age 85.

Although a complete and precise diagnosis list is essential, the functional impact of each diagnosis should be evaluated. Specific diagnoses often have little relation to functional status, and the length of the diagnosis list provides little insight into the specific needs and capabilities of the elderly pa-

tient. Too often a long diagnosis list provides physicians a bias that the patient is multipy impaired and frail, although this may not be the case at all. Thus, diagnoses themselves are often a weak criterion for assessing the health care needs of the elderly.

An important advance in recognition of the need for data regarding functional status in the elderly came from the relationship of functional status to diagnoses and morbidity. As reviewed by Manton,[27] the World Health Organization has proposed a model that describes the linkages among mortality, disability, and morbidity. Although it is clear that the overall mortality experience of the elderly population has an underlying curve or morbidity experience in which individuals accumulate diseases and losses in specific capabilities, the specific interactions between the development of diseases and the subsequent development of disability have not been elucidated. It is particularly important to recognize that many different pathologic processes may result in, or contribute to, identical functional impairments. Within a given elderly individual, several coincident pathologic processes interact in a complex fashion to result in disability. This interaction is often strongly influenced by other factors, particularly in the psychosocial sphere.

A major policy issue relates to the importance of clarifying the relationship between changes in the mortality experience of the elderly population and coincident changes in the underlying morbidity and disability experiences. A controversial issue of major importance for health policy is whether future increases in longevity will be associated with prolongation of dependency or whether active life expectancy will increase ("compression of morbidity"[12]) as health promotion and disease prevention strategies become increasingly effective. The initial claim that as mortality declines morbidity will also decline has recently been challenged by studies suggesting that the increased life span of the "old old" is not accompanied by decreased morbidity and may actually result in more dramatic increases in the need for health care services.

AN APPROACH TO COMPREHENSIVE FUNCTIONAL ASSESSMENT OF THE ELDERLY

Evaluation of the elderly patient must focus on what the patient can do, relative to what the patient should be able or wishes to do and on identification of recent functional deficits that may be reversible. Because elderly persons are especially vulnerable to loss of functional capacity arising from the interaction of medical problems with adverse economic, psychologic, and social pressures, data must be collected in all these domains.

The history taking and physical examination can be difficult in the elderly, as compared with younger patients. Dementia (in 10% of the elderly), impaired hearing (in 22%), and visual handicaps (in 15%) limit communication. Effective history taking demands increased skill, time, reliance on significant others, and use of medical records that place the patient's current symptoms in perspective. Physical examination may be time consuming and tedious, especially in the office setting, because of decreased mobility and the increased length of time required for the patient to disrobe.

One must obtain a thorough medication history and be aware of the special vulnerability of the elderly to the development of adverse effects from medication. Special consideration should be given to the detection of thyroid, breast, and cervical cancer; occult bleeding; hypertension; postural hypotension; disease in the oral cavity that may impair nutritional status; wax impaction in the ears that may limit hearing; and serious auditory or ophthalmic disorders. Attention should be paid to bowel function and the possible presence of varying degrees of urinary incontinence and sleep disturbance. Specific questions regarding postural stability are mandatory in view of the high prevalence and serious consequences of falls in the elderly.

A reliable, easily administered, brief examination of mental status provides valuable data regarding the mental status of elderly persons whose apparently slight cognitive impairment may be incorrectly labeled as "normal" for their age.[20] Patients with well-developed social skills who are not subjected to objective mental status testing will often not appear to have as much of a defect in mental function as is actually present. In such cases, the health care provider may not identify mental failure or dementia as a specific problem, and potentially reversible underlying causes, such as drug intoxication, hypothyroidism, azotemia, vitamin B_{12} deficiency, or depression may not be sought (see Chapter 3).

A third dimension of functional assessment is evaluation of the patient's social and economic status. The health care of elderly persons, perhaps more than any other age group, is influenced by the social support system available to them. The network of current and potential informal supports, such as family or friends, has an important role in modulating the clinical impact of underlying disease and is often the major determinant in decisions to institutionalize elderly people. For every impaired aged person in a nursing home there are approximately two equally impaired elderly people living in the community who remain there by virtue of the critical role of informal support systems. These informal support systems provide approximately 80% of their long-term care.

THE ROLE OF THE GERIATRIC NEUROLOGIST IN THE 1990s

The role of the neurologist in our society, traditionally that of the consultant, is undergoing a major change as neurologists increasingly assume responsibility for the continuing care of patients with chronic neurologic disorders. When such disorders constitute the principal health problem of patients, the neurologist becomes the *principal care physician,* a term espoused by Dr. William Landau and others. This term is appropriately descriptive of the neurologist's role in the care of such patients, although it is a term not yet accepted by the public health policy community. The role of the neurologist as a principal care physician is most clear-cut in geriatric neurology and best illustrated in patients with dementia, PD, and stroke. As the principal care physician, the geriatric neurologist must not only diagnose and prescribe medication, but must also counsel the patient and family in regard to the patient's prognosis and daily health care; special treatment facilities available in the community including day care programs, home health and attendant services, residential and nursing facilities; legal and fiscal planning (e.g., durable power of attorney for health and finances); local support groups; and other community resources. An obligation of a neurologist assuming the role of the principal care physician is to follow the patient at regular intervals in order to anticipate and prevent crises, rather than simply react to them.

In some major academic centers and teaching hospitals, there is a multidisciplinary geriatric "team" consisting of internists (geriatricians), neurologists, psychiatrists, psychologists, nurse practitioners, social workers, occupational or physical therapists, and nutritionists. The existence of a team implies that examination and information about a patient will be gathered by several members of the team, not only from the patient but also from the family or caregiver and often including a home visit. The home visit permits the visiting home doctor to identify problems in interpersonal relationships within the family as well as environmental problems and to inspect the medicine cabinet and determine what drugs not usually considered as medication are being taken. The information obtained is then reviewed by the team as a whole who make diagnostic and management decisions. This model often works very effectively if the team is flexible and well coordinated. The patient and family are then provided with accurate diagnoses, a management plan, and access to community resources. Such multidisciplinary geriatric teams, although highly visible, are few in number in the United States. In most situations, the principal care physician must undertake to provide the equivalent service, in part by assuming several of these roles as an individual and by helping to identify others within the community who can direct the patient and the patient's family to the available resources, which are often more extensive than generally realized.

CONCLUSION

The significant increase in life expectancy that began in the 19th century has affected the prevalence and clinical presentations of disease processes in the elderly population. It is important not only to differentiate "normal" aging from specific disease processes but also to recognize the two types of normal aging—"successful" versus "usual" aging. Physicians must become aware of the physiologic variables that do not change with age, those diseases that become more or less likely or severe with advanced age, and those physiologic changes of aging that alter the typical presentation of a disease. It is also important to recognize normal age-related physiologic changes that may mimic specific diseases or that have direct adverse clinical consequences. Appropriate diagnosis can also be hindered by underreporting of illness, coexistence of multiple pathologic conditions, and atypical presentation of diseases.

Maintaining functional capability in the elderly must be emphasized, and thus a comprehensive functional assessment—including history taking and physical examination, thorough medication history, brief mental status examination, and evaluation of socioeconomic status—is essential. When chronic neurologic disorders, such as dementia, PD, and stroke, constitute the principal health problem of elderly patients, the geriatric neurologist often acts as the principal care physician, and therefore must counsel the patient and family in a wide range of areas, direct them to appropriate community resources, and anticipate and prevent crises.

REFERENCES

1. Anderson, WF: The Prevention of Illness in the Elderly: The Ruthergien Experiment in Medicine in Old Age. Proceedings of a conference held at the Royal College of Physicians of London. Pitman, London, 1966.
2. Antel, JP, Weinrich, M, and Arnason, BGW: Circulating suppressor cells in man as a function of age. Clin Immunol Immunopathol 9:134–141, 1978.
3. Besdine, RW: Geriatric medicine: An overview. Annu Rev Gerontol Geriatr 1:135–153, 1980.
4. Brody, JA and Foley, DJ: Epidemiologic Considerations. In Schneider, EL (ed): The Teaching Nursing Home. Raven Press, New York, 1985, p 9.
5. Brody, JA and Schneider, EL: 1986 Disease and disorders of aging: An hypothesis. J Chronic Dis 39:871–876, 1986.
6. Chiba, K, Trevor, A, and Castagnoli, N: Metabolism of the neurotoxic tertiary amine, MPTP, by brain monamine oxidase. Biochem Biophys Res Commun 120:574–578, 1984.
7. Clarke, JM: The Bradshaw Lecture: Nervous affections of the sixth and seventh decades of life. Lancet 2:1016–1021, 1915.
7a. Comfort, A: The Biology of Senescence, ed 3. Elsevier, New York, 1979.
8. Critchley, M: The neurology of old age. Lancet 2:1119, 1221, 1331-1336, 1931.
9. Cross, RJ, Markesbury, WR, Brooks, WH, and Roszman, TL: Hypothalamic immune interactions. I. The acute effect of anterior hypothalamic lesions on the immune response. Brain Res 196:79–87, 1980.
10. Cutler, RG: Evolution of longevity in primates. J Hum Evol 5:169–202, 1976.
11. Cutler, RG: Evolution of human longevity: A critical overview. Mech Ageing Dev 9:337–354, 1979.
12. Fries, JF: Aging, natural death, and the compression of morbidity. N Engl J Med 303:130–135, 1980.
13. Garraway, WM, Whishnant, JP, Furlan, AJ, Phillips, LH, Kurland, LT, and O'Fallon, WM: The declining incidence of stroke. N Engl J Med 300:449–452, 1979.
14. Gillis, S, Kozak, R, Durante, M, and Weksler, ME: Immunological studies of aging: Decreased production of and responses to T cell growth factor by lymphocytes from aged humans. J Clin Invest 67:937–942, 1981.
14a. Gompertz, B: On the nature of the function expressive of the law of human mortality, and on a new mode of determining the value of life contingencies. Philos Trans R Soc Lond 513, June 9, 1825.
15. Gordon, J and Shurtleff, D: Means at each examination and interexamination variation of specified characteristics. In Kannel, WB and Gordon, T (eds): The Framingham Study: An Epidemiologic Investigation of Cardiovascular Disease. US Dept of Health, Education, and Welfare publication. NIH 74-478. US Government Printing Office, Washington, DC, 1973.
16. Gupta, M, Gupta, BK, Thomas, IR, Bruemmer, V, Sladek, JR, and Felten, DL: Aged mice are more sensitive to 1-methyl-4-phenyl-

1,2,3,6-tetrahydropyridine treatment than young adults. Neurosci Lett 70:326–331, 1986.

17. Hannan, JH: The Flushings of the Menopause. Bailliere, Tindall, and Cox, London, 1967, p 1.

18. Hope-Simpson, RE: The nature of herpes zoster: A long-term study and a new hypothesis. Proc R Soc Med 58:9–20, 1965.

19. Jarvis, MF and Wagner, GC: Age-dependent effects of 1-methyl-4-phenyl-1,2,3,6-tetrahydropyridine (MPTP). Neuropharmacology 24:581–583, 1985.

20. Kane, RA and Kane, RL: Assessing the Elderly: A Practical Guide to Measurement. Lexington Books, Lexington, MA, 1981.

21. Katzman, R: Overview: Demography, Definitions and Problems. In Katzman, R and Terry, RD (eds): The Neurology of Aging. FA Davis, Philadelphia, 1983, p 1.

22. Langston, JW, Ballard, P, Tetrud, JW, and Irwin, I: Chronic parkinsonism in humans due to a product of meperidine-analog synthesis. Science 219:979–980, 1983.

23. Langston, JW: Current theories on the cause of Parkinson's disease. J Neurol Neurosurg Psychiatry (special suppl):13–17, 1989.

24. McFarland, D: The Aged in the 21st Century: A Demographer's View. In Jarvik, LF (ed): Aging into the 21st Century: Middle Agers Today. Gardner Press, New York, 1978, p 214.

25. McGeer, PL, Itagaki, S, Akiyama, H, and McGeer, EG: Rate of cell death in parkinsonism indicates active neuropathological process. Ann Neurol 24:574–576, 1988.

26. McWhirter, N: Guinness Book of World Records, ed 27. Sterling, New York, 1989, p 24.

27. Manton, KG: Changing concepts of morbidity and mortality in the elderly population. Milbank Mem Fund Q 60:183–244, 1982.

28. Miller, AE, Neighbour, PA, Katzman, R, Aronson, M, and Lipkowitz, R: Immunological studies in senile dementia of the Alzheimer type: Evidence for enhanced suppressor cell activity. Ann Neurol 10:506–510, 1981.

29. O'Rourke, MF: Arterial hemodynamics in hypertension. Circ Res (suppl 2)27:123–133, 1970.

30. Pathy, MS: Clinical presentation of myocardial infarction in the elderly. Br Heart J 29:190–199, 1967.

31. Riley, MW and Foner, A: Decline of Functioning: Aging and Society. Russell Sage Foundation, New York, 1980, p 230.

32. Robinson, DS, Nies, A, Davis, JM, Bunney, WE, Davis, JN, Colburn, RW, Bourne, HR, and Shaw, DM: Ageing monoamines and monoamine-oxidase levels. Lancet 1:290–291, 1972.

33. Rosenwaike, I, Yaffe, N, and Sagi, PC: The recent decline in mortality in the extreme aged: An analysis of statistical data. Am J Public Health 70:1074–1080, 1980.

34. Strolin-Beneditti, MS and Keane, PE: Differential changes in monoamine oxidase A and B activity in the aging rat brain. J Neurochem 35:1026–1032, 1980.

35. Tetrud, JW and Langston, JW: L-Deprenyl as a possible protective agent in Parkinson's disease. J Neural Transm (suppl)25:1–20, 1987.

36. Vital Statistics of the US, 1975. Vol II, Mortality, Part A. US Dept of Health and Human Services, Public Health Service.

37. Vital Statistics Report. Final Mortality Statistics, 1978. US Dept of Health and Human Services, Public Health Service 29:1, 1980.

38. Vital Statistics Report, 1986. Vol II, Mortality. US Dept of Health and Human Services, Public Health Service, 1989.

39. Weale, RA: The Aging Eye. Harper & Rowe, New York, 1963.

40. Wilson, LA, Lawson, IR, and Brass, W: Multiple disorders in the elderly. Lancet 2:841–843, 1962.

Chapter 2

NORMAL AGING OF THE NERVOUS SYSTEM

Robert Katzman, M.D., and Robert Terry, M.D.

COGNITIVE CHANGES IN AGING
CLINICAL MEASURES IN NORMAL
  AGING
MORPHOLOGIC CHANGES IN
  NORMAL AGING
NEUROTRANSMITTERS

I am seventy-nine and would like to go on. It is still good to be alive, and I appreciate it every day. I am still curious about life, and I want to know how things will work out. It frustrates me to think my death will come, long before all kinds of interesting ideas now being formulated will be carried out. . . . I was an empire-builder in my own sphere of neurology, and knowing what I accomplished keeps me going now. Also, I know that I have been lucky in having been able to show what talent I had. I went out and I did something in the world. I was able to improve things. I know I didn't have all the answers, but I had some. I helped. . . . Some people get radical changes in the brain when they are old, and they are the geriatric tragedies. I have remained wonderfully well in this respect, but I have to admit that there comes a moment in research work when you simply can't do it, no matter how brilliantly you did it once. You have to tell yourself, No, you cannot do this work because you are old. You must not deceive yourself in these matters. Being old is the reason why you cannot take things in as you used to. . . . I'd read a paper when I was young and get the guts out

of it in an hour or less. Now I would have to read it three or four times and take days. My ability to acquire new knowledge is small or impossible, and I get into a remarkable mess over what I could do, and what I now cannot do. But I continue to work. There is a tendency to underestimate the energies of old age, which are considerable. You won't do what you could do, but yet you find that you need to do far more than society allows you to do.[21]

Normal aging of the nervous system, defined as *aging changes that occur in individuals free of overt diseases of the nervous system*, is characterized by slow, sometimes continuous changes in specific functions. A variety of studies have shown that there is little or no change with age in certain functions, such as store of information. In contrast, there is a continual loss in the speed of learning, speed of processing new information, and speed of reaction to simple or complex stimuli. There is a loss of sensory functions, especially vibration sense. Muscle strength and motor efficiency decrease. At advanced age, changes in posture and gait frequently develop. Minor changes in electroencephalogram (EEG), evoked responses, and perhaps cerebral blood flow may occur. Anatomically and biochemically, aging of the brain is characterized by the loss of a minor to moderate percentage of nerve cells in specific regions of the brain, loss of dendritic arborization, loss of enzymes involved in the synthesis of transmitters, and a moderate but definite loss of receptors for specific neurotransmitters.

These changes, although significant, are not functionally important in terms of ordinary living, social activities, or performance in occupation (an obvious exception being the athlete), until past the 75th year. Our concept of who is old has changed as more and more individuals have reached older ages free of disabling diseases. Mandatory retirement at age 65 has been abandoned: This arbitrary age has been pushed to 70 and will undoubtedly be raised further in coming decades. To an increasing extent, persons in their late 60s still have living parents, and as mortality in those over 85 continues to plunge, this phenomenon will increase, reducing the tendency to identify those in their late 60s with age. Gerontologists have recognized this phenomenon by subdividing the elderly into the *young-old,* under age 75, and the *old-old,* over age 75. But even in the old-old group, there are many individuals who maintain not only active, independent lives, but creative ones. There are numerous examples of artists, lawyers, musicians, physicians, politicians, and writers continuing to be productive in their careers in their 80s and 90s. The encroachment of specific disease processes is what produces much of the incapacity attributed to aging. This chapter examines the bases for these summary statements concerning normal aging.

COGNITIVE CHANGES IN AGING

The most intensively studied and best-documented aspects of normal aging are changes in intellect, memory, and other psychologic variables. These topics have occupied the attention of psychologists for several decades; the literature abounds with lively arguments concerning measurement techniques and the relative validity of cross-sectional versus longitudinal studies. But there now seems to be a growing consensus on which we can base the following general principles:

1. Intellectual performance as measured by tests of verbal abilities in vocabulary, information, and comprehension reaches a peak between age 20 and 30 and is then maintained throughout life, at least until the mid-80s, in the absence of disease.

2. Performance on timed tasks, including those requiring abstraction such as the Digit Symbol Substitution (DSS) test, and on other tasks requiring speed in processing information reaches a peak about age 20 and then declines slowly throughout life. Although part of this change may be attributed to alterations in motor or perceptual abilities, there now is unequivocal evidence that the speed of central processing is impaired with age. This change is noticed by almost all persons reaching their 70s. Yet, there is still an overlap, that is some 70-year-olds perform better than some 20-year-olds. This change probably affects the efficiency with which older adults can perform all realatively complex cerebral tasks, regardless of their nature (thinking, perceiving, remembering, and so on).

The Relative Preservation of Verbal Skills

Psychologists agree almost unanimously that scores on performance tests, especially of timed tasks, decline more rapidly with age than do scores on verbal tests. Disagreement exists, however, as to whether there is any loss of ability as a function of age on verbal tests until at least the mid-70s in healthy individuals. This disagreement is based on the differences in results obtained in cross-sectional studies, which, with one exception, show a small but significant and apparently continuous decline after age 30, and in results obtained in longitudinal studies, many of which show no decline until the 70s. One study showed no evidence of decline even to the early 80s.[7,11,12,88,153,182−184]

One of the most important, comprehensive, and statistically well-organized cross-sectional studies of intelligence was the 1955 standardization of the Wechsler Adult Intelligence Scale (WAIS).[217,218] The WAIS consists of a verbal scale and a performance scale. The verbal scale is based on tests of vocabulary, information, comprehension, arithmetic, similarities, and digit span; the performance scale is based on timed tests of picture completion, block design, picture arrangement, object assembly, and digit symbol substitution (DSS). In the 1955 standardization, a negative correlation between age in subjects over 25 and score was found, the correlation for the verbal scale being $r = -0.233$, whereas the correlation for the performance scale with age was $r = -0.509$.[218] In general, over the period from age 25 to 74 the mean in the verbal subtest scores fell less than 1 standard deviation (SD) (referred to the 25- to 30-year-old group), the mean scores on DSS fell 2 SD, and the mean score on the other performance subtests about 1 SD. Thus, the decline with age in the performance subtests was greater than in the verbal subtests, but most of this difference was attributed to the test most sensitive to changes in speed.

The WAIS standardization, however, confounds education and age. The stratified sample of 2175 subjects was chosen to reflect the US population in a number of important variables including age, education, and socioeconomic status. As a necessary consequence of this selection process, the formal education of younger and older subjects differed dramatically: over 65% of subjects 55 to 64 years of age had less than an eighth grade education compared with 18% of those 18 to 19 years of age.[217] Wechsler recognized that performance on many of the tests correlated with formal education, but he believed that age decrements were nonetheless real in the absence of proof to the contrary from longitudinal studies.[218]

There are now a number of longitudinal studies in which the subjects have been followed for periods of 7 to 41 years. For the most part, these studies show no decline with age in tests of vocabulary, information, comprehension, and other verbal skills until well past age 70, suggesting that the Wechsler findings did result from educational differences and were, therefore, cohort effects rather than aging effects. In a classic study[153] in 1950 and 1961, subjects originally tested in 1919 with the Army Alpha test as freshmen at Iowa State College were reexamined. From baseline at age 18 to 20 to retest at age 48 to 50, test scores *improved* in seven out of eight subtests, the improvement being significant at the $P < 0.01$ level in four subtests: information, practical judgment, synonym-antonym, and disarranged sentences. During the period from age 50 to 61, test results were stable. Similarly, when parents of gifted children were tested in 1940 and 1952 with a synonym-antonym test, an improvement in scores was obtained at the second testing when subjects were 36 to 53 years old.[14]

Similar findings were obtained in the National Institute of Mental Health (NIMH) longitudinal study in which a group of older male volunteers (primarily professional) were followed between 1956 and 1967.[88] The average age of the subjects was 70 at the first testing session and 81 at the last. The sample was small (only 19 remained in 1967), but the subjects were well studied. The results were striking: Vocabulary (and picture arrangement) scores actually improved over this 11-year period, six other WAIS subtests remained unchanged, as did the Raven Matrices, while the DSS subtests showed a decline (not statistically significant) and various other timed tests showed a significant decline (Table 2–1).

These longitudinal studies have been

Table 2–1 NIMH LONGITUDINAL STUDY

	Scores on Subtests	
	1956	*1967*
TESTS IMPROVED		
WAIS vocabulary	12.8	14.1*
Picture arrangement	6.4	7.7*
TESTS, NO CHANGE		
WAIS information	13.1	13.0
Comprehension	13.0	13.2
Similarities	10.2	11.6
Digit Span	9.4	9.2
Picture completion	7.9	8.8
Block design	8.3	8.2
Raven matrices	29.4	29.6
TESTS WITH DECLINE		
WAIS arithmetic	12.0	10.9
Digit symbol substitution	6.7	6.0
Draw-a-person	24.2	21.4*
Addition rate	0.9	0.8*
Arithmetic alternation rate	0.4	0.3*
Speed of copying words	35.0	29.1

*$P < 0.05$.
Source: From Granick,[88] p. 18, with permission.

criticized because of a high dropout rate. In the NIMH study, for example, only 19 of the 47 subjects originally tested in 1956 were available for retesting in 1967; 24 had died and 4 were unavailable for other reasons. Death is a hazard intrinsic to research into aging. Another criticism of these studies is that the subjects were of superior intelligence. There is evidence that attrition in longitudinal studies may be selective, leaving intellectually superior subjects in the study.[190] However, similar results have been obtained in other longitudinal studies using subject groups with different backgrounds, including a stratified sample of 380 individuals aged 50 to 75, representative of the population of Hamburg, Germany (using a German-language version of the WAIS)[165]; a sample of lower-middle-class residents of Bonn, Germany[207]; and a stratified sample of members of the Puget Sound Health Maintenance Organization.[182–185]

The last-named study is especially important because it combined a 14-year longitudinal study of 16 individuals with a cross-sectional study of another 2000 subjects at different intervals of time; together these studies constituted a cross-sequential paradigm. Neither the longitudinal study nor comparison in different years of independent samples *born* in the same period showed decrements in verbal and other abilities measured on the Primary Mental Abilities Test (with the sole exception of the timed-word fluency subtest); cross-sectional studies alone did show loss of function in all tests with age. Schaie and colleagues [181–184] concluded that the results of the cross-sectional studies reflected differing generations, cohorts, and years of birth, all with attendant educational and other cultural features characteristic of a group born in a given decade. Changes in test abilities between older cohorts and younger cohorts represent cultural or educational differences, not aging.

Schaie was so impressed with the maintenance of abilities in older subjects tested over the 14-year period that he described his results as "the myth of intellectual decline" with aging.[179] This bold assertion brought on a storm of objections from other psychologists who challenged his statistical analyses, as well as his reliance on a longitudinal study in which there were many dropouts.[97] Reanalysis of the data, using different statistical approaches to meet these objections, has resulted in essentially the same conclusion.[184,185]

Although it can be argued that in longitudinal studies, intact subjects are more willing to volunteer for reassessment of function, the conclusion must hold that a substantial proportion of subjects from a variety of socioeconomic backgrounds do not show a decline with aging, at least until age 70, in those functions measured by subtests of vocabulary, and in intellectual ability. These stable intellectual functions have been termed "crystallized" intelligence in contrast to other psychologic functions that may change more readily and are consequently labeled "fluid" intelligence.[34]

A loss in verbal performance by the mid-70s has been found in two longitudinal studies. In the Duke Aging Study, 98 subjects, aged 60 to 79, were followed for a 10-year period.[65] Subjects initially aged 60 to 69 showed no change in full-scale WAIS scores until past age 70, and then began to show some decrement primarily in the performance score; those initially aged 70 to 79 showed continuous decline in both verbal and performance scores. Similarly, a decline in function after age 75 in verbal tests was found in a subset of 35 subjects from the Kalman Twin Study, all of whom were restudied in 1955 and 1967 (Table 2-2).[20] Scores on the vocabulary and similarity subtests showed no change between 1947 (mean age 65) and 1955 (mean age 75), but did show a decrement between age 75 and 85. DSS showed an even greater loss.

These results contrast with those obtained in the NIMH study. In the latter study, subjects with early "senile" changes were excluded; this was not done in the Duke and twin studies. Thus, the loss of ability within these cohorts measured over time may reflect the earliest stages of beginning cognitive dysfunction associated, for example, with cerebral infarcts or Alzheimer

disease (AD). By the age of 85, over 25% of the population will have frank dementia. A longer follow-up of a much greater number of elderly would have to be carried out to determine whether this late cognitive decline is part of normal aging of the brain affecting most of the population, or warning of impending disaster affecting a significant but definable proportion of the sample. Preliminary evidence in support of this latter concept has been found in the Bronx Aging Study.[7] In a group of 434 ambulatory, nondemented lower-middle-class volunteers initially aged 75 to 85 years, 295 showed no change in WAIS scores over a 4-year period; the remaining individuals developed frank dementia or cognitive changes suggestive of early dementia.

Changes in comprehension of complex information in the elderly may be greater than changes on WAIS verbal scores. This was tested by using complex sentences, such as "the giraffe that bumped into the cow kicked the hippo," and making subjects enact the sentence using figures.[72] Subjects 74 to 80 years of age made about twice as many errors as subjects 18 to 25, or 63 to 69 years of age, although all groups had been matched in WAIS vocabulary scores and education. However, the distribution of errors among subjects in the 74- to 80-year-old age group was bi-

Table 2-2 EVIDENCE OF DECLINE IN FUNCTION AFTER AGE 75 IN VERBAL TESTS OF 35 SUBJECTS (KALMAN TWIN STUDY)

	Gender	1947	1955	1967
Vocabulary	M	27.10	27.20	24.30*
	F	29.05	29.14	27.82
Similarities	M	10.09	10.18	6.73*
	F	10.00	10.33	8.73*
Block design	M	13.29	13.00	6.29*
	F	15.33	14.72	10.72*
Digit symbol	M	27.75	23.30*	13.25*
Substitution	F	33.83	30.53*	20.10

*P <0.05.

Note: This sample closely reflected the New York State population for the age; only 29% of the subjects had had any secondary education.

Source: Adapted from Blum, Jarvick, and Clark,[20] p 173.

modal; roughly half performed as well as the younger subjects.

A word should be said about the concept of preterminal decline. If one looks at test scores of individuals in longitudinal studies who die during the study[11] or shortly thereafter,[163,164] one finds that their IQ scores (verbal as well as performance) are lower than the scores of those who survived. This phenomenon has been called *preterminal decline,* with the implication that either the brain has somehow been forewarned that death will occur or has become involved in the cascading decline of function as postulated in the "one horse shay" concept of late-age death. Alternatively, however, it does not seem unlikely that some of these individuals had been in the earliest stages of development of AD, a process that is surely malignant.

The Speed of Behavior and the Speed of Central Processing

One of the most significant changes in the function of the nervous system that can be attributed to the aging of otherwise normal individuals is a slowing in a variety of behaviors. Slowing occurs in such simple motor tasks as running and rate of finger tapping; in sensory perceptions as monitored by latency of sensory evoked response; and in reaction time and more complex tasks requiring central processing.[17-19,220,221] Birren has suggested that these observed changes reflect "a general central nervous system mediated process" that "has impact across a wide range of behaviors."[17]

Consistent with this is the finding that the only unequivocal changes that occurred over the 11-year period of the NIMH longitudinal study were in timed tests, such as speed of copying words, addition rate, and arithmetic alternation rate (see Table 2–1). It is generally accepted that the WAIS subtest most likely to deteriorate with normal aging is the DSS subtest, a timed task on the WAIS.

The speed of motor activities, as expressed in athletic endeavors, usually reaches a peak in the late teens or 20s and then shows a progressive decline with age. This is evident in racing as well as events that require strength or coordination. Older athletes continue to participate meaningfully in "master" events (as senior athletic contests are euphemistically called), but the time required for completion of races increases year by year. In the 1980 New York marathon, the newspapers carried feature articles on the 76-year-old contestant who completed the race in 3 hours, 50 minutes, but the winner was a 21-year-old runner whose time was 2 hours, 10 minutes. Fries[76] has shown that record times for the marathon rise linearly with age. Similar changes occur in every timed event.[37]

Longitudinal data confirm these changes. For example, Payton Jordan, who qualified for the 1936 Olympic trials in the 200 meter with a time of 21.1 seconds, has the master's record for this distance for ages 60 and 61 at 24.9 seconds and 25.0 seconds, respectively.[177] Thus, his time increased almost 20% yet is still incredibly fast. The record at age 70 for this event is 30.1, and at age 80, 41.2 seconds.[37]

It is evident that times for older athletes are much better than what would be achieved by younger, nonathletic individuals. Older active men perform better on reaction time and measurement of rate of arm movement than do younger nonathletic or sedentary individuals.[23,197] Studies of rate of simple movements in nonathletic subjects show a roughly linear change with age after the teens or 20s; for example, a movement of the arm aimed at a target, a side-to-side movement of a lever, tapping two targets alternately, or the speed of copying words or digits or tracing figures showed a 30% increase in time between subjects in their 20s and 60s.[220]

In some instances, older subjects make fewer errors at the expense of speed. In the tapping test, for example, the increase in time required by older subjects was accompanied by greater accuracy in hitting the target. Similarly, the increased time required by older subjects is compensated by a decrease in errors made in the tracing task.

The results attained in studies of writing speed are quite variable, depending on the population that is used. In one study, an increase in times of digit copying from 0.6 seconds per digit for 20-year-olds to 2.0 seconds per digit for 80-year-olds in a nursing home was found.[16] However, another study revealed that still employed clerks in their 60s could copy at a rate of 0.7 seconds per digit, essentially unchanged from their younger coworkers, although professionals and laborers showed a decrease in writing speed.[124] It is therfore important to note that the speed of copying words was significantly decreased over an 11-year period in the NIMH longitudinal study (see Table 2–1).

The *rate* of muscle contraction, which is the time between the arrival of the nerve impulse to the muscle and the effective contraction, may decrease with age. In a simple reaction time test requiring the lifting of a finger, the time of contraction increased from 65 per second in subjects aged 18 to 30, to 75 per second in subjects aged 65 to 80, but total reaction time increased 54 per second in the older subjects.[219] The *time* of muscle contraction contributed to, but was not the predominant cause of, the slowing of response that occurred during aging.

During aging, the rate at which nerve impulses are propagated along peripheral nerves may slow.[125] Does this contribute to the motor slowing observed in athletes, or to the changes in reaction times in older subjects? The best evidence is that only a small fraction of the age changes in reaction time are due to these peripheral nerve changes. Thus, the maximum conduction velocity of ulnar nerves measured from axilla to wrist decreased continuously with age from a value of 57.7 ± 2.1 m/sec in 25 subjects aged 20 to 29, to a value of 48.5 ± 1.8 m/sec in 25 subjects aged 80 to 89.[146] This slowing of conduction in the motor nerve could account for only 4% of the changes that occur in digital reaction time over the same age span.

A somewhat greater change occurs in the conduction velocity of sensory nerves during aging. For example, in the median nerve, maximum conduction velocity falls from about 42 m/sec at age 20, to about 31 m/sec at age 85.[122] This may contribute as much as 10% to the slowing of voluntary reaction time that occurs when the stimulus is a touch of the finger or foot.

Perceptual processing is slowed during aging. That this slowing is due primarily to an increase in the time required for central processing of sensory information is shown by experiments using backward masking.[96,119,120,210,212,213] In this technique, two visual stimuli are presented milliseconds apart. Depending on the strength and length of each stimulus and the length of the interstimulus interval, the second stimulus may block perception of the first. The interstimulus interval that will allow backward masking is increased 20% to 70% (depending on stimulus variables) in subjects in their 60s and 70s compared with 20-year-olds. This occurs whether both stimuli are presented to one eye (monoptic)[120] or whether target and masking stimuli are presented to different eyes (dichoptic stimulation),[210] thus assuring that the process is central and not retinal. Training will improve discrimination somewhat in both older and younger subjects, but the relative difference between the age groups remains.[96]

Additional evidence confirming an increase in central processing time for sensory stimulation is the finding that late (over 100 ms) components of visual, auditory, and somatosensory evoked potentials have increased latency in older individuals. These studies are described more fully later in this chapter.

The major component in simple reaction time that slows with age is the time of central processing. Birren and Botwinick[16] found that the age difference in reaction to an auditory stimulus was approximately the same whether the motor response was an involvement of jaw, finger, or foot; hence, the length of the path to the effector site played little role.

Choice reaction time, which presumably requires additional time for central decision making, is increased to a greater degree in older subjects than simple reaction time. The difference between simple and choice reaction time in subjects aged 18 to 24 was 18%; in subjects 55 to 64, it was 64%.[220] Numerous examples have been reported indicating that the more complex the task, the greater the age effect.[19,118,220,221] Central decision time is also increased in older subjects asked to mentally rotate geometric figures to determine if they are congruent.[78]

The rate at which both older (average age 70) and younger (average age 21) subjects can perform specific tasks can be speeded through practice.[100] There does not appear, however, to be any general transfer effect; for example, the ability to copy words faster will not lead to an improvement in performance in other timed tasks.

Learning and Memory

Forgetfulness is one of the most frequently acknowledged complaints of the elderly. It is a socially acceptable complaint, sometimes even used for secondary gain.[181] This complaint, however, is based on reality. Both cross-sectional and longitudinal studies show that most—although not all—individuals develop some degree of impairment of learning and memory as they age, especially after age 70.

Learning and memory are complex processes that are not fully understood. However, it is known that not all aspects of these processes are equally affected by aging.[187] Within the memory system as it is generally conceived, information is held for varying lengths of time, from seconds to permanent, even lifetime storage. Therefore, one way of looking at age-related memory performance is through tasks reflecting short- or long-term memory functions. Some aspects of short-term, or primary, memory remain relatively unchanged during normal aging. In the standard digit span test, most older as well as younger individuals can recall a list of five to seven digits immediately without difficulty (see Table 2–1).[20,23] Similarly, both 20-year-olds and 70-year-olds can learn a 10-word list (if it is meaningful),[43] and in free recall both groups show the recency effect, that is, superior recall for the last-heard items.[44] Somewhat longer sequences are also learned well by older subjects if the end point is recognition rather than recall.[45]

SHORT-TERM MEMORY

Overwhelming evidence that some short-term memory tasks show consistent (although not universal) impairment in older subjects, however, has prompted analyses of the types of tasks that do show decrements with aging. In contrast to memory tests such as those noted above, which involve simple repetition of items, older individuals have particular difficulty when required to simultaneously store and manipulate or reorganize material.[44] Repeating a digit span backward is more sensitive to age than repeating digits forward, for instance. Accumulation of evidence that performance on a memory task often suffers more in the old than in the young when a secondary concurrent task is added[27] supports the proposal that the act of dividing attention leads to decrements in performance in older people.[46] Recent preliminary reports indicate, however, that the nature of the processing task is crucial to the outcome rather than the division of attention per se. For instance, increases in sentence complexity led to slower response and reduced recall in older subjects whereas increase in the concurrent memory load affected young and old equally.[143]

WORKING MEMORY

The concept of a "working memory" has been proposed that differs from short-term memory in its emphasis on the processing as well as the storage of information held for a short period of time.[8,9,79] Applied to the data on aging, working memory provides an alternative explanation for the vulnerability that has been documented. A critical feature of this theoretical model is an attentional supervisory system called the *central executive,* which is "capable of selecting strategies and integrating information from several different sources." Baddeley[8] makes a cogent argument for the central executive as an origin of age effects in memory, arguing that stresses on the central executive system compromise the efficiency of working memory, which thereupon places constraints on a wide range of nonmemory tasks.[9] One line of research into the capacity of working memory has yielded evidence suggesting that capacity of working memory may be reduced in aging,[8,26,203] although study results are not in uniform agreement and measures of capacity are not well-defined. Other experimentation aimed at identification of the locus of age-related effects in working memory[143,224] has prompted the suggestion that the ability to process incoming information, especially when it is complex, is more vulnerable in aging than is the holding and rehearsal of information.[143] Research in working memory is pertinent to both the subjective experience of aging individuals and studies of everyday memory lapses,[162] which highlight the role of attentional control in holding and acting on information.

LONG-TERM MEMORY

Long-term memory has been subdivided into separate but interacting domains on the basis of, for example, the kind of information that is stored or how it is accessed. One recent classification posits three systems, *episodic, semantic,* and *procedural.*[208] Episodic memory refers to personally experienced events contextually bound to time and place. Semantic memory is one's cumulative knowledge of the world, of language, and of concepts. Whereas an age-related decline in episodic memory is widely reported, semantic memory generally is stable or improves across the decades.

Episodic Memory. With increasing age, subjects show consistent, although not universal, impairment in episodic memory as tested by subsequent recall or recognition following presentation of, for example, word lists, pictures, or brief stories. Learning, storage, or retrieval of recently learned information more complex than simple digit span is diminished in the elderly. If one asks subjects to memorize a long ("supra span") list of digits, for example, 15 digits, then both old and young subjects will have difficulty and on the first trial be able to recall only two or three digits correctly.[61] After repeated presentations of the list, memory improves— but it improves more rapidly in younger than in older subjects (Fig. 2–1).

Older subjects will have difficulty with both verbal (including associate learning, recall of test items) and visual (e.g., recognition or reproduction of designs) material.[1,29,50,103,107] Among the verbal tasks, however, greatest difficulty is found if the items to be learned are nonsense items. For example, in one of the classic studies of learning and memory in the elderly, the ability of English-speaking elderly to learn Turkish words was found to be more impaired than their ability to remember paired associates.[80] Older subjects show less impairment in learning lists of English words if they are given the opportunity to sort the words into meaningful groups.[106]

Semantic Memory. The memory system that is most resistant to change with age, *semantic* memory, is critically linked to meaningfulness. Seman-

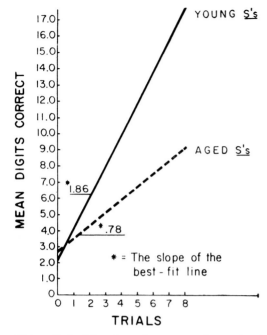

Figure 2–1. Mean learning curves of young and aged subjects for supra-span digits plotted by mean slope and y intercept. (From Drachman and Leavitt,[60] with permission.)

tic memory performance is traditionally measured by tests of vocabulary, confrontation naming, factual information, and reading. In vocabulary and information tests, older adults sometimes show improved performance over prior testing or will score significantly higher than younger adults.[141,179] In the aforementioned study with the Army Alpha Test,[153] which compared baseline measurements at age 18 to 20 with retesting at older ages, verbal scores had improved at age 48 to 50 and remained stable thereafter to age 61. A recent study employed longitudinal data to examine changes at both the subtest and item level of the Wechsler intelligence scales.[178] Vocabulary subtest scores improved overall between the ages of 18 and 54 (improvement on seven items and decline on two) but showed little change in the cohort followed to age 61 (improvement on two items and decline on two).

Walsh and Baldwin[211] found that older subjects (mean age, 67.3 years)

learned and retained a set of 16 ideas as well as younger subjects (mean age, 18.7 years). To make sure that they had not obtained an anomalous set of subjects, they also tested both groups on free recall of a 25-item word list and found, as expected, that the older group recalled only 55% as many words as the younger group. Both groups were able to integrate linguistic information into well-remembered ideas equally well, even though ordinary tests showed the older subjects to have impaired "short-term memory." Elderly subjects can produce as many names under a timed condition within a category (e.g., fruits, vegetables, girls' names) as younger subjects.[60] Retention of this capability in normal aging is important because it is often impaired in patients with dementia.

Overlearning can mitigate age differences in storage and retrieval. It takes longer for older subjects to learn a word list. Yet, if subjects are asked to learn a word list to the same criterion of accuracy, however many trials it takes, and then are retested 1 week later, older subjects will retain the same proportion of words as younger subjects.[105] Indeed, retrieval of well-learned material from very long-term memory can be impressive in the elderly; for example, subjects over 63 were able to remember 80% of a portion of catechism on which they had been tested 36 years earlier and that had not been practiced.[192]

Procedural Memory. Together, episodic and semantic memory, memory for episodes and facts, constitute declarative memory. This is distinct from "memory that is contained within learned skills or modifiable cognitive operations," called *procedural* memory.[199] Procedural memory does not rely on intentional remembering and does not show age-related differences. Procedural memory,[208] also called *implicit* memory,[87] refers to situations in which performance on perceptual-motor skills or cognitive operations is facilitated or enhanced by recent experience without necessarily intention or conscious awareness on the part of the individual. Just as vocabulary tests are used to measure explicit semantic memory, experimental paradigms such as lexical decision tap implicit semantic knowledge. In lexical decision, for instance, the subject sees a letter string and must decide if it is a word or a nonword (e.g., Nurse/Narse). The preceding word is varied and the reaction time of the target word is measured. On this task, younger and older people show similar response latencies and equivalent accuracy and facilitation for word meanings.[98,99] In other common experimental tasks, accuracy may improve in word completion or naming a picture, or speed in identifying a word or picture. Performances of older and younger adults are equivalent on these and other procedural tasks[127] even when recall or recognition of test items is poorer in the older subjects.

Squire[199] (pp 160–164) argues that the distinction between the procedural (implicit) and declarative (explicit) memory systems has a biologic basis. The distinctness of procedural memory is supported by the finding that procedural memory is not affected by the administration of scopolamine, whereas recall, recognition, and cued recall are.[145] This is pertinent to demented patients with cholinergic impairment such as occurs in AD.

EVERYDAY MEMORY

With age, individuals often experience an increase in error or failure of memory involving names ("the capital letters go first") and actions, past or planned ("prospective memory" or "remembering to recall").[92] A recent cross-sectional study of naming in "optimally healthy" subjects aged 30 to 80 years,[3] using the Boston Naming Test,[115] reported that naming ability remained stable until the subjects reached their 70s, at which point it declined significantly. The measures of neither primary nor secondary memory were significantly related to the naming scores.

The frequent complaint of difficulty

in name and word retrieval[31] was investigated in a study employing a task of naming the precise word that fit a given definition.[25] The older subjects (mean age 73; range 66 to 80) were both slower and less accurate in word retrieval, but the age difference was eliminated by providing the initial two letters of the target word. Conversely, performance of older subjects was inhibited by the presence of a semantically related but incorrect word (e.g., dragon when the target was unicorn). The authors of this study speculate that failure in word retrieval involves processing from the semantic (meaning) network to the lexical (word) network. They propose that successful communication in the opposite direction, from word network to meaning network, as evident in the data on vocabulary scores and lexical decision, is intact in normal aging.

An important feature of naming errors and retrieval failures in normal aging would seem to be randomness. Several studies of AD patients with anomia have demonstrated consistency of errors in identical items across tests (e.g., in both visual naming and verbal association) suggesting an actual loss of semantic information in this condition rather than an inability to access an intact semantic network.[77]

The evidence that learning and memory are impaired in elderly subjects is based primarily on cross-sectional studies comparing 70-year-olds with 20-year-olds. Many investigators have taken care to match subjects on educational experience and vocabulary scores to increase the comparability of groups. However, it is still possible that "age" decrements are in part due to more subtle cultural changes. For example, older subjects are more likely to have been taught only rote memory when in school, whereas younger subjects may have been taught a variety of mnemonic devices. Thus, in paired associate learning, only 36% of 70-year-old subjects used self-originated verbal or imagery connecting, whereas 68% of high school subjects did so.[104] Also, younger subjects were often college students and thus more likely to be still in "training" with respect to memorizing,[181] although in at least one study, the older subjects were recruited from among a group that had returned to college. Therefore, the possibility must be considered that observed changes in performance on memory tests might be in part culturally derived. Fortunately, a few longitudinal studies have included memory tests. These studies show that, in general, aging is accompanied by memory loss, but that some individuals show no change over extended periods. Gilbert[81] was able to retest 14 subjects who had taken the Babock-Levy Test of Mental Efficiency about 35 years earlier. The average age at the time of retest was 65 years; age ranged from 60 to 74 years. As expected from the results of other studies, vocabulary scores were unchanged or showed a slight improvement. However, scores on the Initial Learning subtest declined from 17.2 to 13.1 ($P < 0.01$), and on the Retention test from 18.8 to 13.2 ($P < 0.01$) over the 35-year period. Within the population of older individuals, decline in memory has been measurable over shorter time periods. For example, 52 volunteers in the Baltimore Longitudinal Study, initially aged 70 to 79, showed a significant reduction in score over a 6-year period on a visual retention test.[6] However, there were wide differences among the subjects, with a minority of subjects performing better on the second trial. A decline in memory scores over a 10-year period in hypertensive elderly subjects, but not among nonhypertensive elderly, was reported in the Duke Aging Study.[222] These investigators tested both short-term memory and a longer-term memory (paragraph recall after 20 minutes).

Incidental learning may be tested by asking subjects to perform various tasks other than memorizing and then asking for recall of the tasks or items in the tasks.[29,222] Such tasks might include counting letters in a set of words, rhyming the words into categories, and thinking of images for the words. Few words are learned by either younger or older subjects if the task is mechanical, as in counting letters. If the task requires more thought, such as sorting into categories or thinking of images, recall will be better in younger than in older subjects.[222] Although this has been attributed to the tendency of older subjects to focus more intensely on a task in hand, the difference between the age groups is about the same as that found in direct tests of short-term memory.

FACTORS IN DECLINE OF MEMORY

Why are short-term learning and memory impaired in older subjects? One factor may be the longer processing time. There is good evidence that the increase in central processing time in aging underlies part of the difficulty older subjects have in learning. The time required for central processing when retrieving items from short-term memory can be measured in a simple and elegant paradigm introduced by Sternberg.[67,200a] Subjects are asked to recognize items immediately after presentation. For example, a subject may be presented with a list of one, two, or four digits, and then asked to determine whether a test digit was part of the list. The time of response increases with only one test item (Fig. 2–2). The slope of the line is a measure of the time spent scanning memory. The intercept of the line is a measure of the time required to initiate the memory search and to respond to it. Both slope and intercept increase in older subjects.[5,67] It has been argued that this increase in time required for a search of items will lead to poorer overall performance on short-term memory tests because more items may be forgotten during the longer search process.[67]

There is also evidence that older subjects take longer to register or encode materials such as abstract designs[1] and are less able to recall information heard at increased rate of speech.[201]

Another factor in the decline of memory with aging may have to do with a

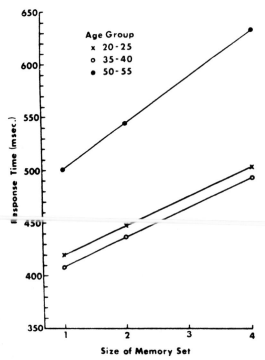

Figure 2–2. Increase in response time as size of memory set is lengthened. The slope of line is a measure of the time spent scanning memory. The intercept of the line is a measure of the time required to initiate the memory search and to respond to it. Both slope and intercept increase in older subjects.[67] (From Katzman, R and Terry, R: Normal aging of the nervous system. In Katzman, R and Terry, R [eds]. The Neurology of Aging, FA Davis, Philadelphia, 1983, p 25, with permission.)

limitation in the mnemonic strategies used. Older subjects are less likely than younger subjects to use such strategies as verbal mediation, repetition, or imagery in trying to memorize word pairs.[104,174] The reduction with aging of the ability to recall concrete words as compared with abstract words has been attributed to a decrement in the spontaneous imaging of the word referent.[167] The memory advantage of pictures over words, well-documented for young adults is attenuated in the elderly.[166] Orienting instructions successfully restore the picture superiority effect, supporting prior evidence that older people fail to carry out mental operations spontaneously that are within their capability. Younger subjects are also better able to group items, "chunk," and integrate word lists.[73,191] If mnemonic devices such as chunking and imaging are taught to older subjects, their performance improves by about 10% to 21%,[104] but such instruction also helps younger subjects, and the net result is that the age difference in short-term learning persists.

CLINICAL MEASURES IN NORMAL AGING

Neurologic Changes in Normal Aging

Beginning with the classic report of McDonald Critchley[47] in 1931, neurologists have described a variety of findings sometimes observed in apparently healthy elderly. These compilations are of value to neurologists concerned with the differential diagnosis in aged subjects. Because it is important to know which findings are most likely to indicate ongoing disease, this topic will be covered in Chapter 4. But our knowledge of the effect of normal aging on neurologic function is quite sparse. Neurologic signs present in small numbers of healthy elderly may represent asymptomatic subclinical disease, for almost half of the cerebral infarcts observed at postmortem examinations showed no symptoms that were recognized during life.[114] Cervical spondylosis, clinically asymptomatic, may give rise to findings on neurologic examination. Neurologic signs secondary to such disease processes have to be sorted out from normal age changes.

Neurologists have not carried out longitudinal studies such that analysis might identify specific diseases related to the development of neurologic signs. There are only a handful of cross-sectional studies that compare well-characterized older subjects with younger ones. In a particularly important study of this sort, investigators measured changes in neurologic function using a semiquantitative neurologic battery in 61 healthy male volunteers, 20 to 80 years of age, with one subject for each year.[158,159] All of the subjects were active, community-residing individuals with at least a high school education. The subjects met rigid standards as to health and personal habits (less than one-half pack of cigarettes per day, less than one cup of coffee per day, no psychoactive drugs). None of the subjects were artists or professional athletes, or otherwise especially proficient in sensory or physical skills. Within this highly selected subject sample, the investigators found that a variety of neurologic functions did decrease with age, the changes occurring in a slow, relatively linear fashion (as determined by a polynomial best-fit analysis) over the 60-year interval.

Despite the care in selecting subjects, this cross-sectional study is subject to the same criticism as cross-sectional studies dealing with cognitive function; that is, some of the differences observed may be due to lifelong differences between generations based on variances in early nutrition or in opportunities for physical development early in life rather than to aging per se. For example, the investigators found a statistically significant decline in right-hand grip strength as a function of age. At age 50 to 59, grip strength was only 84% of that of subjects age 20 to 29, and by the eighth decade of life, it had fallen to 77% of the 20- to 29-year-old value.[158] Yet the single available longitudinal study of grip strength involving 187 male alumni of Columbia College showed no decline in grip strength; in fact, the men restudied after 37 years were found to be slightly stronger! In this sample, right-hand grip strength averaged 52.6 ± 0.7 kg at age 57.1 years.[48]

Nevertheless, the data of Potvin and associates[158,159] are very useful as they allow us to compare the relative decrement of different functions in the same sample. Examples of these changes are shown in Table 2–3.

These observations become especially useful when one considers the neurologic symptomatology of the "normal" aged. This is pithily described by Malcolm Cowley, an author and editor who celebrated his 80th year by writing in his perceptive essay, "The View From 80"[42] "age is not different from earlier life as long as you are sitting down."

What happens when one stands up? Posture may be flexed and immobile rather than erect and active. It resembles that seen in parkinsonian patients and may be due to loss of some dopaminergic neurons and striatal dopamine receptors, a topic that will be discussed in detail later. But it should be noted that nonneurologists have a different view of these postural changes. Hazzard and Bierman[94] note:

The stature is typically stooped forward, reflecting chiefly the dorsal kyphosis or "dowager's hump," but also loss of the normal lumbar lordosis. There is also loss of height due to thinning and sometimes anterior wedging and collapse of the intervertebral discs. The vertebral bodies themselves may be compressed as the skeleton becomes demineralized to the point of osteoporosis, a phenomenon especially pronounced in women. In addition, the normally obtuse angle between the neck and the shaft of the femur may become more acute, accentuating the bent over posture (and increasing the risk of fracture at this point).

The challenge of walking is often a difficult one for an 80-year-old. The gait may be somewhat shuffling, resembling parkinsonism, yet no evidence of rigidity or tremor will be present. These changes may result in part from the alterations that occur in the nigrostriatal dopaminergic system in normal aging. Again, Hazzard and Bierman note that the development of painful osteoarthritis may also give rise to a stiff and awkward gait. Frequently the gait is unsteady in a nonspecific fashion; less often there is frank apraxia.

The problem in sorting out the conditions underlying the gait problems of the elderly is the overabundance of possible etiologies. In addition to bony and arthritic degeneration and changes in the basal ganglia, there is often some

Table 2–3 RELATIVE DECREMENT OF VARIOUS FUNCTIONS, AGES 25 TO 75*

Function	Little or No Change	<20%	20%–40%	40%–60%	>60%
Vocabulary	X				
Information	X				
Comprehension	X				
Digits forward	X				
Touch sensation, fingers and toes†	X				
Two-point discrimination, finger†	X				
Raven Progressive Matrices:					
Tying bow		X			
Manipulating safety pin		X			
Simple reaction time		X			
Hand tapping		X			
Finger dexterity		X			
Foot tapping		X			
Tandem stepping		X			
Rising from chair with support			X		
Putting on shirt			X		
Managing large button			X		
Zipping garment			X		
Cutting with knife			X		
Speed of handwriting			X		
Digit symbol substitution			X		
Foot dorsiflexion			X		
One leg standing, eyes open			X		
Vibration sense, upper extremities				X	
Leg flexion				X	
Vibration sense, lower extremities					X
One leg standing, eyes closed					X

*Cross-sectional study.[158]
†Longitudinal studies; see text.

degree of atrophy of frontal lobes, sometimes large infarcts involving motor pathways. Furthermore, the possibility of proprioceptive loss in the lower extremities must not be ignored.

Here the data of Potvin and associates[158,159] are informative. Their septuagenarians did not have a gait problem. Tandem stepping was as brisk in the 70- to 80-year-old cohort as in the 20- to 30-year-old group. Standing on one leg was markedly impaired, however, and the ability to stand on one leg with eyes closed was essentially lost by the oldest subjects. We have tested for this finding and can confirm that there are 80-year-old subjects still able to jog and do calisthenics who can no longer maintain themselves on one leg with eyes closed. Why? Is this a vestibular-cerebellar problem? Other tests of cerebellar function (including tandem gait) are normal. Is this proprioceptive

loss? Position sense as normally tested is intact, but clinical testing of position sense is crude. When vibration sense is tested with a loud 128-Hz tuning fork on the malleolus, the subject can perceive the vibration. When vibration sense threshold is tested, however, the loss in normal aging is almost as great as the loss of the ability to stand on one leg. The serious vibration sense loss has been confirmed by a number of investigators. Another change to be expected involves the large proprioceptive fibers that results in a loss of the ankle jerk. This is a less common but still frequent change during aging. Thus, one might speculate that these lower-extremity difficulties are due to the loss of some of the large diameter myelinated dorsal root fibers whose bipolar axons extend from the toes to the medulla. This neuron, required to maintain the metabolism of one of the longest processes in the body, may be among those most vulnerable to aging.

Malcolm Cowley was quite aware of the difficulty of maintaining oneself on one foot, and noted that one of the criteria of being old was "when he can't stand on one leg and has trouble pulling on his pants."[42]

We have now covered three of the most important areas of dysfunction that accompany normal aging[42]:

1. "When everything takes longer to do . . . when it becomes an achievement to do thoughtfully, step by step, what he once did instinctively"—loss of speed of motor activities, slowing in the rate of central information processing.

2. "When it becomes harder to bear in mind two things at once. . . . When he forgets names"—memory.

3. "When he can't stand on one leg. . . . When he hesitates on the landing"—impairment in stature, proprioception gait.

Another major area of dysfunction is related to the hypothalamus and related structures. Changes in diurnal rhythms and sleep and visual and auditory perception are discussed in Chapter 13.

Age as a Hyperadrenergic State

Many of the changes that normally accompany aging—for example, changes in vascular and cardiac reflexes, galvanic skin response, potency, micturition, and pupillary response—may result in part from alterations in autonomic nervous system activity, whether in central regulation or owing to peripheral changes. The nature of these autonomic shifts is poorly understood; this is an area where much descriptive work needs to be done. A body of evidence suggests, however, that sympathetic hyperactivity is commonly present and that "old age may represent a hyperadrenergic state."[175] There is direct evidence that basal plasma norepinephrine measured in supine subjects is often, but not always, elevated in older subjects.[36,113,123] Older subjects experience a greater and more sustained increase in plasma norepinephrine when they stand or exercise.[226] It has been postulated that this sympathetic hyperactivity underlies the mild increase in plasma glucose that is often seen in normal elderly patients.[175]

This sympathetic hyperactivity interferes with cognitive functioning in older subjects, especially under the stress of psychologic testing.[64] During a learning and memory task, older subjects experienced a greater rise in free fatty acids and heart rate, and a greater change in galvanic skin response—all indicative of sympathetic overactivity—than did younger subjects. Performance of the older subjects was poorer than in the younger. When the sympathetic system was blocked by use of the β-adrenergic receptor antagonist, propranolol, the older subjects' performances improved. On the other hand, large doses of propranolol taken regularly may impair cognition.

Cerebral Blood Flow and Cerebral Metabolism

It is now accepted that the metabolic activity of the brain, measured in terms of either oxygen or glucose metabolism, reflects neuronal activity. Moreover, cerebral blood flow (CBF) reflects and is controlled by the metabolic needs of the brain in normal subjects (e.g., subjects without occlusion or severe stenosis of blood vessels) and in normal circumstances (subjects must respire normally because CBF is sensitive to fluctuation in carbon dioxide levels in the blood). Thus, measurement of CBF ought to be an ideal method for following changes in neuronal activity with aging.

Unfortunately, reports of CBF in normal elderly subjects are inconsistent. From a physiologic point of view, the preferred method of increasing blood flow is the nitrous oxide technique developed by Seymour Kety.[117] This method uses the arterial–jugular vein difference in nitrous oxide concentration to estimate brain uptake of this relatively inert and freely diffusible gas. Measurement of jugular venous concentration requires catheterization of the vein, and although it is a safe procedure, it is considered invasive and is seldom employed today; hence, there are no recent data for this method. The issue that arose from earlier studies is straightforward.[195,196] One study reported that in 13 normotensive older subjects (57 to 99 years in age, mean 80 years), CBF averaged 47.7 mL/min per 100 g of brain and oxygen metabolism, cerebral metabolic rate of oxygen consumption ($CMRo_2$), averaged 2.7 mL/min per 100 g of brain compared with values in younger subjects of 57.5 (CBF) and 3.2 ($CMRo_2$).[70,71]

However, no changes in CBF or $CMRo_2$ were found in 26 healthy males aged 65 to 81 (mean 71.0) in the 1956 NIMH study. The CBF (57.9 ± 2.1 mL/100 g per minute) and the $CMRo_2$ (3.33 ± 0.08 mL/100 g per minute) obtained were almost identical to those obtained in 15 normal young subjects, mean age 20.8 years.[49] Eight of the 26 older subjects were retested after CBF had fallen to 44.4 ± 3.4 mL/100 g per minute. Although two of the eight subjects had developed EEG slowing and one had developed a chronic brain syndrome, the CBF had also fallen significantly in four of the remaining five still healthy subjects. These data suggest that in healthy 70-year-olds, CBF may be intact, but that during the eighth decade changes are likely to occur in the absence of overt disease.

A noninvasive technique for measuring CBF utilizing xenon 133 (^{133}Xe) inhalation has received wide acceptance because ^{133}Xe can be inhaled and its gamma emission measured by detectors placed over the scalp.[148,150] By use of compartmental analysis, it is possible to estimate gray matter flow (fast components) and white matter flow (slow component), and eliminate much of the artifact from blood flow through extracranial tissues (a very slow rate of flow). The method has proved useful,

although problems persist concerning its interpretation (how much gray matter flow is cortical, how much is from basal ganglia or thalamus) and practice (lung disease impairing absorption of ^{133}Xe would interfere with the analysis). When this method was applied to 48 elderly community volunteers (79.9 ± 6.9 years) who participated in the Duke longitudinal study, the value of gray matter flow over the parietal regions (47.4 ± 10.2 mL per 100 g per minute) was about 24% lower than that obtained in younger controls.[216] This reduction is similar to that found with the Kety technique in the 80-year-old group. The authors then divided the group into those with CBF above the group median and those below. These two groups did not differ in race, education, socioeconomic background, or presence of cardiovascular disease. The group with the lower CBF did, however, have significantly slower EEG frequencies (8.53 ± 0.73 vs 9.33 ± 0.64 Hz) and WAIS performance scores (23.7 ± 11.4 vs 31.8 ± 13.7), suggesting the possibility that structural changes in the brain had occurred.[214]

Electrophysiologic Changes

EEG

Aging is often accompanied by a slowing of the alpha frequency in the EEG. EEG frequencies and patterns change markedly during maturation through the late teens, but after age 20 become quite stable.[133] In adults the EEG is often dominated by sinusoidal electrical activity with a frequency between 8 and 12 Hz (or cycles per second), the so-called alpha activity, occurring at greatest amplitude in occipital leads. In subjects 20 to 40 years of age this mean alpha frequency is almost exactly 10 Hz. Cross-sectional studies show that the alpha frequency changes at a very slow rate throughout life, such that the mean frequency is 9.5 Hz at age 70. This is followed by an accelerated decrease to 9.0 Hz in the ninth decade and to 8.5 Hz after age 90, but then no further change in normal persons aged 100.[101,102,147,151,152,214] The changes in EEG frequency are especially prominent if one examines the limiting frequencies of the alpha range, that is, 8 and 12 Hz. Twelve hertz activity was found in 3.9% of subjects 20 to 39 and in only 1.72% of subjects 60 to 89; conversely, 8-Hz activity occurred in 3.7% of 20- to 39-year-olds, and in 25.9% of 60- to 89-year-olds.[75] Thus, there is a marked shift within the spectrum of EEG frequencies with aging, even though the actual mean frequency change is small.

It should be noted that these changes in EEG frequencies are statistical; many individuals retain 9.5- or 10-Hz alpha activity into the ninth decade. By age 100, only one out of seven neurologically normal subjects still had an alpha frequency between 9 and 10 Hz, one had a frequency of 9 Hz, four were between 8 and 9 Hz; and one had a frequency of 7.5 Hz.[101]

Slowing of the EEG alpha frequency with aging has been confirmed in two longitudinal studies. In the Duke Aging Study, EEGs were followed over a 42-month period in 46 volunteers; during this relatively short period, there was a small shift in mean alpha frequency from 9.50 to 9.28 Hz ($P < 0.005$).[215] In the NIMH longitudinal study, changes in EEG were followed in 19 normal subjects whose average age at the beginning of the study was 70.5 and whose average alpha frequency was 9 Hz. After 11 years, with an average age of 81.5, 10 subjects showed no change in EEG frequency, and 5 showed slowing of 0.5 to 1.0 Hz to an alpha frequency of 8 Hz. Four subjects showed much greater changes, developing either predominantly slower activity in the 7- to 8-Hz range, or hemispheral focal slowing. All 4 of these subjects had also developed a chronic brain syndrome (the psychiatric synonym for dementia), whereas the other 15 subjects had remained relatively intact.

The mechanism underlying the slowing of alpha frequency with age is un-known. Some investigators have attempted to correlate the change in alpha frequency with a decrease in cerebral blood flow, but cerebral blood flow correlates with EEG only if one includes subjects with frank cognitive impairment who have major EEG and blood flow changes. Among normal elderly subjects there is no correlation.[126,149] Another speculation attributes these EEG changes to the loss of choline acetyltransferase, a marker of cholinergic activity (the cholinergic antagonist, atropine, regularly slows the EEG if given in high enough doses).

EVOKED RESPONSE

Although one might suppose that the rich physiologic phenomenology explored by the use of scalp-recorded evoked responses would be especially helpful in understanding the aging brain, relatively few advances have resulted from this approach. This reflects both the great demand on investigator time required for carrying out and interpreting an evoked-response study and the complexity of interpretation. These barriers will no doubt be overcome and the full potential of this methodology realized as clinical applications increase, techniques become more automated, and routine and interpretation are better understood.

Most evoked-response studies are concerned with the brain potentials arising as a consequence of repetitive sensory stimuli—visual, auditory, or somatosensory. Other classes of event-related potentials are those that occur in response to novel or random stimuli (for example, a positive wave at 300 ms, the P300),[59] in anticipation of a stimulus (contingent negative variation),[35] with success in making a correct choice when discriminating sensory stimuli or that occur preceding speech or movement. Available data with respect to aging concern the classic sensory evoked response, but much of current research is concerned with the more complex event-related potentials that may be directly related to cognitive processes and might be expected to change in aging and dementia.

The earliest components of sensory-evoked response represent the direct relay of impulses to the sensory cortex; later components reflect activity in appropriate association areas. In general, during normal aging, some early components (those occurring less than 100 ms after the stimulus) are increased in amplitude, whereas later components are decreased in amplitude. Latency of early components may be unchanged or minimally increased during aging, but latency in later components is markedly increased.[35,62,193,202] Because these later components are presumed to be associated with information processing, the increase in their latency is consistent with the hypothesis that the speed of processing is reduced in normal aging.

This interpretation, now cited in reviews, must be viewed skeptically at present. Consider, for example, the responses evoked by visual stimulation produced by a reversing checkerboard pattern of constant luminance. This form of pattern reversal stimulation has been found to be very useful clinically because it can be used to detect small asymptomatic demyelinating lesions of the optic nerve. When scalp-recorded potentials evoked by pattern reversal defined luminance are compared in normal younger and older subjects, it is found that there is a small increase in the latency of early potentials, and a greater increase in later potentials—changes consistent with a delay in central processing. However, these findings can also be explained in part by changes that occur in the pupil and lens in normal aging. At the luminance used in these experiments, the pupil in 70-year-olds is on the average one fourth less in diameter than in 20-year-olds.[41] This will result in only one half as much light reaching the retina. Moreover, light transmission is further decreased in older subjects because of the subclinical opacification of the lens that occurs in normal aging.[176] This decrease in light reaching the retina will alter the latency of the evoked-response poten-

tials. For example, at 20 log luminance U, the latency of the 100-ms positive peak (P100) is increased from 102 ms in 20-year-olds to 108 ms in 70-year-olds; but if luminance is decreased to 1.0 U, then latency in 20-year-olds goes up to 112 ms.[188] Thus, an unknown fraction of the age change may be due to changes in lens and pupil rather than brain. Also, it has been found that the size of the checkerboard patterns alters the age effect,[189,194] with greater decrements occurring in older subjects if the checks are small, again consistent with the possibility that the lens and pupil may alter the evoked response. Similar peripheral changes can occur in other sensory systems, for example, in the auditory-evoked response.

To solve this problem, new methods must be developed to permit equalizing the stimulus to the primary sensory neuron. One may assume, however, that suprathreshold stimuli, for example, a flashing stroboscopic light, would minimize the effects of pupil size and lens changes.

A delay of all components of the occipital-evoked response to a flashing light in 34 older subjects, aged 56 to 81, compared with 24 younger subjects, aged 20 to 29, was found in one study.[62] However, the delay ranged from 6 ms for the first negative potential (N40) to 12 ms for the third positive potential (P180). Amplitudes of potential recorded in the first 100 ms were on the average two to three times greater in the older subjects.

In a study of later components of the visual-evoked response, a profound decrease in amplitude and increase in latencies in subjects age 71 to 81 was found, compared with subjects aged 20 to 30.[193] The differences were greater in response to novel stimuli than to the standard stimuli. An increase in latency of over 80 ms was observed in a positive component with 481 ± 15.7 ms in the older subjects. Subjects aged 60 to 68 years had intermediate latencies.

A very similar pattern has been found for the auditory-evoked response. An early (less than 50 ms) potential had about the same latency in young (age 20 to 28) and older (age 74 to 87) subjects, but the amplitude was greater in the older subjects.[74,156,157] Later potentials, beginning with a positive potential over 100 ms, were increased in the older subjects, the greatest change occurring in the third positive peak, which was recorded at 300 ms in young subjects and at 420 ms in older subjects.[84] Latency for this component increased almost 2 ms per year, and the change was apparently continuous through adult life.

A detailed analysis of age-related changes in somatosensory-evoked response has been reported.[56,129] In one investigation, 19 subjects aged 80 to 90 were compared with 25 younger subjects aged 20 to 30. Brief (0.2-ms) electrical impulses (5 to 10 mA) were administered through silver ring electrodes attached to the second and third fingers. Potentials were recorded from multiple sites. The arms were warmed so that conduction times would not be affected by the lower body temperature of the older subjects. Conduction through the afferent nerves was at a rate of 71.7 ± 4.0 m/s in younger and 61.2 m/s in older subjects, a slowing of only 0.16 m/s per year. Results were similar to those reported by Norris.[146] There was no age-related change in conduction from neck to cortex. The early negative potential at the cortex, N22, was much greater in amplitude in older subjects, just as had been found for the early components of auditory and visual-evoked response. Subsequent but still early components of the somatosensory-evoked response (precentral P25, postcentral N35, P65) had longer latency in the older subjects. However, a large-amplitude parietal component (W wave, P30, N35, P45) was present in 90% of older subjects and only 48% of younger subjects, suggesting that pattern of activation of association cortex had shifted with age.

Event-related potentials (e.g., P300, N400, and contingent negative variation) are increasingly used to monitor cognitive function. In general, the latency of these potentials increases during aging, but analysis of these changes is still in an early state.[57,140,154,188] In this regard a potential of particular interest is the N_A, a negative potential that immediately precedes the N200 when properly elicited. N_A is related to a pattern recognition process, whereas N200 reflects discrimination and classification of data. One paradigm[168,169] used to elicit N_A is a simple reaction time experiment in which the stimulus is a set of dimly lit letters and the subject is asked to visually discriminate a stimulus, for example, a vowel embedded in a series of consonants. If it is correct that a major effect of aging is to delay N_A and that subsequent delays in N200, P300, and N400 reflect this initial perceptual task, then this would be an important finding, certainly one that is in accord with intuitive perceptions of the aging process and with neuropsychologic findings. Again, however, one must consider the effect of aging on primary ocular and retinal reception and take great care to rule out change at these locations as the cause of the delay in N_A.

Brain Atrophy and CT Scans

Atrophy of the brain occurring in normal aging is well documented in CT studies. Visual inspection of CT scans of normal older subjects suggests that both cortical atrophy[91,111] and ventricular enlargement exist.[13,83,91,110,111,170,225] However, it is easier to document the ventricular enlargement quantitatively. Estimates of sulcal widening are difficult to quantify, both because of the wide variation in gyral pattern that occurs in normal individuals and because measurement of subarachnoid space on CT scans is subject to artifacts consequent to the high density of adjacent skull. Measurement of ventricular size is straightforward by either planimetry or computer computations. Enlargement of the ventricular system occurs with age. When the maximum area of the ventricular system on an appropriate CT cut is compared with the entire intracranial volume, an increase from

Table 2–4 RATIO OF CEREBRAL VOLUME TO CRANIAL VOLUME DURING NORMAL AGING*

Age	N	Ratio
20–29	21	92 ± 3
30–39	19	93 ± 2
40–49	24	92 ± 4
50–59	44	90 ± 4
60–69	37	87 ± 5
70–79	40	83 ± 6
80–89	9	82 ± 6

*In 204 Japanese subjects, volume estimated by classifying pixels as bone (500 to 1500 h), CSF (−21 to +21 h), or brain (221 to 499 h).

3% to 4% in subjects aged 20 to 49 to an area of 14% to 17% in normal subjects aged 80 to 89 is found.[13,110,111] This change is visually striking and must be taken into account when interpreting CT scans of older patients, because there is much overlap in ventricular size between that found in normal subjects and in patients with AD. However, the measurements described are taken on the CT cut where ventricular area is maximal. If the volume of ventricular plus subarachnoid cerebrospinal fluid (CSF) within the part of the cranium containing the cerebral hemispheres is computed on serial CT cuts, the change with aging, although significant, is less dramatic.[225] In Japanese subjects aged 20 to 49 the ratio of cerebral volume to cranial volumes averages 92%, at age 60 to 69, 87%, and at age 80 to 89, 82%. This amounts to about an 11% decline in cerebral volume from the third to fourth decades, corresponding well to the reported decline in brain weight over this period (Table 2–4).

MORPHOLOGIC CHANGES IN NORMAL AGING

Gross Parenchymal Alterations

Although the brain undoubtedly shrinks in the course of normal aging, the degree of atrophy and its major locations are less than certain. There

have been numerous studies and surveys of studies[54] aimed at these aspects, but all seem to neglect one or more problems. The greatest of these difficulties is, of course, the very large normal variation in brain size. Brain weight ranged from 930 to 1350 g in a recent small series of 70- to 89-year-old patients who had been known to be neurologically and psychologically intact, and then found to be neurohistologically normal.[206] With that sort of variation at the end of life, a very large series is needed to plot with any degree of confidence the changes throughout the life span. Large series have indeed been published, but these have all neglected at least two other points. The first is that psychologic studies on the patients during life were lacking, and therefore the population can be assumed to have included specimens with a variety of disease processes that might well have affected brain weight. Second, as Corsellis has pointed out,[39] there has been a significant secular effect (about 3.6%) during the life span of the populations comprised by these surveys, such that patients who were born in the early years of this century, or even before, had a lower normal brain weight than those born more recently.

A technique devised by Davis and Wright[52] allows the examiner to measure the ratio between the volume of brain and that of the cranial vault. They applied the method to a series of moderate size and showed that the ratio was constant at about 0.92 until age 55, after which it fell toward 0.83 at age 90. This comprises sound evidence of significant age-related atrophy in the individual, but even this very promising technique does not address ventricular size, which also increases modestly.

Cerebellar changes are normally less apparent than those of the cerebrum. Most of the loss of brain weight accompanying age would seem to be the result of changes in the forebrain. Adequate studies of this topographic phenomenon, however, have not been performed.

Ideally, the implied questions could

be satisfactorily answered only by a large and probably collaborative prospective study in which patients would be thoroughly examined for mental status and neurologic normality. At autopsy, fresh brain weight and volume would be measured and compared with the volume of the cranial vault. Measurements of the cerebellum, brain stem, individual cerebral hemispheres and ventricles, and weight after fixation would also be helpful. Fresh, frozen, and fixed tissue samples from such a series would have use in a broad variety of subsequent investigations.

The cortical ribbon also shrinks in the course of normal aging, but measuring this variable adequately presents great technologic problems. The observer is often struck by the focal nature of this cortical atrophy. One or two gyri, perhaps in widely separate parts of the cerebrum, may participate while intervening tissue appears normal. In any instance, the shrinkage is quite subtle. Corsellis and his colleagues have compared the ratio between total cortex and white matter as a function of normal aging.[39] Their data display interesting changes, in that in the young mature brain the gray to white ratio is 1:28, declining to 1:13 in the sixth decade. Subsequent to that age, the ratio rises to 1:55 by the 10th decade. That is, in the first 50 years, one loses relatively more gray matter than white, with a reversal of this relationship during the subsequent 50 years. Several explanations might be offered for this phenomenon, but none is by any means certain at this time. One possibility is that during the first five decades the brain might lose predominantly small cortical neurons without extracortical connection, and later the loss could increasingly involve large neurons with long, myelinated axons, and thus affect white matter more than gray. A generalized loss of extracellular fluid might also account for excess shrinkage of the white matter.[22]

Although an impression of ventricular size can be gained from autopsy examination, quantification of the ventricular system is very difficult indeed. Postmortem molds can be made of the ventricles, but even when accurately formed these may not reliably reflect the premortem size. Nevertheless, one can safely say that there is mild to moderate dilatation of the lateral and third ventricles during the course of normal aging. The aqueduct and fourth ventricle participate to a lesser degree. More reliable measurements of the antemortem size may be gained through CT and magnetic resonance imaging (MRI) on patients who have been carefully studied for mental and neurologic status.[55]

Vascular Changes

Only intraparenchymatous changes will be discussed, because atherosclerosis is such a large subject as to have been extensively reviewed elsewhere. The intracerebral arterioles and venules demonstrate increased coiling and looping as the brain ages. The venules appear coarsened, developing sinusoidal enlargements and knoblike protuberances.[69] These alterations can be studied in human autopsy material by staining the luminal contents with the benzidine reaction or the vascular walls with reagents for its reticulin or basement membrane components.

Hunziker and associates[108] have shown that in the aged brain there is increased capillary diameter and length per unit volume compared with younger specimens. Furthermore, they state that the average distance between capillaries decreases in the elderly. This could be the result of parenchymal atrophy with consequent condensation of the capillaries. They suggest that any decrease in cerebral blood flow might be adaptive, or at least that it is compensated by the changes in microvascular architecture.

Careful microscopic study reveals the presence of amyloid in blood vessels in several organs of many aged humans, and the small arteries and arterioles of the brain are occasionally also involved. The amyloid is usually confined to the media and adventitia and is arranged in a segmental fashion with sharp delineation of normal and abnormal zones. It is somewhat more common in the occipital region than elsewhere but is also seen in association with angiomas. Although it may be associated with the neuritic plaque (NP), it is not necessarily so. The nature of the vascular amyloid is identical to the β/A4 amyloid of AD (see Chapter 8).

Cell Counts

Neurons of the CNS are by no means uniformly susceptible to age-related death (Tables 2–5 to 2–9).

Several cranial nerve nuclei have been found to maintain their populations throughout the normal life span.[121] The inferior olivary nucleus also has a stable population according to Monagle and Brody,[142] but Meier-Ruge and associates[139] have reported about a 20% loss in that nucleus. The locus ceruleus (LC)[209] and the substantia nigra (SN)[135] undergo very significant neuronal loss, although most of the nigral loss appears to be in the first three or four decades, with a gradual decline after that time. Cerebellar Purkinje cells fall out at an apparently linear rate, such that about 25% are gone by old age, according to Corsellis.[40] Cerebellar granule cells have not actually been counted, but it is the common impression that their density lessens during the course of normal aging. Bugiani and associates[30] have counted large and small neurons in the putamen and found that both cell types decline in number throughout the years. They re-

port that about 25% of each neuron type is gone by age 65 and suggest that this equal loss maintains a physiologic balance, lessening the impact of what might otherwise be more significant.

The cerebral neocortex is thought to be very susceptible to age-related neuronal decrement. Brody's widely accepted figures come from his study[28] of 20 normal specimens ranging from newborn to 95 years old, in which he manually counted neurons at several locations in precentral and postcentral gyri, superior and inferior temporal gyri, and the visual cortex. He found that the superior temporal region was most severely involved, and here the loss approached 59%. Other locations were somewhat less affected. Small neurons of the second and fourth cortical layers showed the greatest loss.

Henderson and colleagues[95] analyzed areas of the brain similar to those worked on by Brody, but they used a computerized image analysis apparatus rather than hand tallies. Their results were not dissimilar in general, although they did note that the greatest loss was among large neurons, where it approximated 60%, rather than in the smaller cells emphasized by Brody. Furthermore, they found only a very small change in glia.

Devaney and Johnson[58] used a technique of cell dispersion from formalin-fixed brain tissue of the visual cortex, and reported that there were about 46 million neurons per g of tissue at age 20, and that this fell to 24 million per g by age 80. Thus, an entirely different technique revealed a comparable 48% decrement of cortical neurons in the course of normal aging.

Table 2–5 NEURON COUNTS IN NORMAL AGING

Age	Precentral	Postcentral	Superior Temporal	Striate
16–21	1479 (5)*	1477 (5)	2122 (3)	2565 (5)
45–48	1307 (2)	1151 (2)	1950 (1)	1828 (2)
70–78	1036 (5)	1386 (4)	1140 (6)	1704 (5)
80–95	937 (3)	1848 (2)	949 (3)	1691 (3)
(80–95)/(16–21)	63%	128%	45%	66%

*Indicates the number of cases.
Source: Adapted from Brody.[28]

Table 2–6 NEURON COUNTS AT AGE 90 COMPARED WITH AGE 20

| Area | Neurons | |
	Small, %	Large, %
Precentral	62	51
Postcentral	59	47
Superior temporal	66	48

Source: Adapted from Henderson, Tomlinson, and Gibson,[95] p 129.

Table 2–8 NEURON COUNTS IN SUBSTANTIA NIGRA

Age	Number
18–30	380,000
50–90	250,000
(50–90)/(18–30)	66%

Source: Adapted from McGeer,[135] p 430.

It is remarkeable that despite the loss of so many cortical neurons the histologist finds so little to mark their passing. There is no neuronophagia, no overt nuclear pyknosis or karyorrhexis, no phagocytosis, and no inflammation. The cytoplasm of old neurons displays less intense cytoplasmic basophilia, but even this alteration is not very marked. Neuronal nuclei and nucleoli are somewhat smaller in the aged.[131] The mechanism by which the cells die is entirely unknown, and this is at least in part because they seem to disappear without a trace, without leaving any hint of pathogenesis.

Autoantibodies[144] might be the cause of natural cell death, but round cell inflammation is lacking. Slow or unconventional virus of the scrapie type always seems to produce a spongy encephalopathy, and this is not found to be significant in normal aging. The hallmarks of ischemia are not present in relevant areas. Environmental toxins might be a causative factor, but which one, and what is the evidence? Evidence that lipofuscin is cytotoxic is sparse indeed. Naturally formed analogues of neurotransmitters might well be neurotoxic, but again evidence for their presence is lacking.

The other possibility is that there really has been little or no actual neuronal death in the normally aged neocortex. Our own cell counts were done with image analysis apparatus on three association areas of about 50 normal specimens.[205] Cases were carefully selected to exclude subjects with functional impairment during life as well as neurologic changes at autopsy. There was no change in neuronal number in a column of cortex 600 μm wide through the full thickness of the cortex. However, since the neuronal density did not change and the brain weight did decrease, there must be an overall loss of cerebral neurons, but this is not directly measurable. Large neurons (those over 90 μm^2) decreased significantly in number, while small neurons increased to an equal extent, indicating that the large ones were shrunken into the smaller size class (Fig. 2–3). These neuronal counts are in agreement with those of Haug[93] but stand in sharp contrast to those of Brody,[28] Henderson and associates,[95] and Devaney and Johnson,[58] and the differences have not been explained.

Table 2–7 NEURON COUNTS IN PUTAMEN

| Age | N* | Neurons | |
		Small	Large
16–49	5	220	2.72
55–65	5	154	1.99
(55–65)/(16–49)		70%	73%

*Number of cases.
Source: Adapted from Bugiani et al,[30] p 288.

Table 2–9 NEURON COUNTS IN LOCUS CERULEUS

Age	Mean Cell Count	N*
0–59	16,840	8
60–69	14,750	7
70–79	11,300	4
80–89	10,620	5
(80–89)/(0–59)	63%	

*Number of cases.
Source: Adapted from Vijayashankar and Brody,[209] p 493.

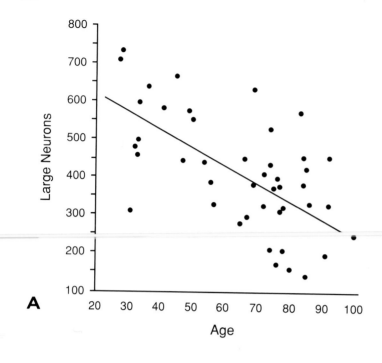

A

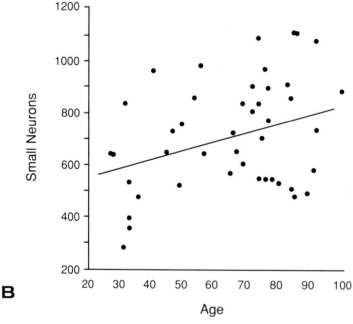

B

Figure 2–3. (A and B). Cell counts were completed with image analysis apparatus on three association areas of about 50 normal specimens.[205] Neurons were counted in a column of cortex 600 μm wide through the full thickness of the cortex. Large neurons (those over 90 μm^2) decreased significantly in number, while small neurons increased to an equal extent, indicating that the large ones were shrunken into the smaller size class. (From Terry et al,[205] pp 533, 534, with permission.)

Dendritic Arbor and Dendritic Spines

Utilizing Golgi preparations of human brain, the Scheibels[186] showed dramatically that in the aged cortex some neurons had lost many elements of their dendritic arbor. The decrement was particularly prominent among basilar neurites of large pyramidal cells. Remaining dendrites from these altered cells often ended bluntly and showed irregularities of diameter along their course. Although these sorts of alterations can sometimes be the result of postmortem change and imperfect fixation,[223] the data are widely accepted as significant features of normal aging. The dendritic loss was often associated with some shrinkage and distortion of the cell body, which in the most severe instances took on a bell shape. The Scheibels found all this to be most significant in the third and fifth layers of cortex. It was indicated that the basilar, or horizontal, dendrites make synaptic contact predominantly with the small neurons of layers 2 and 4. These local connections, they suggested, subserve higher cortical functions in that bundles of horizontal dendrites act as a sort of computer program in terms of clustering and ordering signals. This mechanism would also be reduced by degeneration of dendrites.

Along with this loss of dendrites, the density of dendritic spines per unit length of neurite also decreases with age.[138] There is, therefore, very probably a significant loss of synapses in the aged cortex, with loss of whole neurons, dendrites, and spines. Complete ultrastructural enumeration of synapses in a full-thickness sample of cortex would be very difficult, and such data are not yet available. Huttenlocher[109] has found in the third layer of frontal cortex a 13% decrease of synapses, comparing 74- to 90-year-olds with the constant counts of the 16- to 72-year-old group. Our own immunocytochemical quantification of a synaptic vesicle-specific protein shows a modest but significant decrease in neocortex with aging.[132]

Coleman and Flood[38] also did Golgi studies on normal aged specimens, and their findings were quite different from those of the other investigators. These authors reported a net increase in the dendritic arbor of pyramidal cells in normal aging. They suggest that this is a plastic response related to neuronal loss.

Lipofuscin

This yellow, insoluble pigment increases in an approximately linear fashion in most neurons in the course of aging. It is particularly prominent in the neurons of the inferior olive where the cells are, by the second decade of life, filled with pigment granules to the extent that their cell bodies are rounded and their nuclei pushed aside. The substance is readily recognized in histologic preparations in that it is alcohol-insoluble, sudanophilic, periodic-acid–Schiff positive, and autofluorescent. It is generally considered to be the result of the breakdown of cytoplasmic membranes, and peroxidation may play a major role in its formation. Studies have shown that as the lipofuscin increases, cytoplasmic RNA declines.[131] Nevertheless, at this time there is no clear evidence that lipofuscin is cytotoxic in any direct sense.

Microscopic Lesions

Detailed descriptions of NFT, NP, granulovacuolar bodies, and so forth, are provided in Chapter 8, but certain aspects of their presence in the normal elderly brain must be discussed here. That they are indeed to be found in the normal brain has been recognized for several decades,[173] and in past years this has given rise to considerable debate as to their significance in disease. There is no doubt that neurofibrillary tangles and neuritic or senile plaques are to be found in small numbers in particular locations in the great majority of the normal elderly.[53,134] Tangles, in particular, are extremely rare in such specimens outside the hippocampus and nearby temporal region. Plaques are to be seen more widespread in the neocortex as well as in the hippocampus, but almost always in very small numbers. In rare circumstances, however, significant numbers of NP may be found in neocortex in specimens where not long before death the patient had been well tested cognitively and found to be essentially intact. Other than these very few cases, the presence of large numbers of plaques per unit area in the neocortex is very strongly indicative of abnormal mentation in life. Plaques in the normal aged brain are often made up of abnormal neurites, glial processes, and amyloid core[160] just as in the demented, but some lack paired helical filaments (PHF) in the neurites and stain negatively with antibodies to PHF associated proteins described in Chapter 8.

A satisfactory explanation for those exceptional cases with many plaques but normal cognition is lacking at this time, and the best that one can probably offer is that dementia, like many other disorders, is a threshold phenomenon. That is, a certain threshold of abnormality must be reached before symptoms or malfunctions arise from that defect. The threshold is probably related to functional reserve and may vary widely among individuals. Katzman and associates[116] reported a number of such cases in which the brain was heavier and there was a greater neuronal density in the neocortex than in a comparably aged group with normal cognition and no cortical plaques. Because of this variability, many pathologists are unwilling to set a precise limit on the number of lesions per microscopic field that would separate normal aging from AD. Nevertheless, there should be no question but that the generalization is a very strong one: Many plaques and even a few tangles in the neocortex indicate dementia. Many other parameters, including neuron and synapse counts, neurotransmitter measurements, and so forth, would be necessary for complete certainty.

Granulovacuolar degeneration of Simchowicz and Hirano bodies are two other intraneuronal lesions commonly found in small numbers in the normal aged brain. A few granulovacuolar bodies are seen with increasing frequency in autopsy specimens after 55 to 65 years of age.[10] These lie within the hippocampal neuronal perikarya, whereas the Hirano body often seems to occupy the neuropil. Neither is present in sufficient quantities to modify chemical assay of the tissue, although it is now known that the latter is made up of actin[82] and the former contains tublin.[161]

Corpora amylacea, on the other hand, are present as intra-astrocytic spheres in such great numbers in aged subpial and subependymal regions that their composition might indeed change tissue concentrations of various substrates. These bodies are composed largely of polysaccharide with small amounts of protein.[200] They have not been enumerated specifically as a function of age, but it is safe to state that almost all elderly specimens show very many of them in the areas indicated above.

NEUROTRANSMITTERS

There are remarkable differences in the results obtained by different investigators concerning the concentration of transmitters and their biosynthetic enzymes in brain tissue during normal aging. It seems probable that subject selection may play an important role in producing such differences. Neurochemists are in general quite aware of pitfalls as to the possible effect of postmortem autolytic changes. This has been studied both in animals and in the human brain. In general, it is found that there is an immediate (during the first hour) postmortem loss but that the levels of many transmitters and enzymes are then quite stable for periods of 12 to 48 hours if reasonable precautions are taken. Exceptions are the neurotransmitter acetylcholine and the enzyme tryptophan hydroxylase, which are much too labile to be measured in human postmortem material.

It would seem probable that unrecognized premortem morbidity and postmortem pathology account for many of these apparent differences in results. Either dementia or Parkinson disease (PD) might not have been noted in the medical record, and the inclusion of such samples might well change the assay results. Furthermore, as Bowen and associates[24] have demonstrated, immediately premortem events such as coma can have a significant effect on some transmitter levels. A coordinated clinical, histopathologic, and neurochemical study is needed to clarify this very confusing area of neurotransmitters and aging.

There is remarkably little information about quantitative changes in neuropeptides in human brain during normal aging. There is a larger body of information concerning aminergic transmitters and enzymes.

Catecholamines

DOPAMINE

Changes in the nigrostriatal dopaminergic system in normal aging are of special interest because of similarities between some changes that occur in normal aging and those that occur in PD. These alterations include parallel slowing of various motor processes.[204] It is uncertain to what extent the flexed posture and gait changes that occur frequently in subjects over 75 without the tremor or cogwheel rigidity of PD may represent a forme fruste of the latter. In PD, of course, the major pathology involves the dopaminergic nigrostriatal pathway; postmortem there may be a 90% loss of dopamine in the caudate and putamen,[63] together with a loss of the dopamine biosynthetic enzymes tyrosine hydroxylase and dopa decarboxylase.[136]

Most investigators agree that the concentration of dopamine declines in normal aging at least in the caudate.[33,85] A reduction has also been reported in several other parts of the brain by Adolfsson and associates,[2] but was not found by Robinson and associates,[172] or by MacKay and coworkers.[130] Tyrosine hydroxylase and dopa decarboxylase, both important in the synthesis of dopamine and of noradrenaline, have been reported by several groups[128,135] to decline with age in striatum, SN, and amygdala, but this was not confirmed by Grote and associates.[90] The brain regions said by some to be so affected in aging are supplied, in terms of dopaminergic endings, largely by cell bodies in the SN. This pigmented nucleus undergoes an age-related loss of neuronal somata according to McGeer,[135] and some reduction of the transmitter levels at the relevant terminals might well be on that basis.

NORADRENALINE

The cerebral noradrenergic system is a diffusely projecting system arising from the locus ceruleus (LC), a pigmented nucleus that sustains about a 35% loss of neuronal somata.[208] One might therefore expect to find a loss in the biosynthetic enzyme dopamine beta hydroxylase, but Grote and associates[90] found this enzyme to be unchanged in striatum during aging.

MONOAMINE OXIDASE

The only aminergic system regarding which there seems to be unanimity is the catabolic enzyme monoamine oxidase (MAO) which, at least in its β-form, increases with age.[32,165] Much of this enzyme is extraneuronal in location, contrasting it with many of the other relevant systems. Robinson and associates[171] have found greater activity in women than in men, and this too is unique among the transmitter-related compounds. Gottfries[86] reported strong positive correlations between age and MAO concentrations especially in pallidum, hippocampus, SN, and frontal cortex. The data on the MPTP model of parkinsonism, described in Chapter 1, and human studies with deprenyl, also described in Chapter 1, raise the possibility that the increase in MAO-B may play a role in the etiology of some cases of PD, thereby providing a possible explanation of the age association of this disorder.

Serotonin

Assays of serotonin (5-hydroxytryptamine or 5-HT) have been reported to show an age-related decrease.[130,171] However, the enzyme responsible for synthesis of 5-HT is tryptophan hydroxylase, and this is too unstable to measure reliably in the human brain.[135]

Gamma-Aminobutyric Acid

Gamma-aminobutyric acid (GABA) is the major inhibitory transmitter in the cerebral hemisphere but has been little studied in the aging human brain. McGeer and McGeer[136] found that glutamic acid decarboxylase (GAD), which synthesizes GABA, is decreased with age, especially in the thalamus. It is interesting that GAD is not reduced in areas where choline acetyltransferase and tyrosine hydroxylase are so affected. It is again to be noted that this enzyme is altered by preterminal coma and by certain antibiotics.[24,137]

Acetylcholine

Cholinergic activity is widespread in human gray matter. Whereas acetylcholine is very rapidly hydrolyzed in postmortem tissue, its synthesizing enzyme, choline acetyltransferase (ChAT), is very stable in the autopsied human brain and is useful for assay up to at least 24 hours postmortem.[51,198] In the caudate and putamen where ChAT is primarily present in interneurons, there is no significant change with aging.[15] In cerebral cortex, McGeer and McGeer[136] found a significant negative correlation of this enzyme's activity with age up to 50 years. Perry and associates[155] and Davies[51] reported a highly significant continuing decrease in ChAT between ages 60 and 90. This loss was particularly prominent in the hippocampus and temporal neocortex. Again, however, the extent of this loss might be exaggerated by the inadvertent inclusion of tissue from patients with unrecognized AD. In fact Allen and associates[4] found relatively little change with aging in markers of cholinergic terminals in neocortex but a marked decrease in putamen, as if the

small interneurons of the putamen were selectively vulnerable during normal aging.

This cholinergic activity is presynaptic in the cortex, and most of it appears to come from cell bodies in deep gray matter. Increasing evidence[112] reviewed by Emson and Lindvall[66] places the cell bodies for this neocortical input in the region of the substantia innominata, ventral to the anterior commissure. Cell counts in this area are entirely lacking with respect to normal human tissue during aging.

CONCLUSION

Normal aging of the nervous system is characterized by slow changes in specific functions, the most intensively studied of which is cognitive function. Although verbal skills appear to remain relatively well-preserved in normal aging, slowing in a variety of behaviors, including simple and more complex motor tasks; perceptual processing; and simple and choice reaction time, is particularly significant. Most older individuals develop some impairment of learning and memory with aging, with age-related declines in episodic memory widely reported, whereas semantic memory remains more stable.

Other clinically measurable neurologic changes in normal aging include alterations in gait and proprioception, probable sympathetic hyperactivity, possible lowering of CBF rate, EEG alpha frequency slowing, evoked response changes, and CT evidence of brain atrophy. Reported morphologic changes include gross parenchymal alterations, vascular changes, neuronal and dendritic decrement, increased levels of lipofuscin, and increased numbers of microscopic lesions such as NFT and NP. Various investigators have obtained divergent results regarding the concentrations of neurotransmitters and their biosynthetic enzymes in brain tissue, and this area will require much further investigation. An important example is the normal increase in the level of (MAO-B) activity in the aging brain, particularly in the basal ganglia, an increase that may be related to the development of PD.

REFERENCES

1. Adamowicz, JK and Hudson, BR: Visual short-term memory, response delay, and age. Percept Motor Skills 46:267–270, 1978.
2. Adolfsson, R, Adolfsson, R, Gottfries, CG, Roos, BE, and Winblad, B: Post-mortem distribution of dopamine and homovanillic acid in human brain, variations related to age, and a review of the literature. J Neural Transm 45:81–105, 1979.
3. Albert, MS, Heller, HS, and Milberg, W: Changes in naming ability with age. Psychol Aging 3:173–178, 1988.
4. Allen, SJ, Benton, JS, Goodhardt, MJ, Haan, EA, Sims, NR, Smith, CCT, Spillane, JA, Bowen, DM, and Davison, AN: Biochemical evidence of selective nerve cell changes in the normal ageing human and rat brain. J Neurochem 41:256–265, 1983.
5. Anders, TR, Fozard, JL, and Lillyquist, TD: Effects of age upon retrieval from short-term memory. Dev Psychol 6:214–217, 1972.
6. Arenberg, D: Differences and changes with age in the Benton visual retention test. J Gerontol 33:534–540, 1978.
7. Aronson, MK, Masur, D, Ooi, WL, Blau, A, Bukenya, MA, Antis, RN, and Frishman, W: Cognitive function in the very old: Stability vs. change. Submitted.
8. Baddeley, AD: Working Memory. Oxford University Press, Oxford, 1986.
9. Baddeley, AD and Hitch, GJ: Working memory. In Bower, G (ed): Recent Advances in Learning and Moti-vation, Vol VIII. Academic Press, New York, 1974, pp 47–90.
10. Ball, MJ and Lo, P: Granulovacuolar degeneration in the aging brain and in dementia. J Neuropathol Exp Neurol 36:474–487, 1977.
11. Baltes, PB, Schaie, KW, and Nardi, AH: Age and experimental mortality in a seven-year longitudinal study of cognitive behavior. Dev Psychol 5:18–26, 1971.
12. Baltes, PB and Willis, SL: The Critical Importance of Appropriate Methodology in the Study of Aging: The Sample Case of Psychometric Intelligence. In Hoffmeister, F and Muller, C (eds): Brain Function in Old Age. Springer-Verlag, Berlin, 1979, pp 164–187.
13. Barron, SA, Jacobs, L, and Kinkel, WR: Changes in the size of normal lateral ventricles during aging determined by computerized tomography. Neurology 26:1011–1013, 1976.
14. Bayley, N and Oden, MH: The maintenance of intellectual ability in gifted adults. J Gerontol 10:91–107, 1955.
15. Bird, ED and Iversen, LL: Huntington's chorea: Post mortem measurement of glutamic acid decarboxylase, choline acetyltransferase and dopamine in basal ganglia. Brain 97:457–472, 1974.
16. Birren, JE and Botwinick, J: Age differences in finger, jaw and foot reaction time to auditory stimuli. J Gerontol 10:429–432, 1955.
17. Birren, JE, Woods, AM, and Williams, MV: Speed of Behavior as an Indicator of Age Changes and the Integrity of the Nervous System. In Hoffmeister, F and Muller, C (eds): Brain Function in Old Age. Springer-Verlag, Berlin, 1979, pp 10–44.
18. Birren, JE: Age Changes in Speed of Behavior: Its Central Nature and Physiological Correlates. In Welford, AT and Birren, JE (eds): Behavior, Aging and the Nervous

System. Charles C Thomas, Springfield, IL, 1963, pp 191–216.

19. Birren, JE: Translations in gerontology—from lab to life. Psychophysiology and speed of response. Am Psychol 29:808–815, 1974.

20. Blum, JE, Jarvick, LF, and Clark, ET: Rate of change on selective tests of intelligence: A twenty-year longitudinal study of aging. J Gerontol 25:171–176, 1970.

21. Blythe, R: The View in Winter: Reflections in Old Age. Penguin Books, New York, 1979, p 220.

22. Bondareff, W and Narotzky, R: Age changes in the neuronal microenvironment. Science 18:1135–1136, 1972.

23. Botwinick, J and Thompson, LW: Age difference in reaction time: An artifact? Gerontologist 8:25–28, 1968.

24. Bowen, DM, Smith, CB, White, P, and Davison, AN: Neurotransmitter-related enzymes and indices of hypoxia in senile dementia and other abiotrophies. Brain 99:459–496, 1976.

25. Bowles, NL and Poon, LW: Aging and retrieval of words in semantic memory. J Gerontol 40:71–77, 1985.

26. Broadbent, DE and Gregory, M: Some confirmatory results on age differences in memory for simultaneous stimulation. Br J Psychol 56:77–80, 1965.

27. Broadbent, DE and Heron, A: Effects of a subsidiary task on performance involving immediate memory in younger and older men. Br J Psychol 53:189–198, 1962.

28. Brody, H: Organization of the cerebral cortex. III. A study of aging in the human cerebral cortex. J Comp Neurol 102:511–556, 1955.

29. Bromley, DB: Some effects of age on short term learning and remembering. J Gerontol 13:398–406, 1958.

30. Bugiani, O, Salvarani, S, Perdelli, F, and Mancardi, GL: Nerve cell loss with aging in the putamen. Eur Neurol 17:286–291, 1978.

31. Burke, DM and Light, LL: Memory and aging: The role of retrieval processes. Psychol Bull 90:513–646, 1981.

32. Carlsson, A, Adolfsson, R, Aquilonius, SM, Gottfries, CG, Oreland, L, Svennerholm, L, and Winblad, B: Biogenic Amines in Human Brain in Normal Aging, Senile Dementia, and Chronic Alcoholism. Adv Biochem Psychopharmacol 23:295–304, 1980.

33. Carlsson, A and Winblad, B: Influence of age and time interval between death and autopsy on dopamine and 3-methoxytyramine levels in human basal ganglia. J Neural Transm 38:271–276, 1976.

34. Cattell, RB: Abilities: Their Structure, Growth, and Action. Houghton-Mifflin, Boston, 1971.

35. Celesia, GG and Daly, RF: Effects of aging on visual evoked responses. Arch Neurol 34:403–407, 1977.

36. Christensen, NJ: Plasma noradrenaline and adrenaline in patients with thyrotoxicosis and myxoedema. Clin Sci Mol Med 42:163–171, 1973.

37. Clark, T: The masters movement; Age conquers some, but it doesn't conquer all. Runner's World p 80, July 1979.

38. Coleman, PD and Flood, DG: Neuron numbers and dendritic extent in normal aging and Alzheimer's disease. Neurobiol Aging 8:521–545, 1987.

39. Corsellis, JAN: Discussion. In Katzman, R, Terry, RD, and Bick, KL (eds): Alzheimer's Disease: Senile Dementia and Related Disorders. Aging Series, Vol 7. Raven Press, New York, 1978, p 397.

40. Corsellis, JAN: Some Observations on the Purkinje Cell Population and on Brain Volume in Human Aging. In Terry, RD and Gershon, S (eds): Neurobiology of Aging. Aging Series, Vol 3. Raven Press, New York, 1976, pp 205–209.

41. Corso, JF: Sensory processes and age effects in normal adults. J Gerontol 26:90–105, 1971.

42. Cowley, M: The View from 80. Viking Press, New York, 1976, p 1.

43. Craik, FIM: Short-Term Memory and the Aging Process. In Talland, GA (ed): Human Aging and Behavior. Academic Press, New York, 1968, pp 131–168.

44. Craik, FIM: Two components in free recall. J Verbal Learning Verbal Behav 7:996–1004, 1968.

45. Craik, FIM: Age differences in recognition memory. Q J Exp Psychol 23:316–323, 1971.

46. Craik, FIM: Age Differences in Human Memory. In Birren, JE and Schaie, KW (eds): Handbook of the Psychology of Aging. Van Nostrand Reinhold, New York, 1977, pp 384–420.

47. Critchley, M: The neurology of old age. Lancet 1:1119, 1221, 1331–1336, 1931.

48. Damon, A: Discrepancies between findings of longitudinal and cross-sectional studies in adult life: Physique and physiology. Hum Dev 8:16–22, 1965.

49. Dastur, DK, Lane, MM, Hansen, DB, Key, SS, Butler, RN, Perlin, S, and Sokoloff, L: Effects of Aging on Cerebral Circulation and Metabolism in Man. In Birren, JE, et al (eds): Human Aging—Biological and Behavioral Study (USPHS Publ No 986). US Dept of Health, Education, and Welfare, Public Health Service, National Institutes of Health, National Institute of Mental Health, Bethesda, Maryland, 1963, pp 59–76.

50. Davies, ADM: Age and the memory-for-designs test. Br J Soc Clin Psychol 6:228–233, 1967.

51. Davies, P: Loss of Choline Acetyltransferase Activity in Normal Aging and in Senile Dementia. In Finch, CE, Potter, DE, and Kenny, AD (eds): Parkinson's Disease—II: Aging and Neuroendocrine Relationships. Plenum Press, New York, 1978, pp 251–256.

52. Davis, PJM and Wright, EA: A new method for measuring cranial cavity volume and its application to the assessment of cerebral atrophy at autopsy. Neuropathol Appl Neurobiol 3:341–358, 1977.

53. Dayan, AD: Quantitative histologic studies on the aged human brain. Acta Neuropathol 16:85–94, 1970.

54. Dekaban, AS and Sadowsky, D: Changes in brain weights during the span of human life: Relation of brain weights to body heights and body weights. Ann Neurol 4:345–356, 1978.

55. DeLeon, MJ, Ferris, SH, George, AE, Reisberg, B, Kricheff, II, and Gershon, S: Computed tomography evaluation of brain-behavior relationships in senile dementia of the Alzheimer's type. Neurobiol Aging 1:69–79, 1980.

56. Desmedt, JE and Cheron, G: Somatosensory evoked potentials to finger stimulation in healthy octogenarians and in young adults: Wave forms, scalp topography and transit times of parietal and frontal components. Electroencephalogr Clin Neurophysiol 50:404–425, 1980.

57. Desmedt, JE and Debecker, J: Wave form and neural mechanism of the decision P350 elicited without pre-stimulus CNV or readiness potential in random sequences of near-threshold auditory clicks and finger stimuli. Electroencephalogr Clin Neurophysiol 47:648–670, 1979.

58. Devaney, KO and Johnson, HA: Neuron loss in the aging visual cortex of man. J Gerontol 35:836–841, 1980.

59. Donchin, E: Augmenting mental chronometry: The P300 as a measure of stimulus evaluation time. Science 197:792–795, 1977.

60. Drachman, DA and Leavitt, J: Memory impairment in the aged:

Storage versus retrieval deficit. J Exp Psychol 92:302–308, 1972.

61. Drachman, DA and Zaks, MS: The "memory cliff" beyond span in immediate recall. Psychol Rep 21:105–112, 1967.

62. Dustman, RE and Beck, EC: The effects of maturation and aging on the wave form of visually evoked potentials. Electroencephalogr Clin Neurophysiol 26:2–11, 1969.

63. Ehringer, H and Hornykiewicz, O: Verteilung von Noradrenalin im Dopamin (3-hydroxytyramin) im Gehirn des Menschen und ihre Verhalten bei Erkrankungen des extrapyramidalen Systems. Klin Wochenschr 38:1236–1239, 1960.

64. Eisdorfer, C, Nowlin, J, and Wilkie, F: Improvement of learning in the aged by modification of autonomic nervous system activity. Science 170:1327–1329, 1970.

65. Eisdorfer, C and Wilkie, F: Intellectual Changes with Advancing Age. In Jarvik, LF, Eisdorfer, C, and Blum, JE (eds): Intellectual Functioning in Adults. Springer-Verlag, New York, 1973, pp 21–29.

66. Emson, PC and Lindvall, P: Distribution of putative neurotransmitters in the neocortex. Neuroscience 4:1–30, 1979.

67. Eriksen, CW, Hamlin, RM, and Daye, C: Aging adults and rate of memory scan. Bull Psychonomic Soc 1:259–260, 1973.

68. Eysenck, MW: Age differences in incidental learning. Dev Psychol 10:936–941, 1974.

69. Fang, HCH: Observations on Aging Characteristics of Cerebral Blood Vessels, Macroscopic and Microscopic Features. In Terry, RD and Gerson, S (eds): Neurobiology of Aging. Aging Series, Vol 3. Raven Press, New York, 1976, pp 155–166.

70. Fazekas, JF, Alman, RW, and Bessman, AN: Cerebral physiology of the aged. Am J Med Sci 223:245–262, 1952.

71. Fazekas, JF, Kleh, J, and Finnerty, F: Influence of age and vascular disease on cerebral hemodynamics and metabolism. Am J Med 18:477–485, 1955.

72. Feier, CD and Gerstman, LJ: Sentence comprehension abilities throughout the adult life span. J Gerontol 35:722–728, 1980.

73. Flowers, CR and Darley, FL: Decline of immediate recall with age. Percept Motor Skills 46:1275–1283, 1978.

74. Ford, JM, Hink, RF, Hopkins, WF, Roth, WT, Pfefferbaum, A, and Koppell, BS: Age effects on event-related potentials in a selective attention task. J Gerontol 34:388–395, 1979.

75. Friedlander, WJ: Electroencephalographic alpha rate in adults as a function of age. Geriatrics 13:29–31, 1958.

76. Fries, JR: Aging, natural death, and the compression of morbidity. N Engl J Med 303:130–135, 1980.

77. Gainotti, G, Daniele, A, and Silveri, MC: Abstracts of the International Neuropsychological Society 12th European Conference, July 5–9, 1989, Antwerp, Belgium, 1989.

78. Gaylord, SA and Marsh, GR: Age differences in the speed of a spatial cognitive process. 30:674–678, 1975.

79. Gick, ML, Craik, FIM, and Morris, RG: Task complexity and age differences in working memory. Mem Cogn 16:353–361, 1988.

80. Gilbert, JG: Memory loss in senescence. J Abnorm Soc Psychol 36:73–86, 1941.

81. Gilbert, JG: Thirty-five year follow-up of intellectual functioning. J Gerontol 28:68–72, 1973.

82. Goldman, JE: The association of actin with Hirano bodies. J Neuropathol Exp Neurol 42:146–152, 1983.

83. Gonzalez, CF, Lantieri, RL, and Nathan, RJ: The CT scan appearance of the brain in the normal el-

derly population: A correlative study. Neuroradiology 16:120–122, 1978.

84. Goodin, DS, Squires, KC, Henderson, BH, and Starr, A: Age-related variations in evoked potentials to auditory stimuli in normal human subjects. Electroencephalogr Clin Neurophysiol 44:447–458, 1978.

85. Gottfries, CG, Adolfsson, R, Oreland, L, Roos, BE, and Winblad, B: Monoamines and Their Metabolism and Monoamine Oxidase Activity Related to Age and to Some Dementia Disorders. In: Drugs and the Elderly. Perspectives in Geriatric Clinical Pharmacology. Proceedings of a symposium held in Ninewells Hospital, University of Dundee, on September 13–14, 1977. Macmillan, London, 1979, pp 189–197.

86. Gottfries, CG: Amine Metabolism in Normal Ageing and in Dementia Disorders. In Roberts, PJ (ed): Biochemistry of Dementia. John Wiley & Sons, New York, 1980, pp 213–239.

87. Graf, P and Schacter, DL: Implicit and explicit memory for new associations in normal and amnesic subjects. J Exp Psychol: Learn Mem Cogn 11:501–518, 1985.

88. Granick, S: Psychological Test Functioning. In Granick, S and Patterson, RD (eds): Human Aging, II. US Dept of Health, Education, and Human Welfare, Rockville, MD, DHEW Publication (HSM) 71-9037, 1971.

89. Green, RF: Age-intelligence relationship between ages sixteen and sixty-four: A rising trend. Dev Psychol 1:618–627, 1969.

90. Grote, SS, Moses, SG, Robins, E, Hudgen, RW, and Croninger, AB: A study of selected catecholamine metabolizing enzymes: A comparison of depressive suicides and alcoholic suicides with controls. J Neurochem 23:791–802, 1974.

91. Gyldensted, C: Measurements of the normal ventricular system and hemispheric sulci of 100 adults with computed tomography. Neuroradiology 14:183–192, 1977.

92. Harris, JE: Remembering to Do Things: A Forgotten Topic. In Harris, JE and Morris, PE (eds): Everyday Memory, Actions and Absent-Mindedness. Academic Press, London, 1984.

93. Haug, H: Are Neurons of the Human Cerebral Cortex Really Lost during Aging? A Morphometric Examination. In Traber, J and Gispen, WH (eds): Senile Dementia of the Alzheimer Type. Springer-Verlag, Berlin/Heidelberg, 1985, pp 150–163.

94. Hazzard, WR and Bierman, EL: Old Age. In Smith, D and Bierman, EL (eds): Biological Ages of Man from Conception Through Old Age, ed 2. WB Saunders, Philadelphia, 1978, pp 229–253.

95. Henderson, G, Tomlinson, BE, and Gibson, PH: Cell counts in human cerebral cortex in normal adults throughout life using an image analysing computer. J Neurol Sci 46:113–136, 1980.

96. Hertzog, CK, Williams, MV, and Walsh, DA: The effect of practice on age differences in central perceptual processing. J Gerontol 31:428–443, 1976.

97. Horn, JL and Donaldson, G: On the myth of intellectual decline in adulthood. Am Psychologist 31:701–719, 1976.

98. Howard, DV: The effects of aging and degree of association on the semantic priming of lexical decision. Exp Aging Res 9:145–151, 1983.

99. Howard, DV, McAndrews, MP, and Lasaga, MI: Semantic priming of lexical decision in young and old adults. J Gerontol 36:707–714, 1981.

100. Hoyer, FW, Hoyer, WJ, Treat, NJ, and Baltes, PB: Training response peaks in young and

elderly. Int J Aging Hum Dev 9:247–253, 1979.

101. Hubbard, O, Sunde, D, and Goldensohn, ES: The EEG in centenarians. Electroencephalogr Clin Neurophysiol 40:407–417, 1976.

102. Hughes, JR and Cayeffa, JJ: The EEG in patients at different ages without organic cerebral disease. Electroencephalogr Clin Neurophysiol 42:776–784, 1977.

103. Hulicka, IM: Age differences in Wechsler Memory Scale scores. J Gen Psychol 109:135–145, 1966.

104. Hulicka, IM and Grossman, JL: Age-group comparisons for the use of mediators in paired associate learning. J Gerontol 22:46–51, 1967.

105. Hulicka, IM and Weiss, RL: Age differences in retention as a function of learning. J Consult Psychol 29:125–129, 1965.

106. Hultsch, DF: Adult age differences in free classification and free recall. Dev Psychol 4:338–342, 1971.

107. Hultsch, DF: Adult age differences in retrieval: Trace-dependent and cue-dependent forgetting. Dev Psychol 11:197–210, 1975.

108. Hunziker, O, Abdel'Al, S, Frey, H, Veteau, MJ, and Meier-Ruge, W: Quantitative studies in the cerebral cortex of aging humans. Gerontology 24:27–31, 1978.

109. Huttenlocher, PR: Synaptic density in human frontal cortex—Developmental changes and effects of aging. Brain Res 163:195–205, 1979.

110. Jacobs, L, Kinkel, WR, Painter, F, Murawski, J, and Heffner, RR: Computed Tomography in Dementia with Special References to Changes in Size of Normal Ventricles during Aging and Normal Pressure Hydrocephalus. In Katzman, R, Terry, RD, and Bick, KL (eds): Alzheimer's Disease: Senile Dementia and Related Disorders. Aging Series, Vol 7. Raven Press, New York, 1978, pp 241–260.

111. Jacoby, RJ, Levy, R, and Dawson, JM: Computed tomography in the elderly: I The normal population. Br J Psychiatry 136:249–255, 1980.

112. Johnston, MV, McKinney, M, and Coyle, JR: Evidence for a cholinergic projection to neocortex from neurons in the basal forebrain. Proc Natl Acad Sci USA 76:5392–5396, 1979.

113. Jones, DH, Hamilton, CA, and Reid, JL: Plasma noradrenaline, age and blood pressure: A population study. Clin Sci Mol Med (Suppl 4)55:73s–75s, 1978.

114. Jorgensen, L and Torvik, A: Ischaemic cerebrovascular disease in an autopsy series. I. Prevalence, location, and predisposing factors in verified thrombo-embolic occlusions, and their significance in the pathogenesis of cerebral infarction. J Neurol Sci 3:490–509, 1966.

115. Kaplan, E, Goodglass, H, and Weintraub, S: Boston Naming Test. Lea & Febiger, Philadelphia, 1976.

116. Katzman, R, Terry, RD, De Teresa, R, Brown, T, Davies, P, Fuld, P, Renbing, X, and Peck, A: Clinical, pathological, and neurochemical changes in dementia: A subgroup with preserved mental status and numerous neocortical plaques. Ann Neurol 23:53–59, 1988.

117. Kety, SS: Human Cerebral Blood Flow and Oxygen Consumption as Related to Aging. In Moore, JE, Merritt, HH, and Masselink, RJ (eds): The Neurologic and Psychiatric Aspects of the Disorders of Aging. Williams & Wilkins, Baltimore, 1955, pp 31–45.

118. Kinsbourne, M: Cognitive Decline with Advancing Age: An Interpretation. In Smith, WL and

Kinsbourne, M (eds): Aging and Dementia. Spectrum Publications, New York, 1977, pp 217–235.

119. Kline, DW and Birren, JE: Age differences in backward dichoptic masking. Exp Aging Res 1:17–25, 1975.

120. Kline, DW and Szafran, J: Age differences in backward monoptic visual noise masking. J Gerontol 3:307–311, 1975.

121. Konigsmark, BW and Murphy, EA: Volume of ventral cochlear nucleus in man: Its relationship to neuronal population and age. J Neuropathol Exp Neurol 31:304–316, 1972.

122. LaFratta, CW and Canestrari, RE: A comparison of sensory and motor nerve conduction velocities as related to age. Arch Phys Med Rehabil 47:286–290, 1966.

123. Lake, CR, Ziegler, MG, Coleman, MD, and Koplin, IJ: Age-adjusted plasma norepinephrine levels are similar in normotensive and hypertensive subjects. N Engl J Med 296:208–209, 1977.

124. LaRiviere, JE and Simonson, E: The effect of age and occupation on speed of writing. J Gerontol 20:415–416, 1965.

125. Laufer, AC and Schweitz, B: Neuromuscular response tests as predictors of sensory-motor performance in aging individuals. Am J Phys Med 47:250–268, 1968.

126. Libow, LS, Obrist, WD, and Sokoloff, L: Cerebral circulatory and electroencephalographic changes in elderly men. In Granick, S and Patterson, RD (eds): Human Aging, II. US Dept of Health, Education, and Welfare, Rockville, MD, DHEW Publication (HSM) 71-9037, 1971.

127. Light, LL and Singh, A: Implicit and explicit memory in young and older adults. J Exp Psychol: Learn Mem Cognit 13:531–541, 1987.

128. Lloyd, K and Hornykiewicz, O: Occurrence and distribution of L-dopa decarboxylase in the human brain. Brain Res 22:426–428, 1970.

129. Luders, H: The effects of aging on the wave form of the somatosensory cortical evoked potential. Electroencephalogr Clin Neurophysiol 29:450–460, 1970.

130. MacKay, AVP, Yates, CM, Wright, A, Hamilton, P, and Davies, P: Regional distribution of monoamines and their metabolites in the human brain. J Neurochem 30:841–848, 1978.

131. Mann, DMA and Sinclair, KGA: The quantitative assessment of lipofuscin pigment, cytoplasmic RNA and nucleolar volume in senile dementia. Neuropathol Appl Neurobiol 4:129–135, 1978.

132. Masliah, E: Personal communication November, 1989.

133. Matousek, M and Peterson, I: Automatic evaluation of EEG background activity by means of age-dependent EEG quotients. Electroencephalogr Clin Neurophysiol 35:603–612, 1973.

134. Matsuyama, H, Namicki, H, and Watanabe, I: Senile Changes in the Brain in the Japanese. Incidence of Alzheimer's Neurofibrillary Change and Senile Plaques. In Luthy, F and Bischoff, A (eds): Proceedings of the Fifth International Congress of Neuropathology. Excerpta Medica Series #100, Amsterdam, 1966, pp 979–980.

135. McGeer, EG: Aging and Neurotransmitter Metabolism in the Human Brain. In Katzman, R, Terry, RD, and Bick, KL (eds): Alzheimer's Disease, Senile Dementia and Related Disorders. Aging Series, Vol 7. Raven Press, New York, 1978, pp 427–440.

136. McGeer, EG and McGeer, PL: Neurotransmitter metabolism in the aging brain. In Terry, RD and Gershon S (eds): Neurobiology of Aging. Aging Series, Vol 3.

Raven Press, New York, 1976, p 389.

137. McGeer, PL and McGeer, EG: Enzymes associated with the metabolism of catecholamines, acetylcholine and GABA in human controls and patients with Parkinson's disease and Huntington's chorea. J Neurochem 26:65–70, 1976.

138. Mehraein, P, Yamada, M, and Tarnowska-Dziduszko, E: Quantitative Study on Dendrites and Dendritic Spines in Alzheimer's Disease and Senile Dementia. In Kreutzberg, GW (ed): Physiology and Pathology of Dendrites. Advances in Neurology, Vol 12. Raven Press, New York, 1975, pp 453–458.

139. Meier-Ruge, W, Hunziker, O, Iwangoff, P, Reichlmeier, K, and Sandoz, P: Alterations of Morphological and Neurochemical Parameters of the Brain Due to Normal Aging. In Nandy, K (ed): Senile Dementia: A Biochemical Approach. Elsevier/North-Holland Biomedical Press, Amsterdam, 1978, pp 33–44.

140. Michalewski, HJ, Thompson, LW, Smith, DBD, Paterson, JV, Bowman, TE, Litzelman, D, and Brent, G: Age differences in the contingent negative variation (CNV): Reduced frontal activity in the elderly. J Gerontol 35:542–549, 1980.

141. Mitchell, DB: How many memory systems? Evidence from aging. J Exp Psychol: Learn Mem Cogn 15:31–49, 1989.

142. Monagle, RD and Brody, H: The effects of age upon the main nucleus of the inferior olive in the human. J Comp Neurol 155:61–66, 1974.

143. Morris, RG, Gick, ML, and Craik, FIM: Processing resources and age differences in working memory. Mem Cogn 16:362–366, 1988.

144. Nandy, K: Brain-Reactive Antibodies in Aging and Senile Dementia. In Katzman, R, Terry, RD, and Bick, KL (eds): Alzheimer's Disease: Senile Dementia and Related Disorders. Aging Series, Vol 7. Raven Press, New York, 1978, pp 503–512.

145. Nissen, MJ, Knopman, DS, and Schacter, DL: Neurochemical dissociation of memory systems. Neurology 37:789–794, 1987.

146. Norris, AH, Shock, NW, and Wagman, IH: Age changes in the maximum conduction velocity of motor fibers of ulnar nerves. J Appl Physiol 5:589–593, 1952/53.

147. Obrist, WD: The electroencephalogram of normal aged adults. Electroencephalogr Clin Neurophysiol 6:235–244, 1954.

148. Obrist, WD: Cerebral Circulatory Changes in Normal Aging and Dementia. In Hoffmeister, F and Muller, C (eds): Brain Function in Old Age. Springer-Verlag, Berlin, 1979, pp 278–287.

149. Obrist, WD, Sokoloff, L, Lassen, NA, Lane, MH, Butler, RN, and Feinberg, I: Relation of EEG to cerebral blood flow and metabolism in old age. Electroencephalogr Clin Neurophysiol 15:610–619, 1963.

150. Obrist, WD, Thompson, HK, Wang, HS, Wilkinson, WE: Regional cerebral blood flow estimated by ^{133}xenon inhalation. Stroke 6:245–256, 1975.

151. Otomo, E: Electroencephalography in old age: Dominant alpha pattern. Electroencephalogr Clin Neurophysiol 21:489–491, 1966.

152. Otomo, E and Tsubaki, T: Electroencephalography in subjects sixty years and over. Electroencephalogr Clin Neurophysiol 20:77–82, 1966.

153. Owens, WA: Age and mental abilities: A second adult follow-up. J Educ Psychol 57:311–325, 1966.

154. Patterson, JV, Michalewski, HJ, and Starr, A: Latency variability of the components of auditory event-related potentials to infrequent stimuli in aging, Alzheimer-type dementia, and depression. Electroencephalogr Clin Neurophysiol 71:450–460, 1988.

155. Perry, EK, Perry, RH, Gibson, PH, Blessed, G, and Tomlinson, BE: A cholinergic connection between normal aging and senile dementia in the human hippocampus. Neurosci Lett 6:85–89, 1977.

156. Pfefferbaum, A, Ford, JM, Roth, WT, Hopkins, WF, and Kopell, BS: Event-related potential changes in healthy aged females. Electroencephalogr Clin Neurophysiol 46:81–86, 1979.

157. Pfefferbaum, A, Ford, JM, Roth, WT, and Kopell, BS: Age differences in P3-reaction time associations. Electroencephalogr Clin Neurophysiol 49:257–265, 1980.

158. Potvin, AR, Syndulko, K, Tourtellotte, WW, Goldberg, Z, Potvin, JH, and Hansch, EC: Quantitative Evaluation of Normal Age-Related Changes in Neurologic Function. In Pirozzolo, FJ and Maletta, GJ (eds): Advances in Neurogerontology, Vol 2. Praeger, New York, 1981, p 13.

159. Potvin, AR, Syndulko, K, Tourtellotte, WW, Lemmon, JA, and Potvin, JH: Human neurologic function and the aging process. J Am Geriatr Soc 28:1–9, 1980.

160. Powers, JM and Spicer, SS: Histochemical similarity of senile plaque amyloid in Apudamyloid. Virchows Arch A (Pathol Anat Histol) 376:107–115, 1978.

161. Price, DL, Altschuler, RJ, Struble, RG, Casanova, MF, Cork, LC, and Murphy, DB: Sequestration of tubulin in neurons in Alzheimer's disease. Brain Res 385:305–310, 1986.

162. Reason, J and Mycielska, K: Absent Minded? The Psychology of Mental Lapses and Everyday Errors. Prentice-Hall, Englewood Cliffs, NJ, 1982.

163. Reimanis, G and Green, RF: Imminence of death and intellectual decrement in the aging. Dev Psychol 5:270–272, 1971.

164. Riegel, KF and Riegel, RM: Development, drop, and death. Dev Psychol 6:306–319, 1972.

165. Riegel, KF, Riegel, RM, and Meyer, G: Socio-psychological factors of aging: A cohort-sequential analysis. Hum Dev 10:27–56, 1967.

166. Rissenberg, M and Glanzer, M: Picture superiority in free recall: The effects of normal aging and primary degenerative dementia. J. Gerontol 41:64–71, 1986.

167. Rissenberg, M and Glanzer, M: Free recall and word finding ability in normal aging and senile dementia of the Alzheimer's type: The effect of item concreteness. J Gerontol 42:318–322, 1987.

168. Ritter, W, Simson, R, Vaughan, HG, Jr, and Macht, M: Manipulation of event-related potential manifestations of information processing stages. Science 218:909–911, 1982.

169. Ritter, W, Simson, R, Vaughan, HG, Jr: Effects of the amount of stimulus information processed on the negative event-related potentials. Electroencephalogr Clin Neurophysiol 69:244–258, 1988.

170. Robert, MA and Caird, FI: Computerized tomography and intellectual impairment in the elderly. J Neurol Neurosurg Psychiatry 39:986–989, 1976.

171. Robinson, DS, Nies, A, Davies, HN, Bunney, WE, Davis, JM, Colburn, RW, Bourne, HR, Shaw, DM, and Coppen, AJ: Ageing, monoamines and monoamine-oxidase levels. Lancet 1:290–291, 1972.

172. Robinson, DS, Sourkes, TL, Nies, A, Harris, LS, Spector, S, Bartlett,

DL, and Kaye, IS: Monoamine metabolism in human brain. Arch Gen Psychiatry 34:89–92, 1977.

173. Rothschild, D and Kasanin, J: Clinicopathologic study of Alzheimer's disease, relationship to senile conditions. Arch Neurol Psychiatry 36:293, 1936.

174. Rowe, EJ and Schnore, MM: Item concreteness and reported strategies impaired-associate learning as a function of age. J Gerontol 26:470–475, 1971.

175. Rowe, JW and Toen, BR: Sympathetic nervous system and aging in man. Endocr Rev 1:167–179, 1980.

176. Said, FS and Weale, RA: The variation with age of the spectral transmissivity of the living human crystalline lens. Gerontologia 3:213–231, 1959.

177. San Filippo, S: The masters movement: Payton Jordon springs to the front. Runner's World, p 85, July 1979.

178. Sands, LP, Terry, H, and Meredith, W: Change and stability in adult intellectual functioning assessed by Wechsler item responses. Psychology Aging 4:79–87, 1989.

179. Schaie, KW: Translations in gerontology—from lab to life. Intellectual functioning. Am Psychol 29:802–807, 1974.

180. Schaie, KW: Cognitive Development in Aging. In Obler, LK and Albert, ML (eds): Language and Communication in the Elderly: Clinical, Therapeutic and Experimental Issues. Lexington Books, Lexington, MA, 1980.

181. Schaie, KW: Intelligence and Problem Solving. In Birren, JE and Sloane, RB (eds): Handbook of Mental Health and Aging. Prentice-Hall, Englewood Cliffs, NJ, 1980, pp 262–284.

182. Schaie, KW, Labouvie, GV, and Buech, BU: Generational and cohort-specific differences in adult cognitive functioning. A four-teen-year study of independent samples. Dev Psychol 9:151–166, 1973.

183. Schaie, KW and Labouvie-Vief, GV: Generational versus ontogenetic components of change in adult cognitive behavior: A fourteen-year cross-sequential study. Dev Psychol 10:305–320, 1974.

184. Schaie, KW and Parham, IA: Cohort-sequential analyses of adult intellectual development. Dev Psychol 13:649–653, 1977.

185. Schaie, KW and Zelinski, E: Psychometric Assessment of Dysfunction in Learning and Memory. In Hoffmeister, F and Mueller, C (eds): Brain Function in Old Age. Springer-Verlag, Berlin, 1979, pp 134–150.

186. Scheibel, ME and Scheibel, AB: Structural Changes in the Aging Brain. In Brody, H, Harman, D, and Ordy, JM (eds): Clinical Morphologic, and Neurochemical Aspects in the Aging Central Nervous System. Aging Series, Vol 1. Raven Press, New York, 1975, pp 11–37.

187. Schjonfield, AED: Learning, Memory, and Aging. In Birren, JE and Sloane, RB (eds): Handbook of Mental Health and Aging. Prentice-Hall, Englewood Cliffs, NJ, 1980, pp 214–244.

188. Shaw, NA and Cant, BR: Age-dependent changes in the latency of the pattern visual evoked potential. Electroencephalogr Clin Neurophysiol 48:237–241, 1980.

189. Shaw, NA and Cant, BR: Age-dependent changes in the amplitude of the pattern visual evoked potential. Electroencephalogr Clin Neurophysiol 51:671–673, 1981.

190. Siegler, IC and Botwinick, J: A long-term longitudinal study of intellectual ability of older adults: The matter of selective subject attrition. J Gerontol 34:242–245, 1979.

191. Simon, E: Depth and elaboration of

processing in relation to age. J Exp Psychol 5:115–124, 1979.

192. Smith, ME: Delayed recall of previously memorized material after fifty years. J Gen Psychol 102:3–4, 1963.

193. Snyder, E and Hillyard, SA: Changes in visual event-related potentials in older persons. In Hoffmeister, F and Muller, C (eds): Brain Function in Old Age. Bayer-Symposium VII. Springer-Verlag, New York, 1979, pp 112–125.

194. Sokol, S, Moskowitz, A, and Towle, VL: Age-related changes in the latency of the visual evoked potential: Influence of check size. Electroencephalogr Clin Neurophysiol 51:559–562, 1981.

195. Sokoloff, L: Cerebral Circulatory and Metabolic Changes Associated with Aging. In Millikan, CH (ed): Cerebrovascular Disease, Vol 41. Williams & Wilkins, Baltimore, 1961, p 237.

196. Sokoloff, L: Effects of Normal Aging on Cerebral Circulation and Energy Metabolism. In Hoffmeister, F and Muller, C (eds): Brain Function in Old Age. Springer-Verlag, Berlin, 1979, pp 367–380.

197. Spirduso, WW and Clifford, P: Replication of age and physical activity effects on reaction and movement time. J Gerontol 33:26–30, 1978.

198. Spokes, EGS and Koch, DJ: Postmortem stability of dopamine, glutamine decarboxylase and choline acetyltransferase in the mouse brain simulating the handling of human autopsy material. J Neurochem 31:381–383, 1978.

199. Squire, LR: Memory and Brain. Oxford University Press, New York, 1987.

200. Stam, FC and Roukema, PA: Histochemical and biochemical aspects of corpora amylacea. Acta Neuropathol (Berl) 25:95–102, 1973.

200a. Sternberg, S: Memory-scanning: Mental processes revealed by reaction-time experiments. Am Sci 57:421–457, 1969.

201. Stine, EL and Wingfield, A: Process and strategy in memory for speech among younger and older adults. Psychol Aging 2:272–279, 1987.

202. Straumanis, JJ, Shagass, C, and Schwartz, M: Visually evoked cerebral response changes associated with chronic brain syndromes and aging. J Gerontol 20:498–506, 1965.

203. Talland, G: Three estimates of the word span and their stability over the adult years. Q J Exp Psychol 17:301–307, 1965.

204. Teräväinen, H and Calne, DB: Motor System in Normal Aging and Parkinson's Disease. In Katzman, R, Terry, RD, and Bick, KL (eds): Alzheimer's Disease: Senile Dementia and Related Disorders. Aging Series, Vol 7. Raven Press, New York, 1978, p 85.

205. Terry, RD, DeTeresa, R, and Hansen, LA: Neocortical cell counts in normal human adult aging. Ann Neurol 21:530–539, 1987.

206. Terry, RD, Peck, A, and DeTeresa, R: Some morphometric aspects of the brain in senile dementia of the Alzheimer type. Ann Neurol 10:184–192, 1981.

207. Thomae, H: Patterns of Aging. S Karger, New York, 1976, p I.

208. Tulving, E: How many memory systems are there? Am Psychol 40:385–398, 1985.

209. Vijayashankar, N and Brody, H: A quantitative study of the pigmented neurons in the nuclei locus coeruleus and subcoeruleus in man as related to aging. J Neuropathol Exp Neurol 38:490–497, 1979.

210. Walsh, DA: Age differences in central perceptual processing: A dichoptic backward masking investigation. J Gerontol 31:178–185, 1976.

211. Walsh, DA and Baldwin, M: Age differences in integrated semantic memory. Dev Psychol 13:509–514, 1977.

212. Walsh, DA and Thompson, LW: Age differences in visual sensory memory. J Gerontol 33:383–387, 1978.

213. Walsh, DA and Till, RE: Age differences in peripheral perceptual processing: A monoptic backward masking investigation. J Exp Psychol 4:232–243, 1978.

214. Wang, HS and Busse, EW: EEG of healthy old persons—A longitudinal study. I. Dominant background activity and occipital rhythm. J Gerontol 24:419–426, 1969.

215. Wang, HS and Busse, EW: EEG of Healthy Old Persons. In Palmore, E (ed): Normal Aging, Vol 2. Duke University Press, Durham, NC, 1974, pp 126–140.

216. Wang, HS, Obrist, WD, and Busse, EW: Neurophysiological Correlates of the Intellectual Function. In Palmore, E (ed): Normal Aging, Vol 2. Duke University Press, Durham, NC, 1974, pp 115–126.

217. Wechsler, D (ed): Manual for the Wechsler Adult Intelligence Scale. The Psychological Corporation, New York, 1955, p 75.

218. Wechsler, D (ed): The Measurement and Appraisal of Adult Intelligence, ed 4. Williams & Wilkins, Baltimore, 1958, p 297.

219. Weiss, AD: The locus of reaction time change with set, motivation, and age. J Gerontol 20:60–64, 1965.

220. Welford, AT: Motor Performance. In Birren, JE and Schaie, KW (eds): Handbook of the Psychology of Aging. Van Nostrand Reinhold, New York, 1977, p 450–496.

221. Welford, AT: Sensory, Perceptual, and Motor Processes in Older Adults. In Birren, JE and Sloane, RB (eds): Handbook of Mental Health and Aging. Prentice-Hall, Englewood Cliffs, NJ, 1980, p 192.

222. Wilkie, F and Eisdorfer, C: Intelligence and blood pressure in the aged. Science 172:959–962, 1971.

223. Williams, RS, Ferrante, RJ, and Caviness, VS, Jr: The Golgi rapid method in clinical neuropathology: The morphologic consequences of suboptimal fixation. J Neuropathol Exp Neurol 37:13–33, 1978.

224. Wingfield, A, Stine, EAL, Lahar, CJ, and Aberdeen, JS: Does the capacity of working memory change with age? Exp Aging Res 14:103–107, 1988.

225. Yamamura, H, Ito, M, Kubota, K, and Matsuzawa, T: Brain atrophy during aging: A quantitative study with computed tomography. J Gerontol 35:492–498, 1980.

226. Ziegler, MG, Lake, CR, and Kopin, IJ: Use of plasma norepinephrine for evaluation of sympathetic neuronal function in man. Life Sci 18:1315–1326, 1976.

Chapter 3

NEUROPSYCHO-PHARMACOLOGY

Carl Salzman, M.D.

Psychotropic drugs are widely used to treat behavioral, emotional, and cognitive disorders of the elderly. This chapter reviews fundamental principles of psychotropic drug activity and use. Emphasis is placed on the pharmacologic effects of drugs as altered by the aging process, as well as on the nonpharmacologic context within which psychotropic drugs are prescribed. The following topics are considered: (1) nonspecificity of psychiatric symptoms in the elderly; (2) nonspecificity of psychotropic drug effect; (3) the effect of concomitant illness on symptomatology and drug effect; (4) the effect of concomitant drug administration on psy-chotropic drug effects, polypharmacy, and drug interaction; (5) compliance problems, overmedication, undermedication; (6) pharmacokinetics of psychotropic drugs, altered metabolism, excretion, and therapeutic blood levels; (7) alterations in central nervous system (CNS) and peripheral nervous system (PNS) function that predispose to side effects and psychotropic side effects; (8) types of psychotropic drugs prescribed to older patients.

NONSPECIFICITY OF PSYCHIATRIC SYMPTOMS IN THE ELDERLY

There are five broad categories of dysfunction in older patients for which psychotropic drugs are commonly prescribed. These are disruptive behavior (agitation) and psychosis, depression, anxiety, sleep disturbance, and cognitive dysfunction. With the exception of drugs for cognitive dysfunction, which are developed primarily for use in older patients, psychotropic drugs used to treat the remaining four categories of symptoms were developed for use in younger adult patients, based on the assumption that symptoms in the elderly represent the same disease processes as in younger adults. For example, major depressive disorder, serious mania, and psychotic depression in the elderly are assumed to be essentially the same pathophysiologic disorders, as well as the same psychopathologic disorders, as in young people. Experienced clinicians are aware, however, that symptom patterns are less well defined in some older patients. It is not unusual, for example, to observe older patients who, in addition to having classic symptoms of schizophrenia or mania, also exhibit affective dysregulation, neurologic disorder, and cognitive impairment at the same time. Depressive disorder and generalized anxiety disorder commonly overlap in the elderly,[59] and there also may be considerable comorbidity and overlap between symptoms of depression, anxiety, and sleep disturbance. Depression and cognitive dysfunction occur so commonly together that researchers have searched for a reliable means of distinguishing one from the other, and in states of primary dementia, affective dysregulation, agitation, anxiety, and sleep disturbance are nearly universal.[27,37]

The definition of specific categories of psychiatric disturbance may become blurred for some elderly patients. Lack of diagnostic specificity, in turn, interferes with therapeutic precision, making it difficult to determine which class of psychotropic compounds to use for an older patient whose symptoms bridge two or more diagnostic categories. It is not surprising, therefore, that treatment response to psychotropic drugs in the elderly may not always be certain, and the accurate prediction of therapeutic effect may not always be possible.

NONSPECIFICITY OF PSYCHOTROPIC DRUG EFFECTS

There are five categories of psychotropic drugs commonly used to treat the five categories of psychiatric disorders in older patients: antipsychotics (including antimanic drugs), used primarily to treat agitation; antidepressants; antianxiety drugs; sedative hypnotics; and drugs for the treatment of cognitive disturbance and memory impairment, sometimes called no-otropics. However, this functional classification of psychotropic drugs developed in younger adults is dependent on a reasonably reliable and valid separation of symptoms into diagnostic categories that may not always apply to older patients.

Psychotropic drugs interact with multiple CNS receptors. In the elderly, these receptors are usually more sensitive to drug effect, resulting in clinically significant side effects (Tables 3–1 and 3–2). For example, the dopamine-blocking property of a neuroleptic drug given to an older patient is therapeutic for psychosis and agitation, but also causes extrapyramidal symptoms. Neuroleptics also block histamine receptors causing sedation, and block α_1-noradrenergic receptors, causing orthostatic hypotension.

Although these secondary properties of psychotropic drugs are usually considered to be unwanted side effects, they may be put to therapeutic use. Low doses of neuroleptics or antidepressants, for example, are commonly used

Table 3–1 PSYCHOTROPIC DRUG EFFECT ON NEUROTRANSMITTER SYSTEMS

| Drugs | Neurotransmitter | | | | | |
	Dopamine	Norepinephrine	Serotonin	Acetylcholine	Histamine	GABA
Antipsychotics	+++			+++	+++	
Lithium		+++	+++			
Antidepressants		+++	+++	+++	+++	
Antianxiety (benzodiazepines)						+++

Key: +++ = neurotransmitter affected.

Table 3–2 PROLONGED NEUROTRANSMISSION FUNCTION

Transmitter	Psychiatric Function	Drug Clinical Effect	Other Functions	Side Effects
Dopamine	Normal thought and processes; integration of cognition, emotion; socially appropriate behavior	Antagonist: antipsychotic, antimanic, antiagitation	Extrapyramidal function	Extrapyramidal symptoms; tardive dyskinesia
Norepinephrine	Regulation of mood and affect	Agonist: antidepression	Stimulant; maintenance of blood pressure	Cardiac arrhythmias and orthostatic blood pressure
Serotonin	Regulation of mood and affect	Agonist: antidepression	Regulate appetite, sexual function, aggression, wakefullness	Carbohydrate craving, sedation, increased aggression
Acetylcholine	Memory and cognition, orientation	Agonist: improve memory, concentration, orientation	Regulates cardiac rate, gland serotonin, lens accommodation, prostate function	Tachycardia, dryness, central anticholinergic syndrome

in general hospital settings to sedate nonpsychiatric patients; neuroleptics and lithium are sometimes used to control agitation; and benzodiazepines may be given to treat a range of nonspecific dysphoric states (Table 3–3).

Nonpsychotropic drugs are also given to older patients for their secondary psychotropic effects. Antihistamines, for example, are commonly given to older patients for sedating purposes. The anticonvulsants carbamazepine and valproate, as well as beta blockers, have had increasing use as treatments for serious affective disorder as well as treatments for serious agitation in demented patients. Calcium channel blockers may be useful in controlling treatment-resistant mania.

It is apparent, therefore, that the use of psychotropic drugs to treat older patients is a less specific and less precise process than their therapeutic classification would suggest. Psychotropic drugs (and other drugs as well) may have a broad range of activity at different neurotransmitter systems and these effects may be employed for therapeutic purposes or may produce side effects, or both.

THE EFFECT OF CONCOMITANT PHYSICAL ILLNESS

In the older patient, physical illness may initially present with psychiatric symptoms or may include psychiatric symptoms as part of the clinical picture. For example, pancreatic carcinoma, hypothyroid and hypoadrenal states, and chronic viral infection are

Table 3–3 THERAPEUTIC USES OF PSYCHOTROPIC DRUGS IN THE ELDERLY

Drug	Therapeutic Uses
Neuroleptics	Antipsychotic, antiagitation, sedation
Antidepressants	Antidepression, antipanic, sedation, stimulation
Lithium	Antimanic, antidepression, antiagitation
Benzodiazepines	Antianxiety, antiagitation, sedation, sleep
Anticonvulsants	Antimanic, antiagitation
Antihistamines	Sedation

well known to produce affective disturbance. Psychiatric disturbance is also common in neurologic illness. Significant depression frequently develops in those who suffer strokes,[7,42] and traumatic brain injury may result in exacerbation of pre-existing character or personality disorders, personality change secondary to the injury, intellectual changes, or the development of psychosis.[69] Head trauma may precipitate manic or depressive states in patients with bipolar illness or may result in the development of a first depressive episode.[43] Posttraumatic psychoses can occur immediately following brain injury or after a latency of many months of normal functioning.[69] Depressive mood disorder following a stroke may be a specific complication of brain damage from the stroke, rather than a reaction to the physical disability.[10] Depression is significantly higher in patients with left hemispheric cerebral vascular accidents, especially those with left anterior strokes.[41] Depression and irritability are among early manifestations of brain tumors and may be the only symptoms before the tumor increases in size and becomes associated with confusion, apathy, seizures, and coma.[69]

The presence of physical or neurologic disorder in an older patient makes the diagnosis of emotional disturbance more complicated as well as adding uncertainty to the selection of appropriate pharmacologic treatment. Although psychotropic drugs may be helpful for many of the emotional disturbances that accompany physical and neurologic disorders, the side effects that a psychotropic drug produces as a result of its broad spectrum of pharmacologic activity may exacerbate symptoms of the disease and limit the drug's usefulness. For example, the anticholinergic properties of neuroleptics given to demented older patients to control agitation may produce a worsening of both the agitation or cognitive impairment as well as the dementia.[3,33] The behavior and cognition of demented patients may also be made worse by the administration of benzodiazepines given to treat anxiety,[35,36] and increased agitation or psychosis has been noted when parkinsonian or demented patients are given antidepressants.[24] One of the most difficult and confusing therapeutic challenges occurs with an elderly patient who simultaneously has schizophrenia, Parkinson disease (PD), and tardive dyskinesia. If the schizophrenia is treated with a neuroleptic, then the PD symptoms get worse, and ultimately

Table 3–4 PSYCHOTROPIC DRUG TREATMENT OF ELDERLY PATIENTS WITH NEUROLEPTIC DISORDER

Disorder	Associated Psychiatric Disturbance	Psychotropic Drug Treatment	Potential Hazards of Psychotropic Drug Treatment
Parkinson disease	Depression	1. Cyclic antidepressants	Increased agitation
Stroke	Depression	1. Cyclic antidepressants	Hypotension, cardiac arrhythmias, risk of additional CVA, confusion, sedation
		2. MAO inhibitors	Hypotension, additional stroke
		3. ECT	Exacerbation of brain injury
Dementia	Depression	1. Antidepressants	Increased agitation, confusion due to anticholinergic effects or nonsedation
	Agitation	1. Neuroleptics	Oversedation, anticholinergic confusion
		2. Benzodiazepines	Disinhibition, agitation
		3. Lithium	Neurotoxicity, confusion
Multiple sclerosis	Mania	1. Lithium	Decreased coordination, cognitive impairment

Key: ECT = electroconvulsive therapy; CVA = cerebrovascular accident.

the tardive dyskinesia may be exacerbated. Alternatively, if the PD symptoms are treated with L-dopa, the schizophrenia and tardive dyskinesia will worsen. Table 3–4 lists treatment of emotional or psychiatric systems of common neurologic disorders with psychotropic drugs, and some of the potential hazards of such treatment.

CONSEQUENCES OF POLYPHARMACY AND DRUG INTERACTIONS IN THE ELDERLY

As physical illness and neurologic disorder predispose the older patient to an increased likelihood of psychotropic drug toxicity, medical treatments of concurrent physical disorders also cause an increased risk of drug interactions.

Many older patients regularly take medications including psychotropic drugs and even depend on them to remain alive. Survey data suggest that one third of general hospital older patients are prescribed psychotropic drugs.[47] More than 50% of older patients in a nursing home take at least one psychoactive medication and 11% take medications from two or more psychotropic drug classes.[1,2] Americans 65 years of age or older, who constitute 12% of the total population, receive 32% of all prescription drugs.[23]

Medical drugs given to older patients may cause two sets of psychiatric problems.[16,22,45,58] First, the drugs may cause psychiatric symptoms or exacerbate pre-existing psychiatric symptoms. Some of these psychiatric symptoms may be subtle and diagnostically confusing. For example, beta blockers may reduce initiative, energy, and motivation in a patient who was previously nondepressed. If not severe, these symptoms may be attributed to the aging process itself, pre-existing psychologic conflict, a concurrent stressful life circumstance, or simply to "the stage of life."

Second, medications given for the treatment of medical disorders may adversely interact with psychotropic drugs,[40,61] producing overt toxicity or interfering with the therapeutic effect of one or both compounds. An adverse drug interaction may result from alterations in absorption, distribution, metabolism, or elimination of drugs, as well as medication-induced changes in CNS sensitivity to drugs.

COMPLIANCE PROBLEMS

Psychotropic drugs, like other drugs, cannot be expected to produce an adequate therapeutic effect if not taken as prescribed. Elderly patients, as a group, are notoriously undercompliant or noncompliant in taking their psychotropic drugs.[33] The usual reasons are forgetfulness, confusion about doses and schedules, and side effects.

Forgetting to take one's daily doses of medication on a regular basis is probably common and in older patients leads to undermedication and suboptimal pharmacologic treatment. However, forgetfulness in older patients may also lead to overmedication. For example, the older patient who awakens in the middle of the night, forgetting that a hypnotic had already been taken, may take a second or even third dose. Accidental overdoses and inadvertent toxicity are not unusual.

Confusion over differing doses and dose schedules is also common in older patients who may take several drugs on a regular daily basis. It is not unusual to see older people at mealtime place several vials of pills before them, trying to remember which should be "taken with food," which is "taken before food," which is "taken once a day," and which is "taken several times a day." Physician's instructions written on the labels of these containers may be too small to be easily read, and verbal instructions are typically long forgotten or confused.

Psychotropic drug side effects also may cause drug noncompliance, which commonly leads to underdosing. Constipation, blurred vision, and dry mouth, for example, may be so distressing that the older patient will take less medication than prescribed.

Noncompliance also may result from an older patient's personal beliefs that extend over the course of a lifetime and represent part of the patient's own value system, family traditions, or characteristic ethnic expression of disability. For example, some older patients may have lived their life with a strong conviction that taking medication is a sign of weakness. Although seemingly accepting of a doctor's prescription of psychotropic drugs, such older people may take less than was prescribed, or not take the medication at all. Other older patients, reflecting an opposite set of traditions, may believe that if one pill helps, then two will help twice as much and twice as fast. Still others may or may not take drugs, depending on the symptoms for which they are prescribed. Some older patients, for example, may believe that depression is due to a failure of "character strength" and medication is concrete evidence of such failure. Memory loss, on the other hand, may be considered by the same individual to be a natural consequence of aging, and medications to improve memory become an acceptable treatment.

Whatever the cause, clinicians prescribing psychotropic drugs to older patients must recognize the potential for overmedication as well as undermedication due to compliance problems. Failure to respond to treatment may be due to undermedicating or pharmacologic failure rather than treatment resistance; unusual or early-appearing side effects may be the result of overdosing rather than excessive sensitivity to psychotropic drugs.

AGE-RELATED ALTERATIONS IN THE PHARMACOKINETICS OF PSYCHOTROPIC DRUGS

The aging process alters the disposition of most psychotropic drugs by decreasing the efficiency of hepatic biotransformation and renal clearance.

Delays in hepatic metabolism are especially notable for neuroleptics, cyclic antidepressants, and the long half-life benzodiazepines.[17,45,48] The elimination half-life for these compounds tends to be two to three times longer in older individuals than in younger adult counterparts. Blood levels of these drugs tend to rise as well, so that therapeutic doses that are appropriate for young adults may produce toxic blood levels when given to the elderly.[51,62] Impaired renal clearance of water-soluble substances such as lithium[20] or the hydroxy metabolites of cyclic antidepressants is also delayed by the aging process, leading to accumulation and elevated blood levels.[68] Impaired renal clearance of lithium, in particular, predisposes the older person to neurotoxicity at standard therapeutic doses and blood levels that would be nontoxic in younger adults.[45] In contrast, short half-life benzodiazepines (e.g., oxazepam, lorazepam, alprazolam, triazolam, temazepam) are only subejct to hepatic conjugation, which is not affected by the aging process, so there is no accumulation or prolongation of elimination half-life of these compounds.[17,45,48]

Pharmacokinetic properties of psychotropic drugs may also be altered by diseases that are common in advanced age, as well as by medications that are commonly taken by older patients. Chronic protein-depleting illnesses, for example, reduce serum albumin, thereby decreasing protein binding of psychotropic drugs and leading to increased toxicity. Medications that interfere with enzymatic metabolism of psychotropic drugs, thereby raising blood levels, include the commonly prescribed drugs cimetidine, methylphenidate, and fluoxetine.

THE EFFECT OF AGE-RELATED CHANGES IN CNS NEUROTRANSMISSION ON PSYCHOTROPIC DRUG EFFECTS

It is generally assumed that alterations in CNS neurotransmission cause increased sensitivity to the therapeutic and toxic effects of psychotropic drugs.[5,46,49,63] For example, age-related reductions in CNS dopamine probably predispose the older patient to an increased frequency and severity of extrapyramidal symptoms that result from neuroleptic dopamine blockade. It has been similarly assumed that because of age-related reductions in CNS acetylcholine, older patients become more susceptible to the anticholinergic effects of neuroleptics and cyclic antidepressants. Reduced α- and β-norepinephrine as well as serotonin receptor function may make older patients more sensitive to the effects of cyclic antidepressants, and alterations in gamma-aminobutyric acid (GABA)–benzodiazepine receptor complex function associated with age may make older patients especially sensitive to benzodiazepines, barbiturates, and alcohol.

These assumptions are corroborated by the clinical observation that older patients are often more sensitive to therapeutic as well as side effects of psychotropic drugs at doses of one third to one half those that are usually given to younger patients. However, the necessity for lower doses does not apply to all older patients; some require therapeutic doses that are equivalent to those given to younger adults. It may well be, therefore, that the CNS of older patients may be either more or less sensitive to psychotropic drug effects.

TYPES OF PSYCHOTROPIC DRUGS PRESCRIBED TO OLDER PATIENTS

Neuroleptics

Neuroleptics (antipsychotic agents) are used in psychiatry predominantly for the treatment of psychotic illness. Older patients, like their younger counterparts, may be treated with neuroleptics for symptoms of schizophrenia, mania, or psychotic depression. More commonly, however, neuroleptics are given to control the severe agitation and disruptive behavior that accompany organic brain disorder.[39,54,57,67] Neuroleptics may also be used in older patients as part of the treatment of severe pain, nausea, hiccups, and sedation.

There are no data suggesting unique therapeutic benefits of any particular neuroleptic. Therefore, neuroleptic drug selection for the older patient rests on an appreciation of differential side effect patterns that are produced by neuroleptic drugs. As shown in Table 3–5, low-potency neuroleptics such as chlorpromazine commonly produce sedation and orthostatic hypotension, but relatively weakly produce extrapyramidal symptoms. Conversely, high-potency neuroleptics such as haloperidol or fluphenazine are very likely to produce severe extrapyramidal symptoms, but are less likely to produce sedation or orthostatic hypotension. Several non-

Table 3–5 RELATIVE INCIDENCE OF SIDE EFFECTS OF NEUROLEPTIC DRUGS

Generic Name	Trade Name	Sedation	Hypotension	Extrapyramidal Symptoms	Anticholinergic Symptoms
Chlorpromazine	Thorazine; Chlor PZ	Marked	Marked	Moderate	Marked
Chlorprothixene	Taractan	Marked	Marked	Moderate	Marked
Thiondazine	Mellaril	Marked	Marked	Mild–moderate	Moderate
Acetophenazine	Tindal	Moderate	Moderate	Moderate	Moderate
Perphenazine	Trilafon	Moderate	Moderate	Moderate	Moderate
Loxapine	Loxitane	Moderate	Moderate	Moderate	Moderate
Molindone	Moban	Moderate	Moderate	Moderate	Moderate
Trifluperazine	Stelazine	Moderate	Moderate	Moderate–marked	Moderate–mild
Thiothixene	Navane	Moderate	Moderate	Moderate–marked	Moderate–mild
Fluphenazine	Prolixin	Mild	Mild	Marked	Mild
Haloperidol	Haldol	Mild	Mild	Marked	Mild

Source: Adapted from Salzman,[47] p 55.

neuroleptic strategies have also been employed to treat severe agitation in psychotic or organically impaired elderly patients. These include buspirone,[4] trazodone,[18,31,64,65] propranolol,[66,70] carbamazepine,[28] and lithium.[19]

Antidepressants

There are two basic classes of antidepressant drugs—cyclic antidepressants,[25,30,34,44,51,52,55,60] and MAO inhibitors.[12–15,26,53,71] Selection of an antidepressant, like selection of a neuroleptic, is based on differential side effect production (Table 3–6). In general, the tertiary amine antidepressants tend to produce the most frequent and most intense side effects. However, not all older patients will develop serious side effects from tertiary amines, and with careful dosing, they may be effective and nontoxic. Nevertheless, as a general prescribing guideline, the secondary amines are recommended for older patients, and, among the secondary amines, nortriptyline and desipramine are usually considered the antidepressants of first choice. Fluoxetine, a new[8,9] antidepressant with atypical structure, has been reported to be effec-

tive for elderly patients,[12,15] but further research is necessary.

Among the MAO inhibitors, there are no comparative data suggesting differences in either therapeutic efficacy or frequency and severity of side effects. Some clinicians prefer phenelzine, believing it to be slightly more therapeutic than the other two MAO inhibitors, tranylcypromine and isocarboxazid. Other clinicians, however, prefer tranylcypromine or isocarboxazid, having observed these two compounds to produce somewhat less orthostatic hypotension than the phenelzine.

Lithium

Lithium is used in psychiatry primarily for the treatment and prevention of symptoms of mania and depression.[20,29] Most elderly manic patients have had previous treatment for their disorder, so it is unusual to begin lithium for the first time in older patients. The aging process significantly affects the use of lithium. Therapeutic as well as toxic effects develop with lower doses (and lower blood levels) than in younger adults. Neurotoxicity may be the first indication of excessive lithium in older

Table 3–6 RELATIVE SIDE EFFECTS OF CYCLIC ANTIDEPRESSANTS IN THE ELDERLY PATIENT

Drug	Sedation	Hypotension	Anticholinergic Side Effects	Altered Cardiac Rate and Rhythm
TERTIARY AMINES				
Imipramine	Mild	Moderate	Moderate–strong	Moderate
Doxepin	Moderate–strong	Moderate	Strong	Moderate
Amitriptyline	Strong	Moderate	Very strong	Strong
Trimipramine	Strong	Moderate	Strong	Strong
SECONDARY AMINES				
Desipramine	Mild	Mild–moderate	Mild	Mild
Nortriptyline	Mild	Mild	Moderate	Mild
Amoxapine	Mild	Moderate	Moderate	Moderate
Protriptyline	Mild	Moderate	Strong	Moderate
Maprotiline	Moderate–strong	Moderate	Moderate	Mild
ATYPICAL				
Trazodone	Moderate	Moderate	Mild (except dry mouth)	Mild–moderate
Fluoxetine	*	None	None	None

*Some patients are stimulated; others experience sedation.

patients, and alterations in consciousness may be seen at lithium blood levels that are relatively nontoxic in younger adults.[20] Excretion of lithium through the renal tubular system is also reduced due to age-related changes in renal function, prolonging the elimination half-life of lithium and raising circulating plasma levels.

Sedative Hypnotics

Nearly all older patients complain of disturbed sleep, most commonly awakening in the middle of the night or early in the morning. Their sleep is neither restful nor refreshing, and daytime sleepiness results in "make-up" sleep in the form of daytime naps. Naps, in turn, interfere with nighttime sleep. Other factors that interfere with nighttime sleep include poor sleep hygiene, drugs, alcohol, physical illness, pain, and impaired respiration.

Three benzodiazepine drugs are commonly used for hypnotic purposes[11,38]: flurazepam (Dalmane), temazepam (Restoril), and triazolam (Halcion). Flurazepam has an unusually long elimination half-life, which is further prolonged by the aging process, and may produce unwanted daytime sedation in the elderly, especially at higher doses. Triazolam, having a very short half-life with no active metabolites, is an ideal benzodiazepine from the pharmacokinetics point of view. Unfortunately, prolonged use of triazolam by older patients may be associated with impaired memory as well as strong drug dependence. Temazepam is also a short half-life benzodiazepine but is more slowly absorbed than either flurazepam or triazolam. For this reason, it must be given earlier in the evening before the hour of sleep.

Although there are no data to support the long-term therapeutic effectiveness of these drugs, surveys of nursing home drug prescription patterns indicate that such long-term use of these drugs is not unusual. Older residents of nursing homes often believe these drugs to be helpful for sleep and are extremely reluctant to terminate their use.[32] However, preliminary data, as well as clinical experience, suggest that chronic use of benzodiazepine hypnotics may be associated with impaired cognitive function in older patients. This may be especially true in those individuals who already suffer from mild to moderate dementia.[56]

Benzodiazepines are the drugs most commonly given to assist the onset of sleep in the elderly, although neuroleptics, antidepressants, and antihistamines are also sometimes used by older patients. Benzodiazepine hypnotics are frequently used in general hospitals, as well as in nursing homes. Although short-term use of benzodiazepine hypnotics may be therapeutic and helpful, the long-term efficacy and safety of these drugs in the elderly must be questioned.

Antianxiety Agents

Benzodiazepines are also the class of drugs that are predominantly used for the treatment of anxiety disorders as well as anxiety symptoms in older patients.[43,59] Classified according to their pharmacologic properties (Table 3–7), there are no data to suggest the therapeutic superiority of any particular benzodiazepine or some type of benzodiazepine over any other. Long half-life benzodiazepines may be given to the compliant older patient for whom once-a-day dosing is preferable and toxicity is not likely. Short half-life benzodiazpines, however, are usually preferred for the elderly because they provide flexible dosing and lack cumulative toxicity.[6,21,50]

Although benzodiazepine pharmacokinetics have been well studied in the elderly, there are remarkably few studies of the appropriate therapeutic use of these drugs for the anxious older patient. Opinion regarding their use seems to be divided among experienced clinicians. For some, the benzodiazepines provide older patients consider-

Table 3–7 CLASSIFICATION OF BENZODIAZEPINES

Elimination Half-Life	Therapeutic Potency	
	High	*Low*
Short–intermediate	Triazolam, alprazolam, lorazepam, midazolam	Oxazepam, temazepam
Long	Clonazepam	Chlordiazepoxide, diazepam, flurazepam, halazepam, corazepate

able symptom relief and, with careful dosing, relatively little toxicity. Others consider benzodiazepines to be especially toxic in the elderly, and avoid their use except for brief, crisis situations. Older patients are divided about the usefulness of these drugs. In a recent survey, older patients who took benzodiazepines on a regular basis did not perceive them to be toxic, harmful, or inappropriate.[32] But some older patients, especially those who are mentally alert and active, express concern about benzodiazepines interfering with memory, attention, and mental agility in general.

Recent research suggests that benzodiazepine antianxiety drugs may contribute to subtle cognitive impairments in older patients.[35,36] Most typically, this is manifested by an impairment of short-term memory identical to the short-term memory problems that occur naturally with age. Consequently neither the older patient nor the older patient's family may attribute such memory loss to the benzodiazepine. Similar cognitive impairment may result from long-term treatment with benzodiazepine hypnotic drugs. Clinical experience as well as pilot research data suggest, however, that when the benzodiazepine is discontinued, there may be a demonstrable improvement in concentration and recall.

CONCLUSION

Information from the studies of neurobiology and geriatric pharmacokinetics and the prescription of psychotropic drugs to older patients has increased rapidly in recent years. Clinicians now can draw upon treatment guidelines that are derived from extensive clinical experiences as well as from controlled research data. These guidelines suggest the following: Diagnostic classifications that are used for younger adult psychiatric patients may be somewhat imprecise and less helpful for older patients. Older patients with psychiatric disorders are also more likely to be suffering from age-related impairments in CNS functioning and from medical-neurologic illness. They are often taking concomitant medications or are not complying with the treatment regimens. Each of these factors alone or in combination with one or more of the others may predispose the older patient to a more uncertain therapeutic outcome and enhanced toxicity. Nevertheless, treatment with neuroleptics, lithium, and antidepressants has become firmly established in geriatric psychiatry and medicine, and overwhelming experience leads to the conclusion that these drugs are considerably more beneficial, when used appropriately, than they are harmful. Use of benzodiazepines, sleep medication, and drugs for cognitive impairment is less therapeutically predictable, and for some patients the risks of treatment may not clearly outweigh the benefits.

Older patients, like their younger counterparts, must be carefully and thoroughly evaluated prior to treatment, and clinical psychopharmacologic decisions, including selection of drug as well as dose range, must be tailored to the individual patient. Although treatment generalizations can be made, there is considerable variability among older patients. Old people may be a homogeneous group as defined by age, but they are quite heterogeneous in the response of their bodies and their brains to psychotropic drugs.

REFERENCES

1. Avorn, J, Dreyer, P, Connelly, KMA, and Soumerai, SB: Use of psychiatric medication and the quality of care in rest homes. N Engl J Med 320:227–232, 1989.
2. Beers, M, Avorn, J, Soumerai, S, Everitt, D, Sherman, DS, and Salem, S: Psychoactive medication use in intermediate care facility residents. JAMA 260:3016–3020, 1988.
3. Branconnier, RJ, DeVitt, DR, Cole, JO, and Spera, KF: Amitriptyline selectively disrupts verbal recall from secondary memory of the normal aged. Neurobiol Aging 3:55–59, 1982.
4. Colenda, CC: Buspirone in treatment of agitated demented patient. Lancet 1:1169, 1988.
5. Creasey, H and Rapoport, SI: The aging human brain. Ann Neurol 17:2–10, 1985.
6. Curran, HV, Allen, D, and Lader, M: The effects of single doses of alprazolam and lorazepam on memory and psychomotor performance in normal humans. J Psychopharmacol 2:81–89, 1987.
7. Feibel, JH and Springer, CJ: Depression and failure to resume social activities after stroke. Arch Phys Med Rehabil 63:276–277, 1982.
8. Feighner, JP, Boyer, WF, Meredith, CH, and Hendrickson, G: An overview of fluoxetine in geriatric depression. Br J Psychiatry 153(Suppl 3):105–108, 1988.
9. Feighner, JP and Cohn, JB: Double-blind comparative trials of fluoxetine and doxepin in geriatric patients with major depressive disorder. J Clin Psychiatry 46:20–25, 1985.
10. Folstein, MF, Maiberger, R, and McHugh, PR: Mood disorder as a specific complication of stroke. J Neurol Neurosurg Psychiatry 40:1018–1020, 1977.
11. Gaillard, JM: Place of benzodiazepines in the treatment of sleep disturbances. Rev Med Suisse Romande 107:717–720, 1987.
12. Georgotas, A, Friedman, E, McCarthy, M, Mann, J, Krakowski, M, Siegel, R, and Ferris, S: Resistant geriatric depressions and therapeutic response to monoamine oxidase inhibitors. Biol Psychiatry 18:195–205, 1983.
13. Georgotas, A, Mann J, and Friedman, E: Platelet monoamine oxidase inhibitors as a potential indicator of favorable response to MAOIs in geriatric depression. Biol Psychiatry 16:997–1001, 1981.
14. Georgotas, A, McCue, RE, Hapworth, W, Friedman, E, Kim, OM, Welkowitz, J, Chang, I, and Cooper, TB: Comparative efficacy and safety of MAOIs versus TCAs in treating depression in the elderly. Biol Psychiatry 21:1155–1166, 1986.
15. Gerner, RH: Antidepressant selection in the elderly. Psychosomatics 25:528–535, 1984.
16. Glassman, R and Salzman, C: Interactions between psychotropic and other drugs. An update. Hosp Commun Psychiatry 48:19–22, 1987.
17. Greenblatt, DJ: Pharmacokinetics of Antianxiety Drugs in the Elderly. In Salzman, C and Lebowitz, B (eds): Anxiety in the Elderly. Springer, New York, 1991, pp 131–148.
18. Greenwald, BS, Marin, DB, and Silverman, SM: Serotoninergic treatment of screaming and banging in dementia. Lancet 2:1464–1465, 1986.
19. Holton, A and George, K: The use of lithium in severely demented patients with behavioral disturbance. Br J Psychiatry 146:99–104, 1985.
20. Jefferson, JW, Greist, JH, Ackerman, DL, and Carroll, JA: Lithium Encyclopedia for Clinical Practice. APPI, Washington, DC, 1987, pp 43–46.

21. Koepke, HH, Gold, RL, Linden, ME, Lion, JR, and Rickels, K: Multicenter controlled study of oxazepam in anxious elderly outpatients. Psychosomatics 23:641–645, 1982.

22. Lamy, PP: The elderly and drug interactions. J Am Geriatr Soc 34:586–692, 1986.

23. Lamy, PP: Prescribing Patterns of Psychotropic Drugs. In Salzman, C (ed): Clinical Geriatric Psychopharmacology, ed 2. Williams & Wilkins, Baltimore, in press.

24. Larson, EB, Kukull, WA, Buchner, D, and Reifler, BV: Adverse drug reactions associated with global cognitive impairment in elderly persons. Ann Intern Med 107:169–173, 1987.

25. Laskshamanan, EB, Mion, CC, and Frengley, JD: Effective low dose tricyclic antidepressant treatment for depressed geriatric rehabilitation patients. J Am Geriatr Soc 34:421–426, 1986.

26. Lazarus, LW, Groves, L, Gierl, B, Pandey, G, Javaid, JI, Lesser, J, Ha, JS, and Davis, J: Efficacy of phenelzine in geriatric depression. Biol Psychiatry 21:699–701, 1986.

27. Lazarus, LW, Newton, N, Cohler, B, Lesser, J, and Schweon, C: Frequency and presentation of depressive symptoms in patients with primary degenerative dementia. Am J Psychiatry 144:41–45, 1987.

28. Leibovici, A and Tariot, N: Carbamazepine treatment of agitation associated with dementia. J Geriatr Psychiatry Neurol 1:110–112, 1988.

29. Liptzin, B: Treatment of Mania. In Salzman, C (ed): Clinical Geriatric Psychopharmacology, 1984, pp 116–131.

30. Peabody, CA, Whiteford, HA, and Hollister, LE: Antidepressants and the elderly. J Am Geriatric Soc 34:869–874, 1986.

31. Pinner, E and Rich, CL: Effects of trazodone on aggressive behavior in seven patients with organic mental disorders. Am J Psychiatry 145:1295–1296, 1988.

32. Pinsker, H and Suljaga-Petchel, K: Use of benzodiazepines in primary-care geriatric patients. J Am Geriatr Soc 32:595–598, 1984.

33. Plasky, P, Marcus, L, and Salzman, C: Effects of psychotropic drugs on memory. Part 2. Hosp Commun Psychiatry 5:501–502, 1988.

34. Plotkin, DA, Gerson, SC, and Jarvik, LF: Antidepressant Drug Treatment in the Elderly. In Meltzer, HY (ed): Psychopharmacology: The Third Generation of Progress. Raven Press, New York, 1987, 1149–1158.

35. Pomara, N, Stanley, B, Block, R, Greenblatt, DJ, Newton, RE, and Gershon, S: Diazepam impairs performance in normal elderly subjects. Psychopharmacol Bull 20:137–139, 1984.

36. Pomara, N, Stanley, B, Block, R, Guido, J, Russ, D, Berchou, R, Stanley, M, Greenblatt, DJ, Newton, RE, and Gershon, S: Adverse effects of single therapeutic doses of diazepam on performance in normal geriatric subjects: Relationships to plasma concentrations. Psychopharmacol Bull 84:342–346, 1984.

37. Reifler, BV, Larson, E, Teri, L, and Paulson, M: Dementia of the Alzheimer's type and depression. Am Geriatr Soc 34:855–859, 1986.

38. Reynolds, CF, Kupfer, DJ, Hoch, CC, and Sewitch, DE: Sleeping pills for the elderly: Are they ever justified? J Clin Psychiatry 46:9–12, 1985.

39. Risse, SC and Barnes, R: Pharmacologic treatment of agitation associated with dementia: Geriatric Seminar. J Am Geriatr Soc 34:368–376, 1986.

40. Rizos, AL, Sargenti, CJ, and Jeste, DV: Psychotropic drug reaction in the patient with late-onset depression or psychosis. Part II. Psychiatr Clin N Am 11:253–278, 1988.

41. Robinson, RG, Kubos, KL, Starr, LB, Rao, K, and Price, TR: Mood changes in stroke patients: Relationship to lesion location. Comp Psychiatry 24:555–566, 1983.

42. Robinson, RG and Price, TR: Post-stroke depressive disorders: A follow-up study of 103 patients. Stroke 13:635–641, 1982.

43. Robinson, RG and Szetela, B: Mood change following left hemisphere brain injury. Ann Neurol 9:447–453, 1981.

44. Rockwell, E, Lam, RW, and Zisook, S: Antidepressant drug studies in the elderly. Psychiatr Clin North Am 11:215–233, 1988.

45. Salzman, C: Key concepts in geriatric psychopharmacology—Altered pharmacokinetics and polypharmacy. Psychiatr Clin North Am 5:181–190, 1982.

46. Salzman, C: Neurotransmission in the Aging Central Nervous System. In Salzman, C (ed): Clinical Geriatric Psychopharmacology. McGraw-Hill, New York, 1984, pp 18–31.

47. Salzman, C: Overview. In Salzman, C (ed): Clinical Geriatric Psychopharmacology. McGraw-Hill, New York, 1984, p 307.

48. Salzman, C: Pharmacokinetics of Psychotropic Drugs and the Aging Process. In Salzman, C (ed): Clinical Geriatric Psychopharmacology. McGraw-Hill, New York, 1984, pp 32–45.

49. Salzman, C: The Aging Process and Response to Psychotropic Drugs. In Salzman, C (ed): Clinical Geriatric Psychopharmacology. McGraw-Hill, New York, 1984, pp 3–17.

50. Salzman, C: Treatment of Anxiety. In Salzman, C (ed): Clinical Geriatric Psychopharmacology. McGraw-Hill, New York, 1984, pp 132–148.

51. Salzman, C: Clinical guideline for the use of antidepressant drugs in geriatric patients. J Clin Psychiatry 46(Suppl):38–44, 1985.

52. Salzman, C: Clinical use of antidepressant blood levels and the electrocardiogram. N Engl J Med 313:512–513, 1985.

53. Salzman, C: Caution urged in using MAOIs with the elderly. Letter to the Editor. Am J Psychiatry 143:118–119, 1986.

54. Salzman, C: Treatment of agitation in the elderly. In Meltzer, HY (ed): Psychopharmacology: The Third Generation of Progress. Raven Press, New York, 1987, pp 1167–1176.

55. Salzman, C: Treatment of the depressed elderly patient. In Altman, HJ (ed): Alzheimer's Disease and Dementia: Problems, Prospects, and Perspectives. Plenum Press, New York, 1987, pp 171–182.

56. Salzman, C: Discontinuing benzodiazepines improves cognition in elderly nursing home residents. Unpublished data, 1988.

57. Salzman, C: Treatment of agitation, anxiety, and depression in dementia. Psychopharmacol Bull 24:39–42, 1988.

58. Salzman, C: Drug Interactions. In Salzman, C (ed): Clinical Geriatric Psychopharmacology, ed 2. Williams & Wilkins, Baltimore, in press.

59. Salzman, C and Lebowitz, B: Anxiety in the Elderly. Springer, New York, 1991.

60. Salzman, C and van der Kolk, BA: Treatment of Depression. In Salzman, C (ed): Clinical Geriatric Psychopharmacology. McGraw-Hill, New York, 1984, pp 77–115.

61. Sargenti, CJ, Rizos, AL, and Jeste, DV: Psychotropic drug reactions in the patient with late-onset psychosis and mood disorder. Part I. Psychiatr Clin North Am 11:235–252, 1988.

62. Schmucker, DL: Drug disposition in the elderly: A review of the critical factors. J Am Geriatr Soc 32:144–149, 1984.

63. Severson, JA: Neurotransmitter receptors and aging. J Am Geriatr Soc 32:24–27, 1984.

64. Simpson, DM and Foster, D: Improvement in organically disturbed behavior with trazodone treatment. J Clin Psychiatry 47:191–193, 1986.

65. Tingle, D: Trazodone in dementia. Letter to the Editor. J Clin Psychiatry 47:482, 1986.

66. Weiler, PG, Mungas, D, and Bernick, C:

Propranolol for the control of disruptive behavior in senile dementia. J Geriatr Psychiatry Neurol 1:226–230, 1988.

67. Wragg, RE and Jeste, DV: Neuroleptics and alternative treatments. Management of behavioral symptoms and psychosis in Alzheimer's disease and related conditions. Psychiatr Clin North Am 11:195–213, 1988.

68. Young, RC, Alexopoulos, GS, Shamoian, CA, Kent, E, Dhar, AK, and Kutt, H: Plasma 10-hydroxynortriptyline and ECG changes in elderly depressed patients. Am J Psychiatry 142:866–868, 1985.

69. Yudofsky, SC and Silver, JM: Psychiatric Aspects of Brain Injury: Trauma, Stroke, and Tremor. In American Psychiatric Association Annual Review #4. American Psychiatric Press Inc, Washington, DC, 1985, pp 142–158.

70. Yudofsky, S, Williams, D, and Gorman, J: Propranolol in the treatment of rage and violent behavior in patients with chronic brain syndromes. Am J Psychiatry 138:218–220, 1981.

71. Zisook, S: A clinical overview of monoamine oxidase inhibitors. Psychosomatics 26:240–246, 1985.

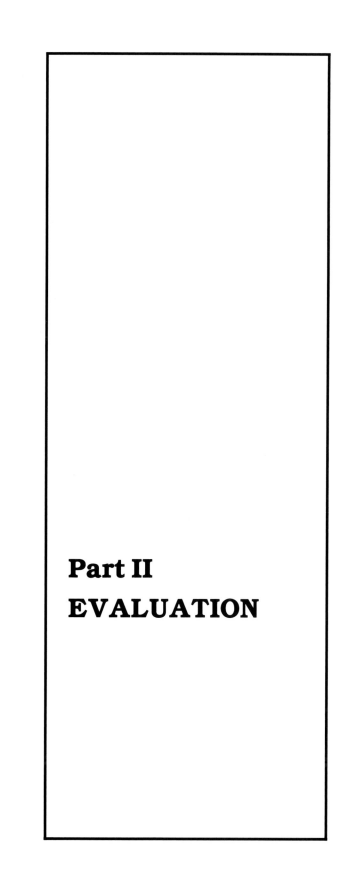

Part II
EVALUATION

Chapter 4

THE NEUROLOGIC CONSULTATION AT AGE 80

Leslie Wolfson, M.D., and
Robert Katzman, M.D.

THE NEUROLOGIC HISTORY AND
NEUROLOGIC EXAMINATION
THE NEUROLOGIST'S ROLE IN
EVALUATION AND MANAGEMENT

This chapter discusses the problems faced by a clinician when assessing the neurologic status of an 80-year-old patient. The physical characteristics of the elderly population today, rather than how they may change in the future, are relevant, and cross-sectional, rather than longitudinal, studies are pertinent.

It should be emphasized that the 80-year-old patient may be subject to any of the neurologic disease processes that normally afflict adults.[62] Thus, we have recently seen the onset of typical myasthenia gravis at age 82. There are age-associated neurologic diseases that are more common in persons in their 80s, but one must not focus on these disorders to the exclusion of other neurologic disorders.

What makes an 80-year-old person special? The octogenarian born in the early 1900s is less apt to have completed more than eight grades of school than are younger persons. She or he is more likely to have been born in a foreign country, with English as a second language. Life expectancy at age 80 is 8.8 years for a woman and 6.9 years for a man.[57] Of every 100 persons reaching age 80, only 68 will reach 85.[57] Chronic diseases of all types are common. Three fourths of all persons aged 80 will be afflicted with at least one chronic disease, and half of those over age 80 will have more than one.[49] On the average, persons dying at this stage of life may have six true medical diagnoses. Malcolm Cowley notes that age 80 is characterized by an accumulation of bottles in the medicine cabinet with "directions to take four a day."[13] Eighty-year-old persons who are disease-free represent a minority of their age group. Therefore, the average patient a neurologist encounters in the course of a consultation is not likely to belong to this healthy minority, but rather to the majority with multiple diseases.

The aging process in essentially healthy, disease-free persons is associated with decrements in many aspects of motor and sensory function (see Chapter 2). When multiple illnesses are superimposed on normal aging, physical reserves used to perform the complex motor activities required for the activities of daily living are compromised (Table 4–1). The loss of functional ability is increasingly common among the very old, frequently leading to a request for neurologic consultation. Specific disorders frequently encountered in the consultation are discussed in Chapter 13.

Table 4–1 FUNCTIONAL STATUS OF "NORMAL" 80-YEAR-OLDS*

	Functional Status		
Activity	**No Difficulty**	**With Difficulty But Does Not Need Help**	**Needs Help**
Getting in and out of bed	78	21	1
Sitting down or standing up from a chair	69	29	1
Toileting, continence	68	31	1
Eating, cutting food, pouring beverages	96	4	0
Preparing own meals	92	1	1
Dressing and undressing	82	17	1
Climbing or descending stairs	50	45	3
Shopping (finding way to store, carrying parcels)	83	9	3
Shopping (making change)	95	3	1
Caring for own finances, balancing checkbook	88	8	0

*Subjects are aged 74–85, ambulatory, community-living volunteers.
Source: Unpublished data, Bronx Aging Study.

THE NEUROLOGIC HISTORY AND NEUROLOGIC EXAMINATION

In general, the skills of neurologic history taking are applicable to the elderly patient. It is important to keep in mind that some patients may be slow in their responses or even mildly demented. For this reason the examiner must be prepared to consult other sources (e.g., family, friends, or medical records) for corroborative information.

When evaluating a history, a note of caution is in order. Some elderly patients will have an indolent response to acute disease, resulting in a seriously ill patient with relatively few signs and symptoms. Most often, there is the muted response to acute infection that results in little, if any, fever or leukocytosis, as well as the absence of more specific signs and symptoms such as headache, nuchal rigidity, or the pain syndromes that are usually suggestive of myocardial infarctions (MIs) or acute abdominal processes. At times, confusional states may substitute for more typical symptom patterns in patients with infections, MIs, or other systemic disorders.

In 1931, Critchley[14] summarized changes he encountered in examining elderly patients overtly free of neurologic disease. Subsequent studies have added to these descriptions,[15,44–46,55] although there is considerable variation from study to study in the frequency of these changes[11,27,36,37,47] (Table 4–2). In addition to differences in the population samples in the studies (hospitalized vs community-based, urban poor vs upper middle class, and so forth), it is likely that examiners differed in their criteria for the abnormalities.

Mental Status

The mental status examination requires special emphasis in the elderly because of the increase in frequency of dementia and delirium with aging. Inpatient services have shown that the presence of the cognitive changes associated with these conditions is grossly underdiagnosed, perhaps due to the reluctance of many physicians to examine mental status.

Because of the importance of diagnosing cognitive impairment as represented by dementia and delirium, formal mental status tests, such as the Mini-Mental State Examination (MMSE)[19] and the Information-Memory-Concentration (IMC)[10,20] examination, were developed against a back-

Table 4–2 FREQUENCY OF NEUROLOGIC FINDINGS IN THE ELDERLY

	Howell et al., [27] 1949	Klawans et al., [36] 1971	Prakash and Stern, [47] 1973	Kokmen et al., [37] 1977	Carter, [11] 1979	Murray et al., Unpublished Data
Age	63–91	65–74	69–84	61–84	70 plus	74–85
Number	200	927	100	51	100	100
Subjects	Active residents of geriatric hospital	Community-based urban poor (receiving old age assistance)	Unselected patients with no neurologic history from geriatric hospital	Community-based volunteers, upper middle class	Hospital inpatients free of neurologic disease	Community-based volunteers, lower middle class
Oculomotor						
Convergence loss	0.56	—	0.12	0.27	0.08	0.10
Pupillary changes	0.36	—	0.34	0.11	0.08	0.09
Motor						
Weakness upper extremities	0.08	0.07	(0.73 atrophy dorsal interossei) (0.63 thenar atrophy)	0.02	(0.5 atrophy of first dorsal interosseus)	0.11
Weakness lower extremities		0.13	(0.23 anterior tibial atrophy)			0.07
Gait abnormalities	—	—	0.22	—	—	0.38
Cerebellar changes —alternating movements	0.20			0.08 (0.16 abnormal F→N)		
Tremor outstretched hands (nonparkinsonian)			0.43			0.12
Reflexes:						
Deep tendon reflex absent						
Biceps jerk	0.13	0.05	0.08	—	0.07	0.08
Knee jerk	0.23	0.12	0.26	—	0.13	
Ankle jerk	0.70	0.76	0.38	0.18	0.44	0.39
Extensor						
Plantar	0.015	0.002	0.03	—	—	
Glabellar			0.35	0.31		0.20
Snout		0.17		0.41		0.12
Palmomental						
Sensation diminished						
Tactile			—	0.27	—	0.07
Pain and temperature				0		0.13
Position	0.15	0.17	0.07	100% showed increase in threshold	0.29	
Vibration	0.25	0.84	0.31		0.57	0.22

ground of decades of research identifying specific test items that are especially sensitive for generalized cognitive impairment.[34] Short versions of these tests that are appropriate to use when examining subjects free of the symptoms of dementia and delirium are available (e.g., six-item test[33]). The clinical evaluation of mental status, however, requires evaluation of functions beyond the formal mental status test. Thus, the examination should contain other elements such as

1. Test of the ability of a patient to follow a three- or four-stage command (e.g., "Close your eyes, touch your right thumb to your left ear, and stick out your tongue").

2. A test of language, including naming of objects and parts of objects, repetition of a phrase, and observation of the fluency, grammar, and amount of spontaneous speech.

3. Ideomotor praxis (e.g., "Please play-act and show me how you would hammer a nail").

4. A simple arithmetic calculation.

5. A test of visual-spatial construction ability (e.g., "Please draw a clock, put the numbers on it, and set the hands at 3:30").

6. A test of verbal fluency (e.g., "How many animals can you name in 1 minute?").

These examination items, together with a short version of a mental status test, such as the six-item mental status test, can be used as a basis for the routine evaluation of elderly subjects who do not have the symptoms of dementia or delirium. If such symptoms are present, then a more complete examination needs to be done, as described in Chapters 7 and 9; in addition, formal neuropsychologic testing is very useful (see Chapter 6).

Still, much can be learned about a patient's mental status during history taking. Most important is the observation of whether the patient is alert. A fluctuating level of awareness might indicate the presence of a delirium and would require immediate follow-through.

During history taking, the examiner can discover whether speech and language are normally fluent and whether any paraphasias are present. If the physician is obtaining a history for the first time from a patient, questions concerning birth date, birth place, age, years of education, and occuption are appropriate and give significant information about long-term and autobiographic memory. Moreover, educational and occupational levels are important information in regard to the interpretation of formal mental status questions.

What levels of performance should be expected of an 80-year-old? Cognitive and verbal ability are usually preserved in the normal elderly, as discussed in Chapter 2. Decrements in central motor processing time and memory with aging are real but are not usually demonstrated on the routine mental status evaluation. Extensive data exist, however, in regard to the formal mental status tests, the MMSE and the IMC. Four or five errors on either test are within normal limits for elderly persons of less than high school education; college graduates should make no more than one or two errors on these tests. If the brief clinical status evaluation described above is used, there should be no more than two errors in the five-part memory phrase of the six-item test or one self-corrected error in the months backward. The subjects should have been able to name at least 10 animals in 1 minute and the other parts of the examination should have been without error. If there is a greater problem than indicated by these guidelines, then a more complete evaluation of cognitive status should be carried out.

Vision

Visual acuity is often compromised in the elderly. Even in elderly subjects with normal acuity measured with a Snellen chart, visual acuity is considerably worse in conditions of low contrast and low luminance.[1,3] This finding is consistent with previous anatomic and functional studies, indicating a deterioration of photoreceptors after age 20.[3,22,48,59] Clinically, however, visual acuity in the elderly is affected primarily by four age-related conditions: presbyopia, cataract, glaucoma, and senile macular degeneration.

Presbyopia, resulting from the decreased ability of the lens to accommodate to near objects, is easily corrected by glasses that magnify; clinically the problem appears to begin in the fifth decade and progresses slowly over decades. In fact, the loss of accommodation of the lens can be considered to be part of a lifelong lenticular developmental process. The lens is reported to continue to grow throughout life, with an increase in bulk of 30% between ages 20 and 60. Changes in accommodation also occur throughout life; accommodation amplitude changes from 7 diopters (D) at age 15 to 3 D at age 30 and 1 D at age 40.[8,25,38] The fact that clinical symptoms do not begin until accommodation is less than 1 D attests to the extraordinary reserve of the visual system. This finding has also been interpreted as an indication that presbyopia is "a sign of continual development, not of deterioration of the accommodative mechanism." Perhaps the loss of accommodative capacity during adult life plays a role in limiting the ability of older athletes in sports requiring a high degree of eye-hand coordination.

Cataracts, representing changes in the lucency of the lens, were a major cause of visual loss in the elderly only 15 years ago. Complications of lens removal were sufficiently significant that only dense cataracts were operated on by many surgeons. New techniques for removal of the lens and implantation of a plastic lens have improved the stituation dramatically; the procedure has become so routine and relatively complication free that the National Eye Institute has reported that the success rate was between 95% and 97% in 1987.[9] Now the procedure is often carried out when visual acuity has only fallen to 20/40; some surgeons are willing to operate on cataracts, producing even less visual loss. The physician may be asked advice in this regard;

clearly the decision depends on the individual situation, that is, the extent to which functional impairment is produced by the early cataract.

The remaining two conditions continue to constitute important causes of blindness in the elderly. The pathophysiology of glaucoma is outside the scope of this book; choice of treatment is in the domain of the ophthalmologist. The obligation of the neurologist and geriatrician is to make sure that patients have a yearly measurement of intraocular pressure if feasible. Drugs used in the treatment of glaucoma, however, may have systemic effects. In particular, although applied locally, beta blockers enter the circulation and, in very susceptible individuals, may affect cognition or produce other side effects that lead to visits to a geriatrician or neurologist.

The success the ophthalmologist has had in treating presbyopia and cataracts, and in controlling glaucoma in some individuals, does not pertain to senile macular degeneration, which continues as a major cause of visual dysfunction in the elderly. Perhaps the best data in regard to the prevalence of conditions that produce visual loss in the elderly are those from the Framingham Longitudinal Study.[35] At ages 75 to 85, 46.1% of the cohort had cataracts, 27.9% senile macular degeneration, 7.2% open-angle glaucoma, and 7.0% diabetic retinopathy. The pathogenesis of senile macular degeneration appears to involve Bruch's membrane early in the course rather than photoreceptors alone.[63] In contrast to presbyacusis, a condition in which noise trauma plays a major role, exposure to sunlight, including ultraviolet light (UVA and UVB), is not related to the development of macular degeneration.[61] There is some evidence, not yet replicated, that vascular risk factors and hyperopia are risk factors for macular degeneration.[23]

Hearing

Some loss of auditory perception, particularly of higher frequency, is an almost invariable consequence of aging. Clinically significant hearing loss is usually defined as a pure tone loss of 40 dB or greater. Such hearing loss is strongly age related.[5,41] There is a hearing loss rate of 4.2% in the period between ages 17 and 44, 11.4% between ages 45 and 64, 23.1% between ages 65 and 74, and 39.8% in individuals over age 75.[52]

Presbyacusis accounts for most of this age-related change in hearing. The major pathology that accounts for presbyacusis is the loss of cochlear hair cells in the organ of Corti.[4,16] There is reasonable, but not exact, agreement between the degree of hair cell loss and the degree of audition loss. In part, this is accounted for by the coexistence of other otologic conditions that impair hearing.[4,21,51] During a systematic study of presbyacusis started in Denmark in 1951, at the occasion of the provision of free medical examinations, hearing aids, and audiologic rehabilitation, a number of cases of otosclerosis and of sequelae of otitis media, as well as presbyacusis, were found.[31] Hence, a careful examination of the ear is important in all individuals undergoing audiologic testing for a hearing aid.

How useful are hearing aids in the elderly? At the time of the 1951 reform in Denmark, hearing aids were widely distributed. In a 15-year follow-up of binaural hearing aids in patients over age 60, published in 1967, 27% were found to use them full-time, 49% used them part-time, and 22% did not use them.[31] This study was important in that the sudden widespread availability of hearing aids produced a relatively unselected cross section of the hearing impaired. With miniaturization of electronics, far superior hearing aids are made today, and if a similar study were possible now, the percentage benefiting from the hearing aid would increase significantly. The problem that remains in some elderly individuals is that functional speech hearing and speech discrimination are not improved adequately, even with today's sophisticated hearing aids.

Speech discrimination is complex. Significant difficulty in speech discrimination may exist without a substantial deficit in auditory acuity.[6,52] The difficulty that older individuals have understanding speech in a room with high background noise, the "cocktail party" problem, is well documented.[58] Loudness discrimination becomes impaired. It is likely that central age-related impairments such as slowing of perception (described in Chapter 2) may impair the understanding of speech, particularly if it is near threshold and rapid. Changes that may occur in brainstem auditory nuclei with aging may affect these perceptual processes.

Pupillary Changes and Eye Movements

In his original papers and in follow-up studies 25 years later, Critchley[14,15] noted that elderly patients had miotic, poorly reactive pupils with poor convergence. Subsequently, Howell,[27] and later Kokmen,[37] reported a bilateral loss of both pupillary light reflex and accommodation that increased with age. Although cross-sectional studies of normal subjects between the third and ninth decades indicate a 20% to 25% decrease in pupillary diameter under constant illumination,[8,40] some evidence suggests that only pupillary size, not reactivity, diminishes with age.[8] Cinephotography using pupillography indicates a progressive decrease in the velocity and degree of constriction as well as pupillary size.[40] Clinically apparent abnormalities in pupil size and reaction, together with poor convergence, occur in 9% to 36% of the normal elderly (see Table 4–2). Pharmacologic studies of pupillary size and constriction in elderly and younger persons suggest that the miosis of the elderly may be related to diminished preganglionic sympathetic tone.[38]

Critchley[14,15] noted diminished upward gaze in elderly patients, as did Kokmen[37] in 20% of his patients. Using a perimeter, Chamberlain[12] demonstrated progressive limitation of upward gaze from 37° at 15 to 34 years of age, to 16° in persons over 75 years of age. Quantitative oculography and more observational studies of pursuit eye movements in young and elderly patients show increased latencies with diminished smooth pursuit velocities and increased saccadic frequency in the elderly.[39,53,55] These increased saccades, which give the appearance of cogwheeling,[30] probably account for the eye movement changes reported by Kokmen in 31% of elderly patients.[37]

Motor Examination

Cross-sectional studies using quantitative measures of strength indicate that healthy subjects in their 70s can be expected to have 60% to 80% of the strength of persons in their 20s.[45,46] This objective loss of power is comparable to the loss encountered in the elderly on neurologic examination. Just as one corrects for age in evaluating the strength of children, one must take age into consideration when evaluating the power of older patients. This decrease of muscle power is often accompanied by loss of muscle bulk. Atrophy of the intrinsic muscles of the hand, especially the dorsal interossei and thenar muscles, without weakness or fasciculations, is present in over half of all elderly subjects.[11,47]

The neurologist must often rely on functional testing or a comparison of muscle groups within the same patient (left vs right, upper vs lower extremities). In our experience, the glutei and iliopsoas are particularly difficult to test, so that functional testing (i.e., the patient rises from a low chair with arms folded, or walks up steps) may be needed to evaluate functional power in these muscle groups. Behavioral studies have documented a fall-off in both reaction time and the speed of performing a task (see Chapter 2). In their quantitative neurologic examination, Potvin and co-workers[45,46] confirmed this, reporting a decrease in coordination and

dexterity as well as a loss of ability to perform such simulated activities of daily living as putting on a shirt or cutting with a knife (see Chapter 2 and Table 2–3). Dysmetria on finger-to-nose testing was noted by Howell[27] and Kokmen.[37] Skre[55] has noted increasing dysdiadochokinesia with age. In our own experience, mild unexplained ataxia is also occasionally encountered in the elderly and is often the only manifestation of cerebellar dysfunction in these patients.

Sensory Examination

Abnormalities in pain and tactile perception in the elderly were reported by Critchley[14,15] "in a number of very aged individuals." A decrease in the perception of light touch has been reported by others,[27,37] although Potvin and associates[45,46] did not find a statistically significant decrement in touch or two-point discrimination in their quantitative neurologic examination. Psychologic studies show, however, that with increasing age, there is an increase in the threshold of tactile sensitivity on the upper extremities and cornea.[60] The evidence also suggests an increase in the threshold of pain and temperature sensitivity with age, but these are most often not demonstrable by neurologic examination.[60]

Vibratory sensitivity shows a significant decrement with age in both quantitative and qualitative studies. There is both a large increase in threshold (2- to 10-fold),[44–46] and a substantial decrease in the number of patients who can perceive the vibratory stimulus.[14,15,27,36] Loss of vibratory perception is much more prominent in the lower extremities, and if there is a mild upper extremity loss, it is usually accompanied by a much greater loss in the lower extremities.[36]

Abnormalities of joint position sense on neurologic examination have been noted by Howell[27] and Klawans[36] in 15% to 20% of elderly patients. Decreases in both two-point discrimination and stereognosis have been reported also in quantitative psychologic studies,[60] but this has not been carefully studied in the context of the neurologic examination.

Reflexes

Critchley[14,15] noted that deep tendon reflexes became progressively more difficult to elicit with advancing age and finally disappear. He found that the first reflex to disappear was the ankle jerk, and that other deep tendon reflexes were compromised much later. Although this point has been confirmed by most investigators,[11,27,36,54] one exception noted that ankle jerks were obtained in 99% of elderly patients if reinforcement was used; this series excluded patients with overt neurologic disease or diabetes.[17]

In our own experience (M. P. Murray and colleagues, unpublished observations) and in the majority of clinical studies of elderly patients,[7] 30% to 45% of those examined have lost their ankle jerks. Despite some disagreement among researchers, patients with absent ankle jerks may occasionally also lose their knee jerks and biceps jerks.[27,36]

Although the 1931 Critchley paper[14] noted that extensor plantar responses were "occasionally" present in the elderly without pathologic reason, a subsequent paper indicated that this was "exceptional." Other authors[27,36,37] have also reported that unexplained extensor plantar responses are rare in elderly patients. However, superficial abdominal reflexes do disappear with age.[14,15,27] Palmomental and snout reflexes are seen in apparently normal elderly individuals, the palmomental occurring in 28% to 60% of the tested volunteers, the snout reflex occurring in 12% to 33%.[28,36] In one series, the incidence of these abnormal reflexes more than doubled between the fifth and ninth decades.[28] The significance of these release signs in elderly patients who are otherwise normal is unclear.

Disturbances of Gait

> I am now between 97 and 98 years old and enjoy good health . . . excepting the complaint I now attempt to describe.
>
> About 10 or 11 years ago, I found that in walking, I was apt to lose my equilibrium and sometimes to stagger . . . particularly if I looked up to see the town clock or how the wind blew, in doing which I have several times nearly fallen to the ground; this complaint gradually increased. (Memoirs of E. A. Holyoke,[26] 1830.)

Dr. Holyoke, a noted Massachusetts physician and centenarian, formulated his own concept as to the etiology of his difficulty:

> My idea of the disease is this . . . I presume that by disease or old age, the brain may be so shrunk or shrivelled as to leave such a vacuity as to allow the brain to vacillate and so produce the staggering and unsteady walking, so common to persons much advanced in age.[26]

We have progressed only moderately since Dr. Holyoke's speculations. Normal walking occurs with the integration of pyramidal, extrapyramidal, and cerebellar outputs in the frontal cortex, thalamus, and upper brainstem. In the case of Dr. Holyoke, a postmortem examination (witnessed by the full membership of the Essex County Medical Society) confirmed the presence of cerebral atrophy, of "excess fluid," just as he had predicted; in addition, the cerebellum was reported to be small.[26] Thus, multiple etiologies were possible. There is no certainty as to which system is the most important contributor to what has been termed the "idiopathic gait problem of the elderly."

Changes in gait occur as one of the most frequent concomitants of aging (see Chapter 10). Furthermore, difficulties with balance as noted by difficulty with tandem gait, one-legged standing, and even standing steadiness, are also noted in the elderly.[45,46]

Gait characteristics of normal elderly males studied by stoplight photography are shown in Figure 4–1.[42] There is slight anteroflexion of the upper torso

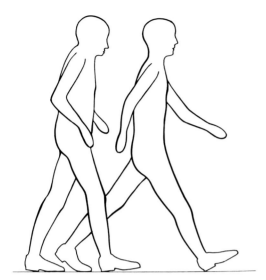

Figure 4–1. With the aid of stoplight photography, the characteristic gait pattern of an elderly male is compared with that of a younger male. Slight anteroflexion of the upper torso with flexion of the arms and knees, diminished armswing, and shorter step length are present. (From Wolfson and Katzman,[62] p 227, with permission.)

with flexion of the arms and knees, diminished arm swing, and shorter step lengths.[42] Although older women have shorter step length, their gait is less easily characterized; the description of this gait as narrow-based with a waddling quality[2,18] is certainly not a consistent finding. Despite these descriptions, *there is no characteristic gait associated with age, although both stride length and walking speed decrease significantly in healthy community-dwelling elderly.*

Deterioration of gait is a frequent cause for neurologic consultation. Gait disturbances are also major contributions to falls, another event frequently leading to neurologic evaluation. These patients' histories should be geared toward delineating the time course of the gait abnormality, dimensions of the current disability, circumstances in which the problem is most prominent (e.g., walking in the dark, steps, and so forth), and other relevant symptoms (e.g., dementia, brainstem and cerebel-

lar symptoms, urinary symptoms, weakness, and sensory symptoms).

In view of the multiple possible loci of neurologic dysfunction underlying gait abnormality, the neurologic examination must be complete, with emphasis on the functional characteristics of gait, turning, balance, arising from a chair, and if feasible, climbing steps. Furthermore, strength, reflexes, and sensory function, especially in the lower extremities, must be evaluated carefully. Several types of gait abnormality are clinically distinct and are identified on clinical grounds, as well as on the basis of associated signs.

Laboratory Evaluation in the Neurologic Consultation of the 80-Year-Old

Most of the elements of the laboratory evaluation carried out in the context of a neurologic consultation are the same whether the patient is 40 or 80 years old. Of course, the laboratory evaluation depends on the nature of the symptoms and signs and consequent differential diagnosis. However, because of the extraordinary efficiency of the automated chemistry laboratory, it is most cost efficient to use a single package that will be appropriate to almost all neurologic patients. We therefore recommend that the neurologist negotiate a laboratory panel that will include a complete blood count and a routine chemical screen, with the addition of a sedimentation rate, thyroid function tests, vitamin B_{12} and folate levels, serologic test for syphilis, and if indicated and permissible, a test for acquired immunodeficiency syndrome (AIDS).[32,34] In addition, of course, special blood (or urine) determinations need to be ordered if exposure to "recreational" drugs or other toxins is suspected, or if a recessive genetic metabolic disorder such as Wilson disease, late-onset Kuf disease, or metachromatic leukodystrophy is suspected. The average 80-year-old is on four or more prescription drugs; their concentration in the blood is often a matter of importance, for example, if a confusional state is present.

Once the mainstay of the neurologist, lumbar puncture is no longer used as often because noninfectious focal processes are more directly diagnosed by computed tomography (CT) or magnetic resonance imaging (MRI). Lumbar puncture is required, however, to demonstrate the presence of subarachnoid hemorrhage, acute or chronic meningitis, or other meningeal processes. Often the organism can be recovered from CSF. Specific changes in immunoglobulins are, of course, found in the CSF of multiple sclerosis (MS) patients, but CSF changes are not consistently present in cases of vasculitis in the elderly.

In regard to imaging, skull x-rays are only rarely indicated. The most frequently performed imaging procedures are CT and MRI. These are indicated in all patients with dementia, delirium, or other cognitive problems, intracerebral strokes, or significant symptoms referable to the brain or brainstem. The CT scan is relatively inexpensive and very rapid and, therefore, the indicated procedure to rule out tumors, abscesses, hydrocephalus, or other focal lesions in the cerebral hemispheres. However, the artifact on CT caused by the radiopacity of bones at the base of the skull is particularly bothersome when searching for posterior fossa lesions; MRI is clearly preferable in such cases. Small vascular lesions are more likely to be visualized on the MRI.

The CT scan has revolutionized the diagnosis of dementia. In the largest pre-CT autopsy series,[29] 7% of persons seen for the diagnosis of dementia were found to have silent brain tumors (4.7%), intracranial masses such as subdural hematomas (1%), or hydrocephalus (1%). The advent of the CT scan has made it possible to readily diagnose, during life, those structural disorders that can produce dementia. In some instances, patterns of cortical atrophy are diagnostic, as in cases with marked frontal-temporal atrophy, suggesting Pick disease, or in cases with caudate atrophy, diagnostic of Huntington disease (HD). With high-resolution CT scanners, it is now possible to diagnose multi-infarct dementia (MID) in an increasing number of individuals who show evidence of areas of focal attenuation on CT scan, consistent with scars of old cerebral infarcts. These scanners make possible the objective diagnosis in some cases of lacunar state. Binswanger disease has been found to present a characteristic picture of focal attenuation in white matter, particularly in periventricular areas[50] (see Chapters 5 and 7).

The T_2 scan on the MRI is quite sensitive in identifying white matter lesions, for example, MS, leukodystrophies, multifocal leukoencephalopathy, and Binswanger disease (also termed *subacute arteriosclerotic encephalopathy*). However, the sensitivity of this technique is so great that bright, intense spots are seen in the white matter of some subjects during normal aging on the T_2 scan. At one time these white matter intensities were routinely diagnosed as subacute arteriosclerotic encephalopathy, but they are now recognized as occurring with minimal changes in the white matter during normal aging, changes that do not correspond to known pathologic entities, although the white matter intensities are more frequent in persons with hypertension or strokes. These will be discussed in great detail in Chapter 5. In regard to spinal cord disease, both the CT myelogram and the MRI have provided much greater resolution of intraparenchymal and extraparenchymal spinal cord lesions. In particular, the syndrome of spinal stenosis is best identified using the CT scan.

Neuropsychologic evaluation assists in establishing the presence of dementia, depression, or both, in determining whether the dementia is cortical, subcortical, or multifocal, and in assessing level of functioning (see Chapter 6). The EEG can contribute both to confirming the presence of an organic process by the presence of generalized slowing, or a focal process by the presence of focal theta or delta activity; its most important function is helping to determine whether seizure activity is present. The utility of the P300 and other event-related potentials is still a matter of clinical investigation.[24,43] The use of positron emission tomography (PET), single-photon emission computed tomography (SPECT), or xenon cerebral blood flows may assist in the differential diagnosis in a limited number of difficult to diagnose dementia cases.

Patients with amyotrophic lateral sclerosis (ALS), myasthenia gravis, or peripheral neuropathy, as well as patients with spinal stenosis or entrapment syndromes, are often referred for neurologic examination. Electromyography and nerve conduction time are as important in establishing an accurate diagnosis in the 80-year-old as in the 40-year-old and are a necessary part of the workup for such conditions.

THE NEUROLOGIST'S ROLE IN EVALUATION AND MANAGEMENT

The neurologist is often pessimistic about consultations in elderly patients but has much to offer. With continuing "compression of senescence" and life expectancy extending gradually toward the 10th decade, the neurologist must be prepared to deal with the problems of the 80-year-old patient. The first responsibility is, of course, to diagnose and care for treatable disease. The neurologist also is responsible for the accurate diagnosis and continued management of diseases considered irreversible. To manage a patient with an irreversible condition, whether the condition be AD, ALS, or a less-threatening disorder, it is necessary to maintain close contact with patient and family or caregiver; for example, in the case of a dementia patient, re-evaluations at about 3-month intervals would be appropriate. In these patients, treatment of concurrent medical and psychiatric problems, attention to environmental

manipulations to maximize remaining function, such as avoiding or altering poorly lit steps without secure handrails, and use of ancillary services, such as physical therapy, add greatly to the quality of life. Socialization may be improved by participation in reminiscence groups. Finally, accurate diagnosis allows for necessary personal and social planning for both patient and family. In many centers, a geriatric "team" has been formed that often includes full- or part-time internists (or family practitioners), neurologists, neuropsychologists, psychiatrists, social workers, nurse practitioners, occupational or recreational therapists, and nutritionists. The geriatric neurologist in solo practice may wish to seek out a nurse practitioner or social worker or community organization to assist in providing these added dimensions of management.

CONCLUSION

The increasingly common loss of functional ability among the "old-old" frequently leads to the request for a neurologic consultation. Because of the greater frequency of dementia and delirium in this age group, the physician must particularly emphasize the formal mental status examination, following careful observation during history taking. Testing of vision and hearing, an age-appropriate motor and sensory examination, and examination of reflexes and gait should also be included. Laboratory evaluation is essentially the same regardless of the patient's age and naturally depends on the signs, symptoms, and differential diagnosis. It is important to be aware that the neurologist's role includes not only diagnosis and management of treatable and irreversible diseases, but also treatment of other medical and psychiatric problems, attention to environmental manipulation, use of ancillary services, and recommendation of additional resources.

REFERENCES

1. Adams, AJ, Wong, LS, Wong, L, and Gould, B: Visual acuity changes with age: Some new perspectives. Am J Optom Physiol Optics 65:403–406, 1988.
2. Azar, GJ and Lawton, AH: Gait and stepping as factors in the frequent falls of elderly women. Gerontologist 4:83–84, 1964.
3. Bagolini, B, Porciatti, V, Falsini, B, Scalia, G, Neroni, M, and Moretti, G: Macular electroretinogram as a function of age of subjects. Documenta Ophthalmologica 70:37–43, 1988.
4. Belal, A: The ageing ear. A clinico-pathological classification. J Laryngol Otol 101:1131–1135, 1987.
5. Bentzen, O: Disorder of Hearing in the Elderly. In Hinchcliffe, R (ed): Hearing and Balance in the Elderly. Churchill Livingstone, London, 1983, pp 123–144.
6. Bergman, M: Central Disorders of Hearing in the Elderly. In Hinchcliffe, R (ed): Hearing and Balance in the Elderly. Churchill Livingstone, London, 1983, pp 145–158.
7. Bhatia, SP and Irvine, RE: Electrical recording of the ankle jerk in old age. Gerontologia Clinica 15:357–360, 1973.
8. Birren, JE, Caperson, RC, and Botwinick, J: Age changes in pupil size. J Gerontol 5:216–221, 1950.
9. Bito, LZ: Presbyopia. Arch Ophthalmol 106:1526–1527, 1988.
10. Blessed, G, Tomlinson, E, and Roth, M: The association between quantitative measures of dementia and of senile change in the cerebral grey matter of elderly subjects. Br J Psychiatry 114:797–811, 1968.
11. Carter, AB: The Neurologic Aspects of Aging. In Rossman, I (ed): Clinical Geriatrics, ed 2. JB Lippincott, Philadelphia, 1979, pp 292–316.
12. Chamberlain, W: Restriction in upward gaze with advancing age. Am J Ophthalmol 71:341–346, 1971.
13. Cowley, M: The View from 80. Viking Press, New York, 1980.
14. Critchley, M: The neurology of old age. Lancet 1:1331–1336, 1931.
15. Critchley, M: Neurologic changes in the aged. J Chronic Dis 3:459–476, 1956.
16. Crowe, S, Guild, S, and Polvogt, L: Observations on the pathology of high tone deafness. Bull Johns Hopkins Hosp 54:315–379, 1934.
17. Ellenberg, M: The deep reflexes in old age. JAMA 174:468–469, 1960.
18. Finley, FR, Cody, KA, and Finizie, RV: Locomotion patterns in elderly women. Arch Phys Med Rehabil 50:140–146, 1969.
19. Folstein, MF, Folstein, SE, and McHugh, PR: Mini-mental state: A practical method for grading the cognitive state of patients for the clinician. J Psychiatr Res 12:189–198, 1975.
20. Fuld, PA: Psychological Testing in the Differential Diagnosis of the Dementias. In Katzman, R, Terry, RD, and Bick, KL (eds): Alzheimer's Disease: Senile Dementia and Related Disorders. Aging Series, Vol 7. Raven Press, New York, 1978, pp 185–193.
21. Gacek, R: Degenerative Hearing Loss in Aging. In Fields, W (ed): Neurological and Sensory Disorders in the Elderly. Stratton International Medical Book Corp, New York, 1975.
22. Gartner, S and Henkind, P: Aging and degeneration of the human macula. 1. Outer nuclear layer and photoreceptors. Br J Ophthalmol 65:23–28, 1981.
23. Goldberg, J, Flowerdew, G, Smith, E, Brody, JA, and Tso, MO: Factors associated with age-related macular degeneration. An analysis of data from the first National Health and Nutrition Examination Survey. Am J Epidemiol 128:700–710, 1988.
24. Goodin, DS and Aminoff, MJ: Electrophysiological differences between demented and nondemented patients with Parkinson's disease. Ann Neurol 21:90–94, 1987.
25. Greene, HA and Madden, DJ: Adult age differences in visual acuity, stere-

opsis and contrast sensitivity. Am J Optom Physiol Optics 64:749–753, 1987.

26. Holyoke, EA: Memoirs of E. A. Holyoke. Essex County Medical Society, Mass, 1830.

27. Howell, TH: Old Age—Some Practical Points in Geriatrics, ed 3. HK Lewis & Co, 1975, pp 38–47.

28. Jacobs, L and Gossman, MD: Three primitive reflexes in normal adults. Neurology 30:184–188, 1980.

29. Jellinger, J: Neuropathological agents and dementia. Acta Neurol Belg 76:83–102, 1976.

30. Jenkyn, LR and Reeves, AG: Neurologic signs in uncomplicated aging (senescence). Semin Neurol 1:21, 1981.

31. Jordan, O, Greisen, O, and Bentzen, O: Treatment with binaural hearing aids. Arch Otolaryngol 85:319–326, 1967.

32. Katzman, R: Clinical approach to dementia. In Smith, JL (ed): Neuro-Ophthalmology Focus, 1980. Masson Publishing USA, New York, 1980, pp 341–346.

33. Katzman, R, Brown, T, Fuld, P, Peck, A, Schechter, R, and Schimmel, H: Validation of a short orientation-memory-concentration test of cognitive impairment. Am J Psychiatry 140:734–739, 1983.

34. Katzman, R and Kawas, C: The Evolution of the Diagnosis of Dementia: Past, Present, and Future. In Poeck, K and Freund, HJ (eds): Neurology: Clinical Aspects of the Dementias. Springer-Verlag, Berlin/Heidelberg, 1986, pp 43–49.

35. Kini, MM, Leibowitz, HM, Colton, T, Nickerson, RJ, Ganley, J, and Dawber, TR: Prevalence of senile cataract, diabetic retinopathy, senile macular degeneration, and open-angle glaucoma in the Framingham Study. Am J Ophthalmol 85:28–34, 1978.

36. Klawans, HL, Tufo, HM, and Ostfeld, AM: Neurologic examination in an elderly population. Dis Nerv Syst 32:274–279, 1971.

37. Kokmen, E, Bossemeyer, RW, Barney, J, and Williams, WJ: Neurological manifestations of aging. J Gerontol 32:411–419, 1977.

38. Korczyn, AD, Laor, N, and Nemet, P: Sympathetic pupillary tone in old age. Arch Ophthalmol 94:1905–1906, 1976.

39. Kuechenmeister, CA, Linton, PH, Mueller, TV, and White, HB: Eye tracking in relation to age, sex, and illness. Arch Gen Psychiatry 34:578–579, 1977.

40. Kumnick, LS: Pupillary psychosensory restitution and aging. J Optom Soc Am 44:735, 1954.

41. Moller, MB: Changes in Hearing Measures with Increasing Age. In Hinchcliffe, R (ed): Hearing and Balance in the Elderly. Churchill Livingstone, London, 1983, pp 97–122.

42. Murray, MP, Kory, RC, and Clarkson, BH: Walking patterns in healthy old men. J Gerontol 24:169–178, 1969.

43. Patterson, JV, Michalewski, HJ, and Starr, A: Latency variability of the components of auditory event-related potentials to infrequent stimuli in aging, Alzheimer-type dementia, and depression. Electroencephalogr Clin Neurophysiol 71:450–460, 1988.

44. Perret, E and Reglis, F: Age and the perceptual threshold for vibratory stimuli. Eur Neurol 4:65–76, 1970.

45. Potvin, AR, Syndulko, K, Tourtellotte, WW, Goldberg, Z, Potvin, JH, and Hansch, EC: Quantitative Evaluation of Normal Age-Related Changes in Neurologic Function. In Pirozzolo, FJ and Maletta, GJ (eds): Advances in Neurogerontology, Vol 2. Praeger, New York, 1980.

46. Potvin, AR, Syndulko, K, Tourtellotte, WW, Lemmon, JA, and Potvin, JH: Human neurologic function and the aging process. J Am Geriatr Soc 28:1–9, 1980.

47. Prakash, C and Stern, G: Neurological signs in the elderly. Age Ageing 2:24–27, 1973.

48. Repka, MX and Quigley, HA: The effect of age on normal human optic

nerve fiber number and diameter. Ophthalmology 96:26–32, 1989.

49. Riley, MW and Foner, A: Decline of functioning. Aging and Society, Russell Sage Foundation, New York, 1968, p 230.

50. Rosenberg, GA, Kornfield, M, Stovring, J, and Bicknell, JM: Subcortical arteriosclerotic encephalopathy (Binswanger): Computerized tomography. Neurology 29:1102–1106, 1979.

51. Rubin, R and Kruger, B: Hearing Loss in the Elderly. In Katzman. R and Terry, R (eds): Neurology of Aging. FA Davis, 1983, pp 123–147.

52. Schow, RL, Christensen, JM, Hutchinson, JM, and Nerbonne, MA: Communication Disorders of the Aged. University Park Press, Baltimore, 1978.

53. Sharpe, JA and Sylvester, TO: Effect of aging on horizontal smooth pursuit. Invest Ophthalmol Vis Sci 17:465–468, 1978.

54. Sixt, E and Landahl, S: Postural disturbances in a 75-year-old population: Prevalence and functional consequences. Age Ageing 16:393–398, 1987.

55. Skre, H: Neurological signs in a normal population. Acta Neurol Scand 48:575–606, 1972.

56. Spooner, JW, Sakala, SM, Baloh, RW: Effect of age on eye tracking. Arch Neurol 37:575–576, 1980.

57. Vital Statistics of the United States. US DHHS Publ No (PHS) 88-1122, Washington, DC, 1986, pp 10–13.

58. Warren, LR, Wagener, JW, and Herman, GE: Binaural analysis in the aging auditory system. J Gerontol 33:731–736, 1978.

59. Weale, RA: The aging retina. Geriatrics 3:425–450, 1985.

60. Welford, AT: Sensory Perceptual and Motor Processes in Older Adults. In Birren, JE and Swane, RD (eds): Handbook of Mental Health and Aging. Prentice-Hall, Englewood Cliffs, NJ, 1980, p 192.

61. West, SK, Rosenthal, FS, Bressler, NM, Bressler, SB, Munoz, B, Fine, SL, and Taylor, HR: Exposure to sunlight and other risk factors for age-related macular degeneration. Arch Ophthalmol 107:875–879, 1989.

62. Wolfson, L and Katzman, R: The Neurologic Consultation at Age 80. In Katzman, R and Terry, RD (eds): The Neurology of Aging. FA Davis, Philadelphia, 1983, pp 221–244.

63. Wright, BE and Henkind, P: Aging Changes and the Eye. In Katzman, R and Terry, RD (eds): The Neurology of Aging. FA Davis, Philadelphia, 1983, pp 149–166.

Chapter 5

STRUCTURAL AND FUNCTIONAL BRAIN IMAGING IN THE ELDERLY

Ranjan Duara, M.D.

CEREBROVASCULAR DISEASES
NORMAL AGING AND DEMENTING
   DISORDERS

CEREBROVASCULAR DISEASES

Today, stroke remains the most common life-threatening neurologic disorder.[215] The incidence of stroke increases with age and is greater in men than in women. In spite of the aging of the general population, death rates from stroke have declined markedly in this century and precipitously so in recent decades.[82]

In a study of 713 strokes at the New York Neurological Institute (1983–1984), 63% were found to be cerebral infarcts and 37% were cerebral hemorrhages.[158] About two thirds of the cerebral infarcts were caused by thrombosis and one third by embolism. Transient ischemic attacks (TIAs) accounted for 11% of all instances of cerebrovascular disease.

Prior to the advent of computed tomography (CT) scanning, the distinction between cerebral hemorrhage and infarction was based on clinical symptoms and signs, examination of the cerebrospinal fluid (CSF), and cerebral angiography. The widespread use of CT scanning has contributed to the more accurate classification of cerebral hemorrhage and, thus, to the epidemiology of the subtypes of stroke.[127]

A classification of cerebrovascular disease useful for radiologic purposes includes

1. TIAs, which are focal ischemic neurologic events that are resolved completely in 24 hours
2. Cerebral infarction resulting from small penetrating arterial or arteriolar occlusive disease (lacunar infarction)
3. Cerebral infarction from large artery occlusion or stenosis
4. Cerebral infarction resulting from embolism (3 and 4 may include hemorrhagic infarction)
5. Cerebral hemorrhage, which may be intraparenchymal, subarachnoid, or subdural

Transient Ischemic Attack(s)

CT STUDIES

In patients with TIAs, the CT scan may show a small infarction (area of radiolucency) that may be deep or superficial in the cerebral hemispheres.[175] Presence of deep infarctions in the basal ganglia is common in patients with TIAs and is not necessarily indicative of the location of the lesion causing the TIAs.[22] However, when the clinical signs and symptoms are closely

89

correlated with the CT lesion location, the assumption can be made of a cause-effect relationship. Occasionally, a postcontrast CT scan may show cortical enhancement compared with the noncontrast CT scan, within days after occurrence of a TIA, suggesting vascular hyperemia resulting from the ischemic event.[119] Occasionally, small hematomas, tumors, or vascular malformations may be found at an appropriate cerebral location on CT done to investigate a TIA.[188] In most instances with TIAs, no abnormality is discovered on CT scans.[128] TIAs resulting from brain stem pathology very rarely if ever are associated with CT scan abnormalities of the appropriate location.[118,175]

MRI STUDIES

In contrast to the CT scan, magnetic resonance imaging (MRI) has shown the frequent presence of ischemic lesions in patients with TIAs. Kinkel and associates[121] showed that 72% of their 29 patients with TIA had abnormalities on MRI but only 22% were abnormal on CT. The abnormalities on MRI were in the periventricular region, the subcortical or cortical regions, and in watershed cortical and subcortical regions. These abnormalities consisted of high signal intensity areas on T_2-weighted sequences. Most of the abnormalities on MRI could not be directly associated with the TIAs because of poor correspondence between their locations and the clinical syndromes. Thus, this high incidence of MRI abnormality in patients with TIA may reflect the increased prevalence of cerebrovascular pathology in this patient group, but not necessarily a strict clinicopathologic correspondence.

Lacunar Infarctions

CT STUDIES

Pathologically, lacunar infarctions range in size (diameter) from 1 to 2 mm to 3 cm and are most frequently found in the distribution of the middle and posterior cerebral, the anterior choroidal, and the basilar arteries.[50,157] On CT scans the frequency (up to 70%) with which lacunes are identified as isolated radiolucent areas is dependent on technical factors that include the resolution of the scanner, the slice thickness, and the proximity of the lacunes to dense bone, as in posterior fossa lesions.[50,121] Kinkel and associates[50] were able to detect 28 lacunes out of 52 identified at autopsy in 24 patients. Those that tended to be missed most frequently were those less than 5 mm in diameter and those located in the posterior fossa, especially the ventral aspect of the cerebellar hemispheres.

MRI STUDIES

Lacunar infarctions are very frequently identified on MRI scans when they cannot be seen on CT scans. Braffman and colleagues[24] studied 36 formalin-fixed brains with postmortem MRI, as well as with CT scans (for 20 of the above brains). Pathologic examination revealed 14 lacunar infarctions, of which all were detected on MRI. By CT, three out of three posterior fossa lacunes were missed, but all the supratentorial lacunes were detected. The lacunes were found to be hyperintense relative to surrounding brain (on T_2-weighted images using short and long echo times [TEs]) (Fig. 5–1 A and B). One lacune that underwent cystic change was isodense to CSF on all pulse sequences. Dilated Virchow Robin (VR) spaces can resemble lacunar infarcts on the long repetition time (TR), long TE sequence, but the long TR, short TE sequence demonstrates that lacunes, but not VR spaces, have higher signal intensity than CSF. Braffman and associates[24] also pointed out that lacunar infarcts cannot be distinguished by MRI signal characteristics from areas of focal gliosis or demyelination. Miyashita and colleagues[156] have shown that gadolinium DTPA-enhanced MRI was effective in showing enhancement in

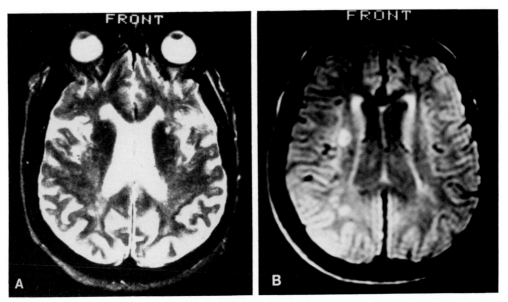

Figure 5–1. Lacunar infarctions. *A*, MRI section (TR = 2.5 seconds, TE = 90 milliseconds) at a mid-ventricular level showing a lacune in the left internal capsule (anterior limb). *B*, MRI section showing a lacunar infarct in the superior part of the right putamen and adjacent white matter. Two to three lacunes are in the right parieto-occipital white matter.

eight of nine recent lacunar infarcts, whereas CT with iodinated contrast medium produced enhancement in only four of these lesions.

Cerebral Infarction (Thrombotic and Embolic)

CT STUDIES

Acute cerebral infarction is manifested as an ill-defined area of hypodensity (Fig. 5–2A) on the CT scan, typically at 1 to 2 days, but occasionally as early as 3 hours after the ictus.[107] Within 3 to 4 days after infarction has occurred, the hypodensity becomes most evident and at this stage edema may produce a mass effect as well. The extent of edema is generally proportional to the size of the infarct.[188] Subsequently, because of macrophage and capillary proliferation, the hypodense infarct becomes less evident and may even become isodense with the rest of the brain (known as the "fogging effect").[13] Complete fogging of the hypodense area is unlikely to occur in large

infarcts but is typically most evident at about 10 days after the ictus. Subsequently, over a period of months, hypodensity becomes prominent again as the infarcted area becomes cystic.[121]

Contrast enhancement occurring after an infarction (Fig. 5–2B) becomes evident at the same time that the lesions start losing their hypodensity. It becomes apparent at 1 to 2 weeks and is maximal at 2 to 3 weeks.[213] These changes in contrast enhancement occur because of dysautoregulation with "luxury perfusion" and also vascular proliferation with altered capillary permeability. Occasionally, early contrast enhancement (within the first 1–2 days) in the gray matter surrounding an infarct may be seen, because of "luxury perfusion." It should be noted that although contrast enhancement improves the diagnostic abilities of CT for infarction, there is the potential danger of neurotoxicity because contrast material leaks into the brain.[187] Worsening of the infarct from contrast injection is especially likely at the stage where vascular permeability is altered.

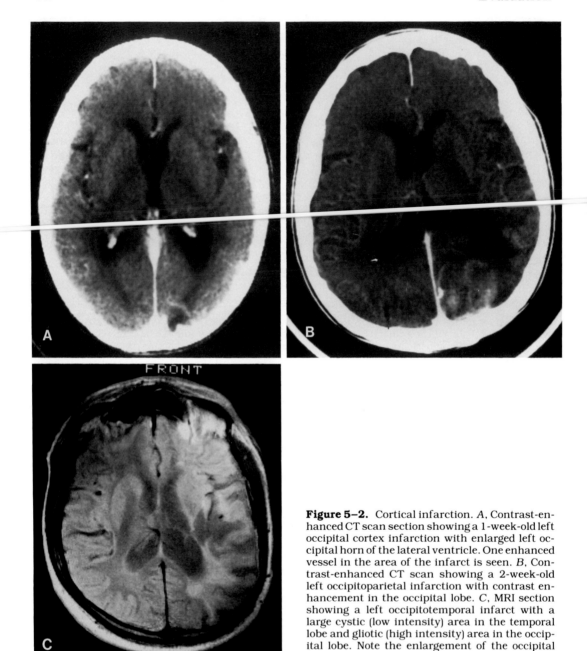

Figure 5–2. Cortical infarction. *A*, Contrast-enhanced CT scan section showing a 1-week-old left occipital cortex infarction with enlarged left occipital horn of the lateral ventricle. One enhanced vessel in the area of the infarct is seen. *B*, Contrast-enhanced CT scan showing a 2-week-old left occipitoparietal infarction with contrast enhancement in the occipital lobe. *C*, MRI section showing a left occipitotemporal infarct with a large cystic (low intensity) area in the temporal lobe and gliotic (high intensity) area in the occipital lobe. Note the enlargement of the occipital horn of the left lateral ventricle.

Infarcts on CT scans may not be visible because of their location close to dense bone and the resulting beam-hardening artifacts, or because of their small size, especially in brain stem locations.[121]

MRI STUDIES

Studies in monkey brain with experimentally induced embolic infarction[205] demonstrated that at 24 and 48 hours after the onset of infarction no changes in CT were present, but significant prolongation of T_1 and T_2 values were evident. These MRI signal changes were in gray and white matter and correlated with increased water content and a decrease in specific gravity of the affected brain tissue. In humans, T_2-weighted MRI images show areas of increased signal intensity in the gray matter within 3 hours and as early as 30 minutes of the ictus.[121] At 24 hours the MRI changes involve the white matter as well. T_1-weighted images show no definite alteration until after CT scan changes appear at 48 hours or more. In the subacute stage (7–21 days) after onset of infarction, T_1-weighted images appear similar to CT images, showing low signal intensity, but the T_2-weighted MRI images demonstrate increased signal intensity beyond the borders of the T_1-weighted abnormality.[121] In the chronic stage of infarction (after 21 days) the T_2-weighted image may show areas of decreased signal intensity, from cavitation, surrounded by thin or extensive bands of increased signal intensity (Fig. 5–2C).

Cerebral Hemorrhage

CT STUDIES

Intracerebral, intraparenchymatous hematomas are best rcognized by CT scanning.[188] Usually the first CT scan after the ictus demonstrates a homogeneous round or oval area of high density on the noncontrast study.[49] A thin rim of low radiodensity appears early around the hematoma and is caused by separation out of serum from the blood clot and from the surrounding infarcted brain tissue.[117] Mass effect from the hematoma is usually proportional to the size of the hematoma in contrast to some brain tumors, which produce most of the mass effect from edema surrounding the lesion.[117] Occasionally, layering of fluid and blood produces high-density–low-density interfaces.[224]

Parenchymatous hemorrhages originate in the basal ganglia-thalamus (Fig. 5–3A) or one of the poles of the frontal, temporal, or occipital lobes and tend to dissect along white matter tracts.[49] About 10% of all hematomas occur in the cerebellar hemispheres, but this site is more frequent in older subjects. Moseley and colleagues[161] demonstrated that in patients over the age of 70 years the relative frequency of cerebellar hematomas was 18% of all parenchymatous hemorrhages. Not uncommonly, on CT, intracerebral hematomas may be seen to be rupturing into the lateral ventricle or the subarachnoid space.

Reduction in the density of the clot starts occurring at the periphery within the first day, and this process continues concentrically so that the average hematoma is isodense with the brain to 3 to 4 weeks.[153] It then becomes hypodense relative to the surrounding brain. Mass effect decreases markedly as the hematoma gets absorbed.

Hemorrhagic infarcts are uncommon entities on CT and consist of mixed hypodense and hyperdense areas in the cortex or deep gray matter.[208] The size of the infarcted area does not change much in time, in contrast to a hematoma, which tends to shrink markedly over a period of weeks after onset.[188]

MRI STUDIES

The evolution of an intraparenchymatous hemorrhage on MRI produces complex changes in the T_1- and T_2-weighted images over time.[51,88] The acute hematoma produces a shortening of T_2 and lengthening of T_1 and hence reduced signal intensity in both T_1- and T_2-weighted images. Surrounding the acute hematoma is an area of increased water content from the separating serum and surrounding brain edema. This is manifested as a rim of low intensity on T_1-weighted images but high intensity on T_2-weighted images. As the hemorrhage becomes subacute, it de-

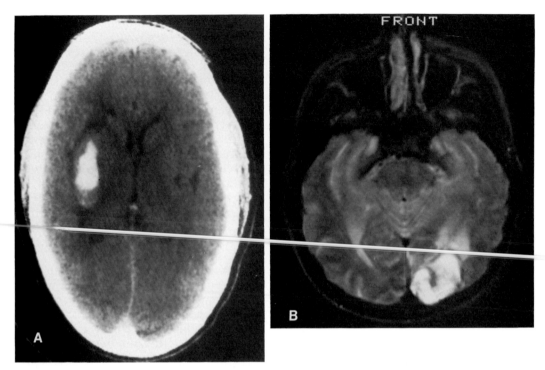

Figure 5–3. Cerebral hemorrhage. *A,* CT scan section showing a hematoma (high-density area) in the right putamen with slight midline shift to the left and obliteration of the right frontal horn. Note also the lacunar infarcts in the left putamen and left claustrum area. *B,* MRI scan section showing a subacute hematoma in the left occipital lobe with areas of low signal intensity (representing deoxyhemoglobin) surrounded by high-signal areas (representing serum). An incomplete thin ring of low-density signal (hemosiderin) is seen surrounding the hematoma. Edema (high signal) extending anteriorly into temporal white matter is also seen.

velops increased signal intensity on both T_1- and T_2-weighted images, starting in the periphery and later encompassing the whole hematoma (Fig. 5–3B). The area surrounding the hematoma in the subacute stage develops decreased signal intensity on T_2 images, perhaps because of the paramagnetic properties of hemosiderin in the surrounding brain (this effect is seen particularly with high-field magnets).[51] Staging of intracerebral hematoma by MRI is probably more accurate than by CT, but the CT scan is superior to MRI in the detection of hematomas,[106] especially in the earliest stages of a hemorrhage when a prompt diagnosis is required for selection of the proper therapy.

Use of CT and MRI in the Differential Diagnosis of Patients with Stroke

Several factors should be considered in choosing between MRI and CT as an investigative instrument in a patient presenting with a stroke syndrome.[39] These include factors relating to sensitivity and specificity of CT and MRI for each stroke syndrome, as outlined in Table 5–1. Other factors are the time available to perform the procedure and the level of cooperation possible from the patient (MRI takes longer). Certain contraindications may exist for the use of MRI (pacemakers, electronic monitoring equipment, cardiorespiratory support equipment) and occasionally for the use of IV contrast-enhanced CT studies (allergy to iodine, potential neurotoxicity). Finally, the expense of each procedure (CT is usually much cheaper than MRI) needs to be considered.

In general, CT should be employed initially in any situation where cerebral hemorrhage (either hematoma or hemorrhagic infarction) is a clinical consideration. In selected instances, MRI may be employed to further evaluate ambiguous or negative findings. MRI has a clear advantage in evaluating patients with lacunar stroke syndromes, TIAs, and posterior fossa strokes of any type other than larger hematomas.

Use of PET and SPECT Studies in Stroke

PET STUDIES

Position emission tomography (PET) studies in cerebrovascular disease have included measurements of regional cerebral blood flow (rCBF), metabolic rate for oxygen (rCMRO$_2$) and oxygen extraction fraction (rOEF), glucose (rCMRglc), and cerebral blood volume (rCBV). As a general principle, in the various stages of cerebral ischemia in experimental animals, as perfusion pressure declines because of disease in or occlusion of a feeding vessel, rCBV increases in that vascular bed because of capillary dilatation. This reduces regional cerebral vascular resistance and maintains rCBF. As perfusion pressure further declines, rCBF declines and rOEF increases, thus maintaining rCMRO$_2$. This condition has been described as the "misery perfusion syndrome."[10,11] A still further decline in cerebral perfusion pressure results in a reduction in rCMRO$_2$ and the beginning of cerebral infarction.[178] Once cerebral infarction has occurred, a paradoxic increase in rCBF may occur as a result of vasodilation in response to acute metabolic acidosis, the so-called luxury perfusion syndrome.[129] Alternatively, a relative excess of rCBF over rCMRO$_2$

may be seen after infarction because rCMRO$_2$ declines much more precipitously than does rCBF in this condition.[135]

PET and single-photon emission computed tomography (SPECT) studies could potentially be usefully employed to assist with decisions regarding intervention if the transition from ischemia to infarction were gradual, or if a chronic stage of ischemia without frank infarction persisted. It appears that such circumstances occur uncommonly but have occasionally been observed in one hemisphere when there is complete ipsilateral carotid occlusion.[75]

In patients with TIAs or unilateral carotid occlusion, subgroups have been identified with increased rCBV and rOEF, and decreased rCBF and normal or decreased rCMRO$_2$.[10,11,86,178] Whether these patients constitute a subgroup who may benefit from extracranial-intracranial bypass surgery is not known at the present time.

In cerebral infarction, rCBF is generally decreased to a greater extent than CMRO$_2$ in the first few days, resulting in an increased rOEF. Following this period rOEF decreases either because a decline in rCMRO$_2$ or a rise in rCBF (luxury perfusion). Finally, within a few weeks there are persistently low values of rCMRO$_2$ with equivalently low values of rCBF and normal rOEF. This pattern of findings has been observed in various studies done in the last decade.[10,11,135,214]

Following focal cerebral infarctions, remote brain regions often manifest decreases in rCBF, rCMRO$_2$, and rCMRglc. The most common finding is that of a contralateral cerebellar hypometabolism following unilateral cerebral infarction. The occurrence of this diaschisis phenomenon seems to be unrelated to the size, location, or age of the infarct.[178] Other sites showing this diaschisis effect are the ipsilateral thalamus, contralateral cortical areas, and ipsilateral basal ganglia structures. In general, a focal vascular event produces much more extensive abnormal-

Table 5–1 NEUROIMAGING FEATURES OF DIFFERENT STROKE SYNDROMES

Stroke Syndrome	Neuroimaging Features		
	Early Features (1st week)	Subacute Features (1–4 weeks)	Late or Chronic Features
TIA	CT: Usually negative scan ± Radiolucent area ± Gray matter enhancement with contrast MRI: ++Single/multiple areas of increased signal on T_2 images (often no correspondence in location of lesion to clinical event).	Same	Same
Lacunar infarct	CT: Radiolucent areas in 70% of lacunes. ± Contrast enhancement. MRI: ++T_2 images show 5- to 30-mm lesions. ++Gadolinium enhancement on MRI.	CT: Radiolucent areas commonly in internal capsule, basal ganglia, thalamus, corona radiata (not often seen in posterior fossa). MRI: +++T_2 images show lesions in same locations as CT radiolucenci es and in posterior fossa as well.	Same

Cerebral infarct (thrombosis-embolism)	CT: + ill-defined radiolucency at 1–2 days. ± Mass effect if edema present (edema severity is proportional to size of infarct). + Hemorrhagic infarcts are identified as patchy areas of increased radiodensity. MRI +++ T_2 images show increased signal by 3 h. ++ T_1 images show decreased signal at 24–48 h. ± Mass effect (hemorrhagic infarcts are poorly identified on MRI).	CT: ++ Well-defined radiolucency at 3–4 days with "fogging" effect at 10–20 days. ++ With contrast enhancement. MRI: +++ T_2 signal hyperintensity. ++ T_1 signal hypointensity.	CT: ++ Reappearance of well-defined radiolucency; no contrast enhancement. MRI: +++ T_2 signal hyperintensity. ± areas of T_2 signal hypointensity. ++ T_1 signal hypointensity.
Parenchymatous hematoma	CT: +++ Oval or round, high-intensity lesion. ++ Rim of radiolucent area. ++ Mass effect. MRI :+++ Oval or round area of decreased intensity on T_1 and T_2 images. ++ Rim of decreased intensity on T_1, but increased intensity on T_2 images. ++ Mass effect.	CT: ++ Intensity decreases over 3–4 weeks from periphery inward. Mass effect decreases markedly. MRI ++ T_1 and T_2 images show increasing signal to hyperintense levels by 3–4 weeks. Rim of T_2 intensity alters to hypointensity. Mass effect declines markedly.	CT ++ Low radiodensity area remains. MRI: ++ Central high-intensity signal on T_2 images. ± Low-intensity signal of surrounding brain on T_2 images.

ity in PET scans than is seen on CT or MRI scans.

SPECT STUDIES

SPECT studies of stroke are less numerous and rigorous than those using PET. Early and extensive perfusion defects are detected by SPECT studies according to Reynaud and associates,[181] but follow-up studies are needed. The sensitivity for detecting stroke is much greater using SPECT than it is using CT or MRI scans, making it a potentially useful clinical tool when TIA or stroke is suspected but not clinically obvious. Remote effects of a focal cerebral infarction are also evident on SPECT studies.[170]

NORMAL AGING AND DEMENTING DISORDERS

Normal Aging

CT STUDIES

CT scan studies have been conducted on large numbers of normal individuals, in some cases, well-characterized normal subjects encompassing the entire age range from young adulthood to late senescence. Consistently, alterations in ventricular size and subarachnoid space on CT scans have been noted with the aging process, though to variable degrees.[132]

For example, Ito and associates[109] found in 130 subjects the CSF volume increased progressively from 40 years of age. Zatz and colleagues[222] found intracranial CSF volume to increase consistently only after the age of 60 years. In both these studies, compartments representing CSF in the ventricular and subarachnoid space were quantified by counting the number of pixels in each space. Schwartz and associates[194] used a similar approach to demonstrate that in subjects 18 to 40, 41 to 60, and 61 to 81 years of age, intracranial CSF volume was 2.5%, 4.9%, and 8.8% of the total intracranial volume, respec-

tively. These volumes differed significantly only in the older two groups and were accompanied by a reduction in gray matter volume for cortical and subcortical structures. White matter volume, however, remained unchanged through the age range. Gado and colleagues[81] estimated the intracranial CSF volume at 4.6% in 47 normal subjects, 25 to 33 years old. They found the corresponding value at 65 to 80 years to be 11% to 12%.[102]

Alterations in the attenuation value (CT number or Hounsfield unit) in the white matter of the centrum semiovale have also been reported to occur,[223] but this was not confirmed by Schwartz and associates[194] or Cala and colleagues.[32] Several studies[84,201] have demonstrated that in "normal" elderly individuals the CT scan may show patchy areas of reduced attenuation in the white matter.

It has been demonstrated that the incidence of these lesions in normal individuals increases with age,[84] and that subjects with such lesions, though not demented, are more likely to show mild cognitive and neurologic changes as compared with those without these lesions.[201]

MRI STUDIES

MRI studies of intracranial fluid volume have not so far been reported, although Condon and colleagues[38] have described a reliable method of measurement. Since the CSF-brain boundary is seen well in both CT and MRI, there is no reason for the results to be different (Figs. 5–4A, B and 5–5A, B.) On the other hand, measurement of white matter volume is relatively easy in MRI images, and one preliminary report suggests no change in volume of white matter with age.[59]

In normal individuals, MRI often reveals focal crescentic or semicircular areas of increased intensity, on T_2-weighted scans, capping the frontal and occipital horns of the lateral ventricles, or pencil-thin bands of hyperintensity along the borders of the body

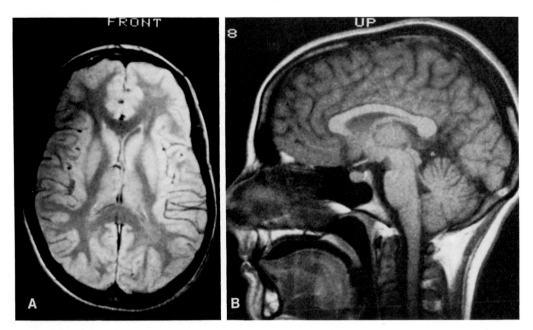

Figure 5–4. Normal young subject. A, MRI horizontal section at level of the basal ganglia. Note the small ventricle size and the lack of increased periventricular signal around frontal horns. B, MRI midsagittal section. Note the small ventricle and cortical sulcal size. Note also the thickness of corpus callosum, midbrain, and pons and width of the aqueduct of Sylvius and of the quadrigeminal plate.

of the lateral ventricles.[203] These periventricular changes increase slightly in width with age; between the third and ninth decades they are present in almost 90% of individuals.[225] The pathologic correlate of these changes is astrocytic gliosis, perhaps resulting from seepage of CSF into the parenchyma.

In contrast to these above-mentioned changes, other areas of increased signal intensity on T_2-weighted scans have been described in normal individuals, usually above the age of 55 years. These lesions are patchy, sometimes punctate, nodular, or confluent areas confined to the white matter, in the centrum semiovale and the subcortical white matter of the frontal, parietal, temporal, and occipital lobes. These white matter lesions (WMLs) clearly increase in incidence with age and with the presence of cerebrovascular disease, particularly hypertension.[7,85] Bowen[20] subdivided these WMLs into subcortical (SCL) and periventricular lesions (PVL) and graded them on a 0 to 3 scale. In 86 clinically normal individ-

uals between the ages of 23 and 84, there was a highly significant positive correlation of PVL and SCL scores with age ($r = 0.40$, $P <0.0005$, for PVLs and $r = 0.39$, $P < 0.0005$ for SCLs). PVLs were found to be most prominent anteriorly and least prominent along the bodies of the lateral ventricles. SCLs, however, were evenly distributed between anterior, central, and posterior locations, but were most prominent at the high ventricular level. The functional significance of these white matter lesions is unclear, although the pathologic bases for these findings are arteriosclerosis, dilated perivascular spaces, vascular ectasia, and gliosis.[6] In preliminary studies examining the metabolic consequences of MRI-identified subcortical white matter signal changes, no corresponding deficits were discovered on fluorodeoxyglucose PET scans.[54] The pathologic correlate of small periventricular zones of increased T_2 signal were found to be subependymal glial accumulation in a zone known as the subcallosal fasicu-

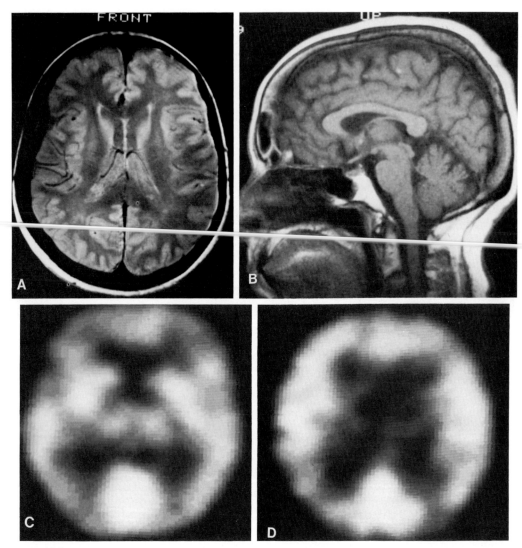

Figure 5–5. Normal elderly subject. *A*, MRI horizontal section at level of the basal ganglia. Note the slightly increased ventricle size and the presence of increased periventricular signal capping frontal horns. *B*, MRI midsagittal section. Note the slight prominence of cortical sulcal size. No change compared to young subjects of corpus callosum, midbrain, pons, aqueduct of Sylvius, and quadrigeminal plate is seen. *C*, PET scan horizontal slice at level of basal ganglia. Note the even distribution of metabolic activity in cortical and subcortical structures and highest activity in the medial occipital cortex. *D*, PET scan horizontal slice at midventricular level. Note the symmetrical cortical metabolic activity with highest activity in occipital area.

lus.[131] In an autopsy study of patients with evidence of focal neurologic disease, Leifer[131] found that more extensive subcortical MRI changes corresponded to wallerian degeneration secondary to infarction, Binswanger disease, or multiple sclerosis.

Normal aging is also associated with the progressive accumulation of iron in the brain, especially in the globus pallidus, red nucleus, zona reticulata of the substantia nigra, the subthalamic nucleus of Luys, and the dentate nucleus of the cerebellum. This distribution of iron content can be seen in normal elderly individuals as dark areas on

T_2-weighted MRI scans, using high magnetic fields, because the paramagnetic properties of iron accelerate T_2 relaxation time.

PET AND SPECT STUDIES

PET and SPECT scan studies of cerebral blood flow (CBF) in normal human aging have shown a significant reduction with increasing age.[48,73,130] Furthermore, all previous studies, using ^{133}Xe and external detectors, have also shown a reduction of CBF with age.[31,152,154,164]

Cerebral glucose metabolism has been shown not to be age-related in the majority of studies using [^{18}F]fluorodeoxyglucose ([18]FDG) or ^{11}C-DG, and PET,[47,55,98,192,221] although Kuhl and associates[116] did report a significant reduction in cerebral metabolic rate for glucose (CMRglc) with age. Studies with oxygen metabolism also have been inconsistent, with some showing a reduction[73,136,167] and one showing no reduction with age.[130] Schlageter and associates[192] found that a trend toward reduction in CMRglc with age was completely eliminated when the effects of brain atrophy were accounted for. Yoshii and colleagues[221] similarly found that in 76 subjects an age-related decrement in CMRglc was present, but when brain atrophy and volume were accounted for, no age-related change in CMRglc was present.

The ratio of frontal metabolism to occipital metabolism shows a tendency to decrease with age.[3,125,221] In the "resting" state most studies demonstrate the highest metabolic rates to be in the calcarine cortex[3,48,55,125,221] (Fig. 5–5C and D). Also, the right hemisphere tends to have slightly higher metabolic rates or blood flow values than the left hemisphere during rest.[3,48,130,141,169,174] This pattern tends to remain unchanged through the age range.[55]

The variability of absolute values of CBF, CMRO$_2$, and particularly CMRglc in normal subjects has been a source of concern. The variability of CMRglc increases with advancing age.[55] The reason for this large variability, which has been reported from many, but not all, centers is probably only partly methodologic. Different techniques used in many different centers have yielded coefficients of variation of up to 30% in normal subjects.[43,55,164] This variability may decrease if individuals are studied in a behaviorally activated condition rather than in the ill-defined resting state.[57] However, Ball and associates[8] reported that activation failed to reduce variability of rCBF. When brain volume, extent of cerebral atrophy, age, sex, and cerebrovascular risk factors were all examined in a single cohort of normal subjects, only brain volume and extent of atrophy were found to contribute significantly to the total variance in CMRglc. Head size was responsible for 17% and cerebral atrophy accounted for 8% of the total variance.[221]

Alzheimer Disease

Alzheimer disease (AD) is a degenerative disorder and is the most common neurologic cause of dementia. It presents insidiously with progressive alterations of memory, higher intellectual functions, language, ability to perform skilled movements (praxis), orientation in the environment, and ability to recognize objects, faces, and places (gnosis).[151] It is the classic example of a cortical dementia, although in the later stages of the disease subcortical features also become evident (apathy and slowness of response), along with extrapyramidal signs (e.g., rigidity), incontinence, and gait apraxia.

CT STUDIES

At least 10 well-controlled CT scan studies have been done to evaluate morphologic alterations affecting the ventricles and the sulci in AD (Table 5–2). These studies are consistent in demonstrating significant alterations, beyond those expected for age, in patients with even the early stages of AD. There is general agreement that for the pur-

Table 5–2 CT SCAN STUDIES OF ALZHEIMER AND OTHER DEMENTIAS

Author/ Year*	Method of Measurement	Control		Patient		Comment on Subjects‡	Results	Comment on Results§
		N	Age in Years†	N	Age in Years†			
Roberts and Caird, 1976[184]	Maximum ventricular area and sulcal width measurement.	17	73 ± 7	49	77 ± 7	All patients considered to have degenerative dementia; three grades of dementia.	Ventricular area enlarged in the demented but no difference in sulcal area.	Correlation of $r = 0.49$ between maximum ventricular area and memory information test score.
Earnest et al, 1979[62]	Width of sulci, linear ratios, and area of ventricles.	17	73 ± 7	29	86 ± 5	Not a true patient group; some were normals. Not a true control group; some were impaired.	Sulci and ventricles larger in the older and more impaired groups.	Correlation up to $r = 0.52$ between psychologic measures and ventricular measures.
deLeon et al, 1980[45]	Subjective ratings. Linear sulcal and ventricular measurements.	—	—	43	70 ± 6	Detailed neurologic and psychiatric evaluation. All considered to have degenerative dementia.	Sixty-five percent of all correlations between ventricular rankings and psychiatric test scores were significant. Third ventricle width showed best correlations.	Subjective ranking or rating was superior to linear measurements.
Jacoby and Levy, 1980[112]	Area of ventricle, Evan's ratio, and subjective rating of sulci.	50	73 ± 6	40	79 ± 7	All considered degenerative dementia (10 had cerebral infarcts on CT).	All measures showed highly significant differences between subject groups.	Highest correlations between ventricular area and memory. CT indices predicted group membership in 83% of cases.
Brinkman et al, 1981[26]	Bifrontal and bicaudate ratios. Area of ventricles, distance from third ventricle to Sylvian fissure (3V-SF), sulcal width measurement.	30	80 ± 7	28	60 ± 9	All considered degenerative dementia (mild dementia; mean WAIS verbal IQ = 88.8). Patients significantly younger than controls.	No differences in bicaudate, bifrontal ratios. Age-corrected ventricular area larger in the demented group; 3V-SF significantly less in demented group; sulcal width larger in controls.	Correlations between verbal and performance IQ and ventricular area–brain ratio was $r = 0.53$, and 0.65, respectively. Ninety-six percent of demented patients and 41% of controls had abnormal findings for at least one measure.
Ito et al, 1981[109]	Pixel counts of cranial, CSF, and brain volumes.	130	20–79			Although all subjects were described as normal, some demented patients were clearly included. Patients were not separated from controls. Significant increase in CSF volume and decrease in brain volume with age. Brain volume was correlated with a mental status score ($r = 0.43$).		

Table 5–2—*Continued*

Author/ Year*	Method of Measurement	Control		Patient		Comment on Subjects‡	Results	Comment on Results§
		N	Age in Years†	N	Age in Years†			
Wu et al, 1981[218]	Linear measurements and subjective rating of ventricular and sulcal size.	31	50–77	24	50–77	Controls have neurologic symptoms, were not demented, and had no focal lesions on CT. Patients were not separated out in any of the analyses.	Highest correlation between CT and behavioral measures was that of orientation and bicaudate-index ($r = 0.52$).	With the exception of the sulcal measurement, all other CT measures correlated significantly with at least one behavioral measure.
Gado et al, 1982[81]	Pixel counts for ventricles, subarachnoid space, and cranial cavity. Linear indices and subjective ratings also obtained.	27	65–83	20	65–81	Controls described as healthy. Patients clinically diagnosed to have mild AD.	Volumetric measures were clearly better than linear measures in separating demented patients from controls, although both gave significant results for ventricular and subarachnoid space.	An unspecified degree of overlap was found between controls and patients using any of the CT measures.
Wilson et al, 1982[212]	Linear and subjective rating of ventricular sulcal size. CT density measures in 14 brain regions.	38	69	42	69	Controls were healthy. All patients were clinically diagnosed to have AD.	On a composite score, patients had more atrophy than controls. High degree of overlap was noted between groups (not quantified). None of the CT density measures was different between groups.	Wechsler Memory Scale scores were correlated with atrophy ($r = 0.39$) only for the combined patients and control group.
LeMay et al, 1986[134]	Perceptual ratings (0–4 scale) for atrophy in 13 regions by three neuroradiologists and linear measurements.	22	65	24	67	Healthy controls. Patients were all diagnosed to have AD, but degree of dementia was not stated.	Perceptual rating, which was superior to linear measures, correctly classified over 80% of subjects. Specific temporal lobe atrophic changes discriminated up to 90% of subjects.	The size of the suprasellar cistern, the width of the interhemispheric fissure, and the Sylvian fissure were the best discriminators.

*See end-of-chapter references.
†Average age or age range.
‡Points to be emphasized regarding controls and patients.
§Points to be emphasized regarding the results.

poses of quantitation, linear measures are inferior to area or volumetric measures of ventricular enlargement. In assessing morphologic changes of ventricle size and cortical atrophy, perceptual ratings by experienced observers have been shown to be quite sensitive and reliable.[134] This last point is important from a clinical standpoint, as most neurologists or radiologists do not make detailed measurements routinely from CT scans. There is general agreement that CT scan linear measures of cortical atrophy, as assessed by an increase in the subarachnoid space, are unreliable and insensitive to the changes in AD.[44,66,218]

Loss of gray-white matter discriminability in AD has been reported[83] but has not yet been confirmed. CT measures of attenuation in Hounsfield or other units have not shown any consistent differences between AD and control subjects, although Albert and colleagues[4] initially reported lower CT numbers in patients with senile dementia. A recent review of CT scan findings in aging and dementia reveals that volumetric analysis of the ventricle and subarachnoid space can achieve a sensitivity of 88% and a specificity of 90% in separating AD from control subjects.[44]

In spite of statistically significant greater ventricular and sulcal size in AD patients, compared to age-matched controls, the usefulness of the CT in discriminating between these two subject groups is limited. Particularly, in the earlier stage of AD there is a great deal of overlap. Many cognitively normal elderly subjects have enlargement of ventricles or relatively prominent cortical atrophy, and many patients with mild AD have unimpressive atrophic features. Therefore, a CT scan demonstrating cerebral atrophy, in any one patient, does not assist in the clinical evaluation of possible dementia. The history, examination, and assessment of the behavior of the patient remain the most important evidence in determining the presence of dementia. In spite of the poor separation of the findings in normal aging and AD, the CT scan is of great utility in excluding certain causes of dementia other than AD (e.g., MID, cerebral tumor, subdural hematoma, normal pressure hydrocephalus [NPH]).

CT scan studies, summarized in Table 5–2, have demonstrated a gross overall relationship between quantitative measures of loss of brain tissue and behavioral deterioration. However, brain atrophy does not explain more than 40% to 45% of the variance in behavioral measures. For example, studies of demented patients, or combined normal and demented patients, have shown correlation coefficients of 0.29 to 0.65 between CT scan measures of

brain atrophy and psychologic function.[45,62,66,109,218] Although methodologic factors, such as the validity of linear measurements in the brain as indices of volumetric change, and the reliability and validity of psychologic measures as indices of brain function, may contribute to a weakening of morphology-behavior correlations in the brain, the relatively weak correlation of CT and psychologic function also reflects the weak correlation of postmortem brain weight and mental status scores in AD patients (see Chapter 7).

Because dementia is a heterogeneous syndrome, patients with AD and MID have ideally not been lumped together in an analysis of structure-function relationships.[66] AD itself may be heterogeneous, however, and there may be specific subtypes distinguishable clinically and with neuroimaging approaches, with corresponding distinct cognitive subtypes. Behavioral heterogeneity in AD is well known.[19,147] Associations of behavioral subtypes of AD with the rate of progression of the disease or genetic forms of the disease have been described.[25,36] The relationship of any of these behavioral subtypes to specific neuroimaging-neuroanatomic features would be of great interest, but remains to be defined. For example, asymmetry of ventricles and of cortical atrophy in AD has not been alluded to in any of the quantitative studies described in Table 5–2. In a review of CT changes in dementing disease, LeMay[132] singles out only Pick disease as showing asymmetric atrophy. In clinical practice, however, obvious asymmetry of ventricles and of cortical atrophy is observed frequently in patients with probable AD.

In recent CT and MRI scan studies it has been emphasized that changes in periventricular white matter in cases clinically diagnosed as having AD occur frequently.[65,67,84,185,201] These periventricular white matter lucencies are usually found to be more common in demented subjects than age-matched controls.[65,84] When patients with AD are classified on the basis of the occurrence of periventricular white matter lucencies on CT scans, those with such lucencies perform worse on cognitive tests than those without,[201] and the severity of the dementia is correlated with the extent of the white matter lucencies. Many patients with clinical features of AD and with lucencies on CT have been found at autopsy to have AD.[64,84,142,209] Corresponding to the white matter lucencies demonstrated on CT, pathologic abnormalities that have been described in these brain regions include demyelination, axonal loss, hyalinization and fibrous thickening of medullary arterioles, and cystic degeneration.[84,142]

MRI STUDIES

MRI is more sensitive than CT to the changes that occur in the brains of patients with dementia.[65,84,106] The abnormalities that are especially amenable to definition by MRI are periventricular and subcortical white matter lesions, atrophy of gray matter structures such as the hippocampus and amygdala, and enlargement of basal cisterns and the sylvian fissure[106] (Figs. 5–6A, B and 5–7A, B). In T_2-weighted images, areas of high signal intensity affecting hippocampal and sylvian cortex have also been described in AD patients.[67]

Brun and Englund[28] and Englund and colleagues[64] in comprehensive studies of neuropathologic alterations and postmortem MRI relaxation times of white matter in patients with AD demonstrated that incomplete white matter infarction was encountered in 60% of patients. This infarction was characterized by the loss of myelin, axons, and oligodendroglial cells, mild reactive astrocytic gliosis, and hyaline fibrosis of arterioles in the deep white matter. These pathologic changes gradually decreased in severity as the cortex was approached. In parallel to these pathologic changes, prolongation of T_1 and T_2 relaxation times occurred. The MRI imaging characteristics that would corre-

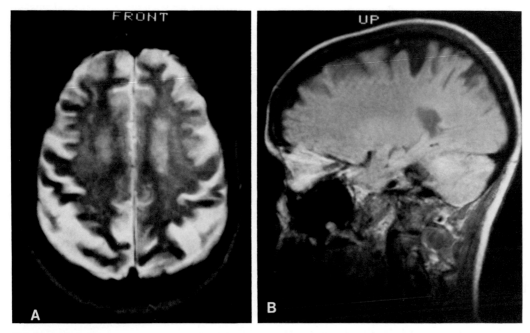

Figure 5–6. Alzheimer disease. *A*, MRI horizontal section (TR = 2.5 seconds TE = 90 milliseconds). Note the increase in sulcal size. (CSF has a bright signal in this MRI sequence.) *B*, MRI parasagittal section. Note the prominence of cortical sulci with evident gyral atrophy at the vertex, especially at the superior parietal region.

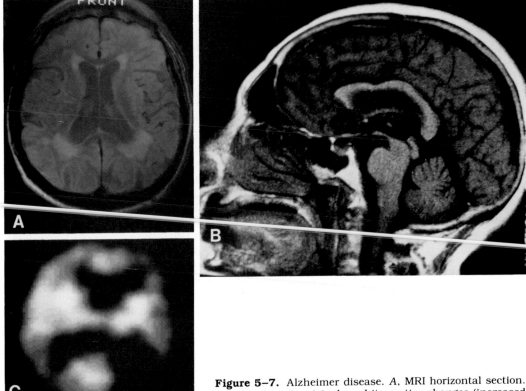

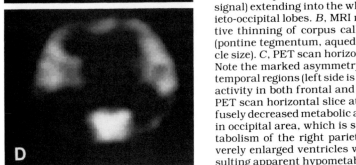

Figure 5–7. Alzheimer disease. *A*, MRI horizontal section. Prominent periventricular white matter changes (increased signal) extending into the white matter of the frontal and parieto-occipital lobes. *B*, MRI midsagittal section. Note the relative thinning of corpus callosum. The brainstem is normal (pontine tegmentum, aqueduct of Sylvius, and fourth ventricle size). *C*, PET scan horizontal slice at level of basal ganglia. Note the marked asymmetry of the inferior parietal/superior temporal regions (left side is more hypometabolic) and reduced activity in both frontal and right parietotemporal regions. *D*, PET scan horizontal slice at basal ganglia level. Note the diffusely decreased metabolic activity of the entire cortex, except in occipital area, which is spared. Especially severe hypometabolism of the right parietotemporal region is present. Severely enlarged ventricles were present in this case with resulting apparent hypometabolism of basal ganglia.

spond to these T_1 and T_2 changes would be decreased signal intensity in T_1-weighted and increased intensity in T_2-weighted images in a predominantly periventricular distribution. Erkinjuntti and associates[65] noted that the MRI showed periventricular "white matter changes" in about one third of their cases with AD. They did not study normal controls, however, so it is not known whether these periventricular changes were in excess of that expected for age. Bowen and associates[20] compared 87 patients with probable and possible AD to 36 age-matched controls and showed a roughly twofold increase in periventricular lesions and a fivefold increase in subcortical white matter lesions in AD subjects. However, Ley and associates[138] did not find any difference in MRI hyperintensities comparing AD patients and age-matched normal individuals.

A study by Fazekas and colleagues[67] described the MRI findings in patients with clinically diagnosed probable and possible AD and compared them with patients with clinically diagnosed MID. A "halo" of periventricular hyperintensity (see Fig. 5–7A) was frequently found in AD patients who did not have any evidence of vascular dementia. This halo is characterized by a smooth margin and is significantly more extensive than the hyperintensity found in controls. Outside of the immediate periventricular area, punctate or partially confluent deep white matter foci of hyperintensity were fairly frequently found in controls, AD, and MID patients. The existence of these foci does not imply vascular dementia. On the other hand, extensive, irregular periventricular hyperintensity and widespread confluent areas of deep white matter hyperintensity were found only in MID or mixed dementia. Since these patients were not confirmed to have AD or MID by pathologic examination, it is not clear how valid these results are. In a recent preliminary report by Bowen and colleagues,[21] extensive periventricular and subcortical white matter disease, that is, the MRI appearance of Binswanger disease, was found in several patients with pathologic evidence of AD alone.

The high sensitivity of MRI for detecting changes in the brain has been both an asset and a source of confusion. The profusion of abnormalities seen on MRI often leaves the clinician unable to categorize a patient because of the present lack of adequate data regarding the normal accompaniments of aging and the specific MRI features of MID. *The additional information contributed by MRI studies in AD patients has not yet resulted in an increase in the specificity of diagnosis.* Thus, at the present time, both CT and MRI are used primarily for excluding other causes of dementia in the diagnosis of AD.

PET SCAN STUDIES

Although the gross morphologic changes in the brain in the early stages of AD are subtle and variable as judged by CT and MRI scanning, alterations in function are more evident. Since a variety of functional parameters in the brain can be examined using PET and SPECT, these methods should be ideal in depicting abnormalities very early in the course of AD. Moreover, function in the brain can be evaluated under a variety of behavioral and pharmacologic conditons. The optimal condition for depicting functional abnormalities in AD may be different in different subtypes or stages of the disease. Very little work has been done thus far in exploiting such functional states to study AD, so as to enhance metabolic or blood flow deficits. Manipulating the functional conditions of a PET study may also be useful in clarifying some aspects of the pathophysiology of AD.

Table 5–3 lists studies done in the "resting state" to study AD by PET. With the exception of a study by Frakowiak and associates,[74] who used ^{15}O-labeled molecular oxygen and carbon dioxide to study CBF, oxygen extraction ratio, and oxygen consumption, all the other studies have been done using ^{18}FDG. The earlier studies[14,46,68,74] focused on alterations in absolute metabolic rate in AD patients, whereas in later studies the regional pattern of change in metabolism has been examined.

In general an inverse correlation has been found between absolute metabolic rates and the severity of dementia, that is, the more severe the dementia, the lower was the global glucose and oxygen metabolic rates and the CBF. The extent of reduction in metabolic rate in severe dementia has been reported to be from 31%[69] to 49%.[14] In the mild and moderate stages of AD, however, often no significant reduction in global absolute metabolic rate has been found.[41,56,99] Many studies have addressed the regional alterations in metabolic rate and the right-left asymmetries in metabolic rate that have been observed in patients with AD. The pattern that has consistently been reported in AD is one of regional deficits in the association neocortices (e.g., parietotemporal, prefrontal) and relative sparing of primary

Table 5–3 POSITRON EMISSION TOMOGRAPHY IN DEMENTIA

Author/ Year*	Type of Study	Control		Patient		Comments on Subjects‡	Results	Comments on Results§
		N	Age†	N	Age†			
Ferris et al, 1980[68]	[^{18}F]FDG (glucose metabolism)	3	63 ± 7	7	73 ± 5	Healthy controls. Patients were diagnosed as having mild (2), moderate (3), and moderate–severe (2) AD.	Metabolic rate in frontal, temporal cortices and caudate, thalamus in patients was 33–37% below control values.	Control group was too small for adequate comparison. Analysis was preliminary. Correlation between behavioral decline and metabolic decline was found.
Frackowiak et al, 1981[74]	Blood flow, oxygen metabolism, and oxygen extraction ratio.	14	61 ± 8	22	66 ± 9	Healthy controls. Patients were diagnosed as degenerative (13) or vascular (9) dementia; severity was moderate (11) and severe (11).	Degenerative and vascular patients had a parallel reduction of rCBF and rCMRO$_2$, with the parietal region being most affected (−33%). Occipital regions were least affected (−19%).	Asymmetries were not studied; however those with severe aphasia had greater left temporal rCMRO$_2$ reduction. Correlation found between dementia severity and flow-metabolism reduction.
deLeon et al, 1983[46]	Glucose metabolism	22	66 ± 7	24	73 ± 7	Healthy controls. Patients were diagnosed as having AD.	Reductions of 17% (caudate) to 24% (parietal) found in AD patients. Membership in AD or control groups could be predicted in 80% of subjects, by regional metabolic rates.	Correlations of up to 0.73 found between memory tests and regional metabolism. Asymmetries were not specifically examined.
Friedland et al, 1983[79]	Glucose metabolism	6	64 ± 8	10	65 ± 7	Healthy controls. Patients diagnosed as having AD.	Prominent asymmetries in some, but anterior-posterior differences were consistent in AD. Frontal-temporoparietal ratio was 1.00 to 1.04 in controls and 1.34 to 1.54 in AD patients.	This study highlighted the regional temporoparietal metabolic deficits in AD and emphasized asymmetries as well. Relative sparing of occipital metabolism also noted.
Foster et al, 1983[69]	Glucose metabolism			13	59	Clinically diagnosed to have AD. Three had prominent language deficits and four had predominant visuoconstructive apraxia.	Metabolic deficits of 19% (left temporoparietal) in the aphasic patients and 31% (right parietal) in apraxic patients.	Correlation between language performance and left temporal metabolism (r = 0.71) and between visuoconstructive tests and right parietal metabolism was as high as r = 0.81.

Table 5-3—*Continued*

Author/ Year*	Type of Study	Control N	Control Age†	Patient N	Patient Age†	Comments on Subjects‡	Results	Comments on Results§
Benson et al, 1983[14]	Glucose metabolism	16		11		Controls were not described. Eight patients had AD (Hachinski scores less than 4). Three had MID ("high" Hachinski scores) but with normal CT scans.	AD patients had 49% and MID patients had 35% reduction in metabolic rate. In AD and MID, parietotemporal association cortex was most affected and primary visual cortex was least affected.	Authors state that, in contrast to the frontoparietal association cortex deficits in AD, there is a variable pattern in MID. (Subject number is small and reliability of diagnosis in MID group is unclear.)
Chase et al, 1984[35]	Glucose metabolism	5	57 ± 2	17	61 ± 2	Patients diagnosed to have AD ("minimal" to severe dementia). All subjects received WAIS IQ subtests. Correlations done on the control and patient groups together.	WAIS IQ scores correlated with overall metabolism (r = 0.68). Verbal IQ correlated best with left temporal (r = 0.76) and performance IQ with right parietal metabolism (r = 0.70).	WAIS Arithmetic subtests correlated best with left inferior parietal-superior temporal metabolism, whereas digit span correlated best with anterior and superior frontal metabolism bilaterally.
Friedland et al, 1984[78]	Glucose metabolism	7	63 ± 3	2	63, 64	Mild and moderate AD. Patients also had CT and MRI evaluation.	MR and CT showed only symmetric ventricular enlargement in one patient, and symmetrical ventricular enlargement and cortical atrophy in the other. Both patients had predominant right-side temporoparietal metabolic deficits.	Author concludes that PET is superior to MRI and CT in diagnosis of AD.
Haxby et al, 1985[99]	Glucose metabolism	26	63 (45–83)	10	64 ± 9	Healthy controls. Patients had mild–moderate dementia. Ten patients and 10 controls were tested with a syntax comprehension test, a drawing test, and memory tests.	Temporal, parietal, and frontal association cortices showed metabolic deficits and asymmetries in AD patients relative to controls. The direction of these asymmetries was related to asymmetries of language and visuospatial function.	There was no difference between patients and controls in absolute metabolic rates. Sensorimotor and visual cortices showed no deficits and asymmetry was not greater in these structures than in controls.

Table 5–3—*Continued*

Author/ Year*	Type of Study	Control		Patient		Comments on Subjects‡	Results	Comments on Results§
		N	Age†	N	Age†			
Kuhl et al, 1985[123]	Glucose metabolism	14	—	14	—	Controls not described. Patients consisted of AD (n = 28), Parkinson dementia (PD) (n = 14) and MID (n = 6). Degree of dementia described as questionable, mild, moderate, and severe.	Parietal-cerebellar metabolic ratio was 0.84 in AD, 0.94 in PD, 1.28 in controls, and 1.29 in MID.	Parietal-cerebellar ratio correlated with severity (r = 0.69) and duration (r = 0.46) of dementia.
Cutler et al, 1985[41]	Glucose metabolism	12	58 ± 4	1	57	Patient had familial AD (father and paternal great aunt had autopsy-proven AD and two other paternal relatives had dementia). PET scan and psychologic testing was repeated twice at 8-mo intervals.	Mild memory loss and normal WAIS IQ subtests were present initially and were not measurably worse subsequently. Metabolic pattern initially normal. Parietal deficits present in second and third scans.	Author shows that very early in the disease, metabolic deficits may not be present. Without objective behavioral deterioration, metabolic deficits appeared in subsequent scans.
Alavi et al, 1986[3]	Glucose metabolism	11		17		Patients had probable AD.	A tendency to left-parietal and temporal metabolic deficits in mild and moderate patients became significant in severe cases.	Reduction was 17% in the left temporal and 42% in the left inferior parietal regions, in severe AD.
Duara et al, 1986[56]	Glucose metabolism	29	63 ± 10	21	64 ± 9	Controls were healthy. Patients had probable AD (10 mild, 7 moderate, and 4 severe cases).	Global metabolism was reduced in severe cases only. In mild AD, deficits occurred in the parietal lobe only, but in moderate and severe cases temporal and frontal lobes were also affected.	Asymmetries occurred in parietal regions only in mild AD and in frontal and parietal regions, in moderate AD. Predominant left-temporal deficits were found in severe AD. Five moderate AD patients showed reduction in WAIS IQ without change in metabolism, on follow-up scans.
McGeer et al, 1986[150]	Glucose metabolism	11	66	14	69	Controls were neurologically normal. Patients had mild (n = 4), moderate (n = 5), and severe dementia (n = 5). MRI or CT scans were also obtained.	Metabolic rates reduced by 32%, 24%, 20%, and 18% in temporal, frontal, parietal, and occipital cortices, respectively.	Asymmetries occurred in all cortical regions in AD patients, greatest in the temporal. Authors conclude that atrophy could not account for the regional hypometabolism seen.

Table 5–3—*Continued*

Author/Year*	Type of Study	Control		Patient		Comments on Subjects‡	Results	Comments on Results§
		N	Age†	N	Age†			
Haxby et al, 1986[100]	Glucose metabolism	29	64 ± 11	22	65 ± 9	Healthy controls. Patients had probable AD (10 mild and 12 moderate cases). Memory, language, and visuospatial function were also assessed.	Mild cases had memory deficits and metabolic asymmetries but without any language or visuospatial deficits. Moderate cases showed metabolic asymmetries with appropriate asymmetries of language vs visuospatial function.	The authors conclude that cortical metabolic dysfunction is evident in early AD, often preceding the appearance of neocortically mediated neuropsychologic dysfunction. In moderate AD, metabolic and neuropsychologic asymmetries are correlated.
Loewenstein et al, 1989[141]	Glucose metabolism	5	68 ± 9	42	73 ± 10	Healthy controls. Patients were divided into those with AD (n = 31) and MID (n = 11). MRI-detected lesions were quantified in MID patients.	71% of AD patients had abnormal scans (outside 95% confidence limits for regional asymmetry or hypometabolism). Forty-eight percent had predominant left-side and 13% predominant right-side hypometabolism. Sixty-four percent of MID patients had abnormal scans; 46% had predominant left- and 9% predominant right-side hypometabolism.	This study quantified the number of patients with abnormal scans for each diagnostic group (AD and MID). In both groups, significantly more had left-side than right-side hypometabolism. MRI lesions were not asymmetrical in MID patients.

*See end-of-chapter references.
†Average age or age range.
‡Points to be emphasized regarding controls and patients.
§Points to be emphasized regarding the results.

sensory and motor cortices, such as perirolandic and medial occipital, as well as the basal ganglia, thalamus, and cerebellar hemisphere (see Fig. 5–7C and D). Association cortex hypometabolism in AD has usually been reported to affect the parietotemporal regions to a greater extent and earlier in the course of the disease than frontal regions, although this is not always the case. In Down syndrome patients, who are known invariably to have the neuropathology of AD by the age of 40 years, metabolic deficits similar to those described in AD have been found to occur when progressive dementia occurs.[189]

The finding of asymmetric metabolic deficits in AD (see Fig. 5–7C) was somewhat surprising when initially reported because the degenerative changes were viewed to be relatively diffuse. In fact, it was expected that asymmetric metabolic deficits would be a differentiating feature of MID.[14] It has been reported that in AD, asymmetric metabolic deficits appear early in the disease course and the side of predominant involvement correlates with the dominant neuropsychologic deficit that is found.

Patients with predominant language deficits manifest predominant left-side metabolic deficits, and those with predominant visuoconstructive deficits manifest predominant right-side metabolic deficits.[69,99] Moreover, it appears that metabolic asymmetries may occur before, and predict the pattern of, "neocortically mediated" neuropsychologic deficits.[100]

The pathophysiology of the metabolic deficits in AD has been the source of some speculation. Two major possibilities exist. First, the pathology in the neocortical association areas in parietal, temporal, and frontal regions gives rise to the metabolic deficits in these same regions. Second, that pathology in other brain regions is manifested primarily as deficits in association neocortical regions, because of transneuronal functional disconnection (diaschisis) effects. Evidence in support of the first hypothesis is that the distribution of neuronal loss in the neocortex of AD patients is similar to the distribution of metabolic deficits, particularly in the early stages of the disease.[27,77] The lack of prominent metabolic deficits in medial temporal cortex[71] where the pathology is known to be most severe in early AD, however, goes against this theory. Degeneration in basal forebrain nuclei or in amygdala-hippocampal regions, both of which are known to project heavily into association neocortex, could result in disconnection of and hypometabolism in these neocortical regions.

McGeer and associates[149] reported on a single case of AD in whom antemortem PET scan findings of glucose hypometabolism were correlated with postmortem neuropathologic findings. On gross pathology the left hemisphere, especially in the parietal regions, showed far greater atrophic changes than the right. Metabolism was also reduced asymmetrically with predominant left-hemisphere hypometabolism. Reduced metabolism correlated best with severity of gliosis and least with the number of plaques in a brain area.

PET has been used to study the blood-brain barrier in AD,[80,191] but no disruption of the barrier has been detected by the methods used. Behavioral activation studies in AD patients[16,57,155] have not as yet yielded any results that have improved diagnostic ability or clarified the pathophysiology of AD.

SPECT STUDIES

Several SPECT imaging studies have been reported thus far in AD patients, with either [^{123}I]iodoamphetamine or ^{99m}Tc-labeled HM-PAO used to obtain measures of CBF. These studies have demonstrated the same distribution of deficits as are evident on PET studies of blood flow or glucose metabolism.*

The greater availability of SPECT cameras and the lack of the necessity for a local cyclotron to produce the isotopes needed for SPECT studies makes SPECT an attractive alternative to PET for assessment of the functional disturbances in dementia, although the poorer spatial resolution and lack of true quantitation of data remain disadvantages. SPECT studies are particularly valuable in the mildly or questionably demented individual, especially where other factors such as depression, medication effects, or cultural factors cast doubt on the diagnosis of organic dementia. A clearly abnormal SPECT study in this situation indicates organicity. Distinctions between the various causes of the organic brain disorder are, however, not easily made by SPECT or by PET.

Parkinson Disease

CT STUDIES

Although dementia is a relatively common finding in Parkinson disease (PD) patients, only one study has thus far been reported comparing CT scans of demented with nondemented PD patients.[199] It was found that there was in-

---

*References 18, 34, 37, 101, 114, 115, 165, 171, 195.

deed an increase in ventricular size in demented PD patients compared with the nondemented who in turn did not have larger ventricles than age-matched normal subjects. Indices of cortical atrophy and ventricular enlargement of CT scans show a greater degree of atrophy in PD patients, in comparison to controls, although severity of atrophy and extrapyramidal symptoms are not correlated.[193] Adam and colleagues[1] studied patients with PD with onset before and after age 65 years and showed that only the later onset patients demonstrated cortical atrophy, which was found to affect the frontal regions most prominently. This result was not obtained, however, by Steiner and associates,[200] who reported that earlier onset patients (before 50 years) demonstrated the greatest degree of both central atrophy (lateral and third ventricular enlargement) and cortical atrophy. They found that patients

in the 60- to 79-year age range differed from controls to a lesser extent, and only in regard to cortical atrophy. Thus, CT scans are not very revealing in nondemented PD patients.

MRI STUDIES

Drayer[53] summarized his experience with high field MRI studies in patients with PD. He described mild ventricular but prominent sulcal enlargement, and signal hypointensity (on T_2-weighted scans), which was outside the average range, in the globus pallidus, red nucleus, substantia nigra, dentate nucleus, and putamen (Fig. 5–8A and B). Patients with PD-plus syndromes (multisystem atrophy), including some with dementia, have been described to have particularly prominent signal hypointensity specifically in the putamen,[52,168] whereas in normal aged individuals and those with idiopathic PD the hy-

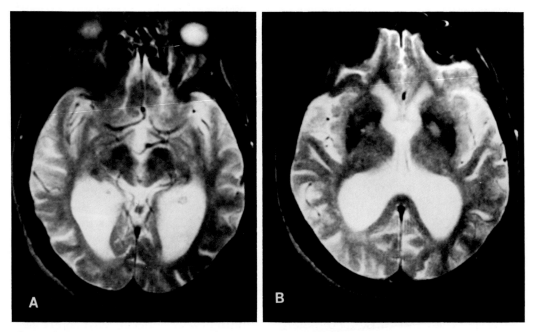

Figure 5–8. Parkinson dementia. *A*, MRI horizontal section at midbrain ventricular level (TR = 2.5 seconds, TE = 90 milliseconds). Note the marked increase in size of temporal horns. There is reduced signal in the red nucleus and substantia nigra regions from iron deposition. (Low signal in substantia nigra merges with the low signal of the cerebral peduncles.) *B*, MRI horizontal section at basal ganglia level (TR = 2.5 seconds, TE = 90 milliseconds). Note the low signal of globus pallidus from iron deposition merging with low signal of the posterior part of putamen.

pointensity in the globus pallidus is more prominent than in the putamen. These signal alterations have been found to correspond to the concentration of iron deposited in these structures.[52] Drayer[53] also described above-average subcortical white matter signal hyperintensity on T_2-weighted images in PD patients. However, Huber and associates[105] used MRI scans to compare age-matched PD patients with and without dementia to normal control patients and were unable to show any differences between the controls and the demented and nondemented groups in the extent of generalized atrophy, atrophy of the corpus callosum, thickness of the substantia nigra, or areas of high signal intensity.

PET STUDIES

PD patients without dementia have been reported to have an 18% reduction in global cerebral glucose metabolism[124] and a 20% reduction in global cerebral blood flow,[216] compared to controls. No consistent focal pattern of deficit has been reported in PD patients,[172] except in those who have concomitant dementia, where parietal lobe reductions in glucose metabolism have been found.[124,126] These deficits in demented PD patients resemble those seen in AD. Pathologic studies suggest that the majority of patients with PD and dementia have some concomitant neuropathologic changes of AD.[179] A single patient presenting with a slowly progressive dementia who had PET scan findings considered typical for AD (i.e., bilateral parietotemporal metabolic defects) was found on autopsy to have pathologic features of PD alone.[190]

SPECT STUDIES

A single report of SPECT studies in seven patients with PD revealed diffusely decreased cortical tracer uptake; PD patients with dementia, however, were not studied.[177]

Pick Disease

The clinical presentation of Pick disease has been considered to have certain typical features by some investigators[40] but not by others.[92] Changes in personality and behavior often occur early in the disease course and may outweigh memory loss; visuospatial dysfunction occurs relatively late. Aphasic features at the onset are common and some patients develop components of the Kluver-Bucy syndrome, such as oral exploratory tendencies, sensory agnosia, and hypersexuality. Nevertheless, many patients with Pick disease are diagnosed as AD antemortem, and it is likely that a proportion have the typical presentation of AD.[104]

Grossly, the brain typically shows lobar atrophy with primarily frontal and temporal involvement and sparing of the parietal lobe (Fig. 5–9A and B). This pattern of atrophy has been reported occasionally among patients with AD.[197] Histologically there is marked neuronal loss, marked astrocytic gliosis, inflated neurons, and Pick bodies. The amygdala, in addition to the cortex and basal ganglia, is severely involved.

CT STUDIES

Several clinicopathologic studies of Pick disease have been reported since the introduction of the CT scanner.* The CT findings in Pick disease have typically been those of frontal and temporal atrophy, evidenced by increased width of the frontal interhemispheric space, the sylvian fissures and the frontal horns of the lateral ventricles. Groen and Hekster[90] studied 14 clinically affected and unaffected adults from three generations of a family with autosomal dominant Pick disease. In three affected members the CT scan findings were generalized atrophy, generalized atrophy with frontal predomi-

---

*References 40, 90, 116, 122, 148, 160, 163, 196, 210.

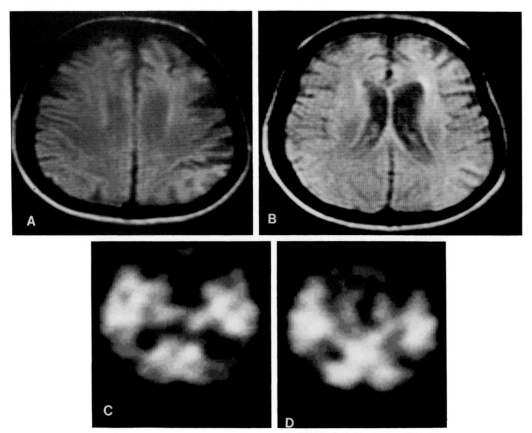

Figure 5-9. Pick disease. *A*, MRI horizontal section at high ventricular level. Note the prominent atrophy of frontal regions bilaterally with sulcal prominence and widening of anterior part of interhemispheric fissure. *B*, MRI horizontal section at midventricular level. Note the sulcal prominence predominantly in the frontal region and the prominence of lateral ventricles especially of the left frontal horn. *C*, PET scan slice at basal ganglia level. Note the marked decrease in bilateral frontal metabolism with preserved basal ganglia activity. *D*, PET scan slice at high ventricular level. Note the marked frontal hypometabolism and the bilateral focal parietal deficits.

nance, and frontotemporal atrophy, respectively. Of 11 clinically unaffected members at risk, 3 showed frontotemporal atrophy in the fifth decade of life. In this family, age of onset was typically in the sixth and seventh decades of life. When typical findings are obtained, CT appears to be a useful procedure to assist in making the antemortem diagnosis of Pick disease.

MRI STUDIES

Thus far MRI has not revealed any findings additional to those obtained with CT in Pick disease. It should be

possible by MRI to demonstrate the extensive subcortical gliosis that is part of the pathology of Pick disease. Future studies with T_2-weighted sequences may demonstrate this finding.

PET STUDIES

Studies of CBF with scalp detectors and [133]xenon inhalation predicted the findings that were obtained with PET and SPECT in Pick disease.[183]

A single clinicopathologic study in a patient with Pick disease confirmed marked (greater than 50%) reduction of cerebral glucose metabolism in the frontal lobes bilaterally.[116] The fronto-parietal ratio was about 26% lower in the Pick disease case than the control value, more than 30% lower than in 12 patients with AD, and more than 4 standard deviations from the mean of the AD value. Of particular interest in this study was the finding that reductions in regional cerebral glucose metabolic rate correlated best with degree of gliosis ($r = 0.78$) and correlated least with the number of Pick bodies or inflated neurons ($r = 0.17$).

PET scans on patients with clinically diagnosed Pick disease have also revealed bilateral or unilateral frontal (Fig. 5–9C and D) and anterior temporal metabolic deficits.[58]

SPECT STUDIES

Neary and colleagues[165] studied nine patients with mental changes suggestive of Pick disease (disordered social conduct, loss of initiative, forgetfulness, disinhibition, impaired abstraction and naming, and sparing of perceptuospatial abilities) by SPECT scanning, using the agent ^{99m}Tc-labeled HM-PAO. Seven of the nine (78%) showed only frontal lobe perfusion defects, one showed a parietofrontal abnormality, and one patient showed only posterior defects. These results were very different from those obtained on patients diagnosed to have AD, in whom 14 of 21 patients (67%) had parietal or parietofrontal defects and 3 (14%) had only frontal defects in perfusion.

Hence, SPECT studies of cerebral perfusion may be useful in confirming abnormalities in the frontal and temporal lobes that are characteristic of Pick disease.

Progressive Supranuclear Palsy

Progressive supranuclear palsy (PSP) is a degenerative disease diagnosed on clinical grounds on the basis of vertical supranuclear gaze paresis (downward gaze), axial rigidity, gait instability, slowing of mentation, and dementia. PSP, as described in Chapter 8, has been considered the model of "subcortical" dementia as contrasted to that of the "cortical" dementia epitomized by AD. Neuroimaging methods, generally, do not contribute toward making the diagnosis but may be helpful in evaluating the presence of concomitant disease and evaluating the pathophysiology of some features of the disease, especially the dementia.

CT STUDIES

The most complete description of the CT changes in PSP has been made by Ambrosetto and associates.[5] The findings include brain stem and quadrigeminal plate atrophy, manifested by enlargement of the quadrigeminal cistern, the ambient cisterns, and the interpeduncular fossa, and dilatation of the aqueduct and the fourth ventricle (Fig. 5–10A). Because of degeneration of the midline thalamic nuclei, the posterior part of the third ventricle is also dilated, producing a characteristic "skittle" shape to this structure, in horizontal sections. Other investigators[97,111,143] have emphasized the dilatation of the lateral ventricles, which also occurs in this disease (Fig. 5–10B). Dubinsky and Jankovic[61] have emphasized the frequency with which multiple infarctions to CT or MRI are evident in patients with PSP (33%), compared to patients with PD (12%). This significantly higher incidence of cerebral infarcts was presumably related to a higher frequency of hypertension, older age at onset of disease and other stroke risk factors. Nevertheless, extrapolating from these CT findings, it is possible that a proportion of patients with the clinical syndrome of PSP have this disorder, not on the basis of degenerative changes, but because of a multi-infarct state.

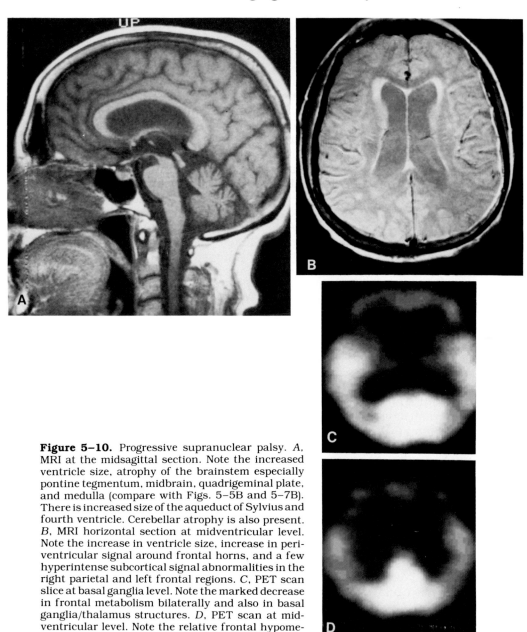

Figure 5–10. Progressive supranuclear palsy. *A*, MRI at the midsagittal section. Note the increased ventricle size, atrophy of the brainstem especially pontine tegmentum, midbrain, quadrigeminal plate, and medulla (compare with Figs. 5–5B and 5–7B). There is increased size of the aqueduct of Sylvius and fourth ventricle. Cerebellar atrophy is also present. *B*, MRI horizontal section at midventricular level. Note the increase in ventricle size, increase in periventricular signal around frontal horns, and a few hyperintense subcortical signal abnormalities in the right parietal and left frontal regions. *C*, PET scan slice at basal ganglia level. Note the marked decrease in frontal metabolism bilaterally and also in basal ganglia/thalamus structures. *D*, PET scan at midventricular level. Note the relative frontal hypometabolism bilaterally.

MRI STUDIES

Abnormalities of signal intensity are frequently found in PSP patients. In a preliminary report, Manon-Espaillat and colleagues,[144] using high-field MRI, showed decreased signal intensity on T_2-weighted scans in the pallidum, putamen, thalamus, pars compacta of the substantia nigra, and superior colliculi. These changes presumably represented increased iron accumulation in these structures and are findings not obtained in patients with idiopathic PD, but are seen also in patients with multisystem atrophy.

PET STUDIES

Decreased frontal lobe glucose metabolism in PSP was reported initially by D'Antona and colleagues.[42] These findings have been confirmed by others.[15] In addition, Baron and associates[12] have shown a loss of striatal dopamine receptors in PSP using PET with radiolabeled ligands.

In comparing metabolic deficits, Foster and colleagues[72] showed that in AD the cerebral cortex was most abnormal followed by thalamic and basal ganglia structures; in PSP, however, there was relatively equivalent hypometabolism of the basal ganglia and thalamic and cortical structures (Fig. 5–10C). Foster and associates[70] have shown that while metabolism in the entire cerebral cortex is reduced, compared to normal individuals, the frontal cortex is most reduced in PSP (Fig. 5–10D). This pattern is quite different from that seen in AD. Another disorder that can be difficult to distinguish clinically from PSP in its early stage is olivopontocerebellar atrophy (OPCA). In OPCA, metabolism is reduced in the cerebellar hemispheres, the vermis, and the brain stem, which are regions that are spared in PSP, but normal values are obtained in the thalamus and cortex.[87] The pathophysiology of frontal cortical hypometabolism in PSP is not well understood. A study by Levasseur and associates[137] showed that patients with bilateral pallidal lesions and behavioral changes have metabolic deficits predominantly in the frontal cortex. Hence, dysfunction in the pallidum may be relevant to the frontal hypometabolism in PSP, perhaps with pallidothalamic and thalamocortical connections mediating the effects.

SPECT STUDIES

Neary and associates[165] studied eight patients with PSP and demonstrated that seven (88%) had frontal perfusion deficits, whereas one (12%) had a normal pattern. This result is in keeping with the PET findings.

Neurotransmitter and Neuroreceptor Studies in Degenerative Dementia

A high level of interest exists in using PET and SPECT to study presynaptic and postsynaptic receptor function in dementing disease, because most degenerative dementias have been associated with dysfunction in one or more neuroreceptor systems. In addition, the findings by quantitative measures that synaptic loss correlates very highly with cognitive dysfunction in AD (see Chapter 8) increases the interest in imaging synaptic receptors. These studies are still in their infancy since quantitative techniques for measuring the synthesis of ligands or receptor number, affinity, and occupancy have not yet been perfected. Nevertheless, some interesting studies have been done and are listed below according to the areas to which they pertain.

NORMAL AGING

Presynaptic dopaminergic function has been studied using [6-^{18}F]fluoro-L-dopa (fluorodopa) and PET in normal subjects 22 to 80 years of age.[146] The fluorodopa uptake rate constant was found to be negatively correlated with age, indicating a reduced incorporation of dopamine precursors by the brain in the elderly.

Wong and colleagues[217] showed that the binding of D_2 dopamine and S_2 serotonin receptors by [^{11}C]3-N-methyl spiperone in the caudate nucleus and frontal cortex, respectively, in humans was reduced as a function of age. These investigators studied 22 men and 22 women and found that the decline in D_2 dopamine receptor binding, but not the serotonin receptor binding declined more steeply in men (46%) than in women (25%) over a five-decade age range.

ALZHEIMER DISEASE

Although no consistent alteration in muscarinic receptors has been found in AD in postmortem tissue, a recent report suggests a decrease in muscarinic receptors in 6 AD patients in parietal cortex, as estimated by binding of [123I]iodoQNB, studied by SPECT.[211] Another SPECT study using 123I-labeled Ro16-0154 to study benzodiazepine receptor binding in the brain also showed reduced binding in AD patients. These results may have been obtained, however, because of tissue loss (atrophy) in the cortex and will require confirmation with appropriate atrophy correction techniques. Nicotinic and serotoninergic receptors are both reduced in the neocortex in AD, and appropriate PET and SPECT markers might be of considerable interest.

PARKINSON DISEASE

Presynaptic uptake of dopamine in the striatum has been studied using [18F]fluorodopa as a tracer.[146] In hemiparkinsonism the accumulation of dopamine was reduced in the striatum (especially putamen) on the side opposite the major motor symptoms. Eidelberg and associates[63] report a correlation between fluorodopa uptake rate constants and clinical scores for dementia, as well as scores for bradykinesia, rigidity, tremor, gait disturbance, and left-right motor symmetry.

Postsynaptic receptor changes can be studied using a variety of agents that have been used to quantify D_2 and D_1 receptor density in the striatum. Preliminary reports in PD patients suggest D_2 receptor supersensitivity, but demented patients were not included in these studies.[173,182]

PROGRESSIVE SUPRANUCLEAR PALSY

Postsynaptic dopaminergic D_2 receptor density studied by the agent [76Br]bromospiperone showed a loss of striatal D_2 receptors in PSP.[12] This finding was in contrast to the supersensitivity of D_2 receptors reported above in PD patients.

Multi-infarct Dementia

The term multi-infarct dementia (MID) appears self-explanatory, that is, a dementia caused by multiple cerebral infarctions. Since the term was coined in 1974 by Hachinski and colleagues,[93] however, the criteria for the diagnosis of this entity, its incidence in the demented population, and its clinical features have been the subject of increasing debate. The application of various types of imaging devices to define this entity more precisely has provided a wealth of information. The data seem to point to a variety of entities under the umbrella of MID.

The existence of the entity of MID is based on the studies of Blessed and colleagues[17] and Tomlinson and associates,[204] who showed that in demented old people, without the neuropathologic features of AD, a strong correlation existed between the volume of brain "softening" (infarction) and the degree of dementia ($r = 0.68$). Moreover, an aggregate volume of at least 50 mL of softening was required to produce the clinical syndrome of dementia. This vascular dementia was diagnosed on pathologic grounds in 9 out of 50 demented subjects (18%). It is remarkable, however, that this classic study has not as yet been replicated.

On neuroimaging studies the pattern of regional ischemic involvement allows a classification of MID patients according to the location of the infarct or ischemic areas. In the first group, those with multiple neocortical infarcts, a frank dementia with a cortical dementia syndrome is likely. In the second group, those with multiple discrete subcortical infarcts, frank dementia does not always occur, but some elements of a subcortical dementia syndrome are often present. The third group includes those with diffuse white matter pathology or Binswanger disease, to be discussed below.

The existence of the entity of MID is not in doubt, but it is said to be both underdiagnosed[166] and overdiagnosed.[30] In a critical and extensive review of the literature, Liston and LaRue[139] conclude that "assuming that strokes have certain reliable neurological manifestations and that strokes are able to cause dementia, then, when demented patients are noted to have a history consistent with one or more strokes, it may be erroneously reasoned that the one led to the other." From a neuroimaging point of view, it is important to realize that although it is valuable to identify cerebral infarcts in a demented patient, the existence of these infarcts does not mean that they necessarily caused or contributed to the dementia.[29]

CT SCAN STUDIES OF MID

The clinical diagnosis of MID is usually confirmed by structural (CT scan, MRI) evidence of infarcts in the brain. Historically, however, Hachinski and colleagues[94] developed criteria for the diagnosis of MID using an ischemic score (IS) (without including neuroimaging findings). Molsa and colleagues[159] reported on 58 demented patients, of which 45 had been classified as AD (n = 28), MID (n = 11), or mixed dementia (n = 6), using the same IS score criteria and without including CT scan findings. The accuracy of clinical diagnosis, on the basis of neuropathologic examination, was 71% for AD, 42% for MID, and 20% for mixed dementia.

Subsequently, a more elaborate study, including the use of CT scans, has been reported by Wade and associates,[209] on 65 patients with dementia. They used an IS of 4 or less, a suggestive history, and a CT scan that was clear of infarcts to diagnose AD. Patients were diagnosed as having MID if they had an IS greater than 4, a history suggestive of cerebral vascular events, and a CT scan that showed infarcts. Patients with mixed features were labeled as mixed dementia. A miscellaneous group, with

diagnoses such as PSP or Creutzfeldt-Jakob disease, was also identified. Pathologic verification was most accurate for 39 patients diagnosed as AD (85% accuracy) and for the 6 patients diagnosed with miscellaneous conditions (83% accuracy). Of 4 patients clinically diagnosed as having MID, 1 did have MID (25% accuracy) and 3 had mixed dementia (a combination of AD and MID). Of 16 patients diagnosed as having mixed dementia, 5 (31%) did have this pathologically, while 5 had AD and 4 had MID. Thus, it appears that the CT scan is most useful for improving the accuracy of the diagnosis of AD by separating AD from MID and mixed dementia. Predictably, the CT scan does not seem to help in distinguishing between MID and mixed dementia.

Other studies have compared the CT scan diagnosis to the Hachinski Ischemic Score classificaion of MID vs AD. Radue and colleagues[180] found that only 38% of patients classified as MID according to the IS ($\geq$6) had CT scan criteria for MID (focal low attenuation areas, focal and asymmetric ventricular enlargement, and asymmetric sylvian fissures). However, if they did have the CT scan criteria, there was a 90% chance of also having IS criteria for MID, Loeb and Gandolfo[140] classified 94 patients with dementia according to the IS. Of 28 patients with IS $\geq$7 (classified as MID), 17 (61%) had CT scan criteria for MID (multiple areas of reduced density attributable to ischemic lesions), whereas 95% of those with CT scan criteria also had IS criteria for MID. Hence, the IS score is not a very good predictor of the CT scan findings, whereas the CT scan is a much better predictor of the IS score.

Erkinjuntti and colleagues[65] classified patients as AD (n = 22) and MID (n = 29) on the basis of clinical criteria alone (i.e., without using the CT scan). They distinguished between cortical and white matter infarcts on CT scans and found that 18 (62%) of the MID cases had infarcts outside the white matter, whereas none of the AD cases had such infarcts. Cystic infarcts and areas of low attenuation in the white matter were present in 26 (90%) of MID cases, and 1 (5%) of the AD cases. With findings that included a combination of white matter lesions and cortical infarcts, 97% of MID and 95% of AD could be correctly classified, according to their clinical criteria. Thus, the correspondence of clinical and CT scan criteria for MID may be reasonably good when stringent clinical criteria are used. A recent report suggests, however, that white matter changes in demented patients are not very specific. Aharon-Peretz and colleagues[2] described white matter changes in the cerebral hemispheres on CT scans in 56% of clinically diagnosed AD and 97% of MID patients. Ventricular dilatation (perhaps an index of severity of white matter disease) was correlated with cognitive status in MID but not in AD cases. From the aforementioned studies it may be surmised that *clinical criteria, including CT scan findings, will not distinguish effectively between pathologically determined MID and mixed dementia*[209] *but will be more effective in separating AD from MID or mixed dementia.*

CT SCAN STUDIES OF BINSWANGER DISEASE

Binswanger disease was considered rare and diagnosed only on autopsy before the advent of the CT scan. In 1979, Rosenberg and associates[186] first documented the characteristic CT findings in an autopsy-proven case of Binswanger disease. Subsequently, it became a relatively common diagnosis, but often an inaccurate one. To quote Kinkel and colleagues,[120] "There remains a large group of patients, usually in the seventh through ninth decades, who develop an identifiable CT pattern of white matter disease of unknown origin. By CT scans, their lesions appear as bilateral, usually symmetric, areas of decreased density of the periventricular white matter and centra semiovale." Of 23 patients diagnosed on CT

scans to have Binswanger disease by Kinkel and associates,[120] eight had nonspecific complaints such as blurred vision and dizziness and no clinical neurologic deficits. Seven cases presented with motor strokes and most of these were demented as well. Eight patients who presented with dementia had gait disturbance and motor deficits, including hemiparesis and paraparesis, as well. One of the severely demented patients came to autopsy and was found to have numerous cystic infarcts (1–6 mm in diameter) in the centra semiovale, basal ganglia, and thalamus; there were early and evolving infarcts in subcortical white matter and gray matter structures. The white matter demonstrated irregular zones of demyelination. Even though the circle of Willis showed minimal atherosclerosis, subcortical arterioles were moderately to severely sclerosed, thus earning the label "subcortical arteriosclerotic encephalopathy (SAE)."

Kinkel and colleagues[120] distinguished the white matter hypodensities seen in Binswanger disease from those seen in NPH. Although the ventricles are frequently enlarged in Binswanger disease, the periventricular hypodensities on CT scans extend further dorsally into the centra semiovale and have a more heterogeneous appearance than in NPH. In some cases, however, the appearances are difficult to tell apart, and in fact the two conditions possibly coexist occasionally.

Other studies on Binswanger disease[33,186] have reported essentially the same experience as that of Kinkel and colleagues.[120] Although many patients with typical CT findings of Binswanger disease are not demented or have mild cognitive disturbance, a positive relationship between the severity of dementia to the extent of CT changes has been described.[89,206] An interesting CT-pathologic study was reported by Lotz and associates,[142] who studied 82 patients, selected only because they had antemortem CT examination and subsequently postmortem examination of the brain. Twenty of these patients had the CT scan appearance of Binswanger disease, of which 18 had histologic evidence of demyelination, axonal loss, and fibrous thickening of the arterial walls in the affected white matter. One patient had metastatic carcinoma, and another, an aqueductal tumor that had produced hydrocephalus; in both these cases the CT lucency was presumbaly caused by edema. In 10 patients with normal white matter by CT, however, there was minimal or no pathologic evidence of Binswanger disease. Thus, it appears that the diagnosis of Binswanger disease on CT scan alone is usually verified on pathologic examination. From a clinician's standpoint, a patient presenting with nonspecific or focal neurologic symptoms, with or without positive neurologic findings, who has the CT scan appearance of Binswanger disease, is likely to be proved to have Binswanger disease on postmortem examination.

MRI STUDIES

A profusion of MRI periventricular lesions occurs in patients at risk for stroke and, therefore, theoretically at risk for MID. It is unclear, however, whether a critical extent and anatomic distribution of these lesions is associated with the development of dementia. Because neuropathologic studies on MID patients with antemortem MRI scans have not yet been reported, the significance of these MRI lesions, with regard to their ability to predict the likelihood of dementia being present, is unknown.

Gerard and Weisberg[85] noted that of patients aged 60 years and above, 10% with no risk factors for stroke, 40% with such risk factors, and 69% with definite evidence of cerebrovascular disease had MRI periventricular high-signal intensity patterns. Marshall and colleagues[145] studied postmortem brains by MRI and then by detailed pathologic examination. In 3 of 21 brains there were multiple foci of periventricular hyperintensity on the MRI image, and these were confirmed histologically to be deep white infarcts, but of smaller size than the MRI abnormality. The gliosis surrounding these infarcts made them appear larger than their true size on the T_2-weighted MRI images. These studies attest to the fact that the MRI is highly sensitive to some of the common neuropathologic effects of aging, that is, white matter infarcts and subsequent gliosis.

Awad and colleagues[7] studied 270 consecutive patients who had MRI scans. They found in this group that in those with an overt diagnosis of dementia, incidental subcortical MRI lesions were not more frequent or severe than in age-matched, nondemented control subjects. They did not distinguish, however, between the different types of dementia and they did not subtype the white matter lesions. On the other hand, Fazekas and associates[67] classified 16 patients with dementia into those with probable AD (n = 7), possible AD (n = 5), and MID (n = 4). The MRI findings in the MID patients differed from that in the AD group. Patients with MID had two distinguishing features, namely, irregular periventricular hyperintensities extending into the deep white matter, and large confluent areas of deep white matter hyperintensity (DWMH) (Fig. 5–11A and B). In AD patients, DWMHs were either punctate or showed only slight evidence of confluence, and periventricular hyperintensities were smooth and halolike in appearance.

Hershey and associates[103] studied patients with known cerebral vascular disease and classified them into those with and those without dementia. The only significant difference on MRI between the 24% of their sample with dementia and the nondemented patients was the greater size of the ventricles in the demented patients.

Opinions currently vary widely with regard to the significance of MRI abnormalities in dementia. With more specific descriptions of the white matter changes in dementing diseases and normal aging as well as with future pathologic correlations, the place of

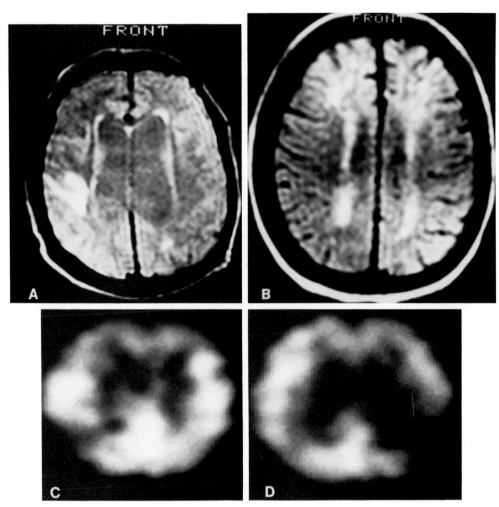

Figure 5–11. Multi-infarct dementia. *A*, MRI horizontal section at midventricular level. Note the high-intensity area in the right parietal region involving the cortex and subcortical white matter and several areas of increased signal in the white matter of the left occipital and left and right frontal lobes, representing infarcts. Mildly increased periventricular signal is also seen. *B*, MRI horizontal section at high ventricular level of the same subject. Note the numerous subcortical white matter areas of increased signal in both frontal lobes extending up to the cortex with moderately increased periventricular signal. *C*, PET scan slice at midventricular level from same subject. Moderate deficits in bilateral frontal and right parietal metabolism. *D*, PET can slice at high ventricular level. Bilateral frontal and large left parietal deficits.

MRI in studying dementia is likely to be better understood. The studies on dementia using MRI have seemingly neglected mention of cortical lesions in spite of the known sensitivity of MRI in detecting such lesions. This may reflect the relatively low prevalence of multiple cortical infarcts. *Binswanger disease, on the other hand, is probably overdiagnosed by MRI in demented patients.* It is clear that patients with AD have prominent periventricular hyperintense areas on relatively T_2-weighted images, more so than age-matched controls. Some investigators have classified these patients with AD within the category of Binswanger disease. Roman[185] went so far as to suggest the label senile dementia of the Binswanger Type. This is an inappropriate

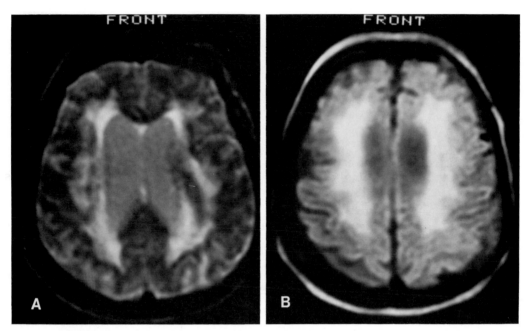

Figure 5–12. Binswanger disease. *A*, MRI at midventricular level (TR = 2.5 seconds, TE = 90 milliseconds). Note the diffuse increase in periventricular signal spreading into the corona radiata and centrum semiovale and extending up to the cortical ribbon in some locations. *B*, MRI at high ventricular level. Note the diffuse increase in signal of the entire white matter regions of this slice. Focal atrophy is also seen in the right frontoparietal cortex.

label. There are well-documented cases of patients with the pathologic features of AD alone who have been shown to have extensive T_2 changes on MRI resembling the T_2 changes seen on MRI in Binswanger disease (Fig. 5–12A and B). These AD patients may show white matter rarefaction on pathologic examination.[21] Hachinski and colleagues[95] have suggested the term "leukoaraiosis" for those white matter changes in AD.

PET STUDIES

In Table 5–3, three studies are listed that have addressed the differences in the PET scan appearances of MID and AD.[14,75,123] Unfortunately, a definitive statement has not been possible regarding reliable differentiating factors in these two conditions. Benson and associates[14] state that in MID the pattern of deficits is asymmetric and variable, compared to the symmetric and diffuse deficits in AD cases. Frackowiak and colleagues[74] were unable to discover any differentiating factors on PET between patients diagnosed to have vascular or degenerative dementia. Of interest from a pathophysiologic point of view is that the occipital cortex was relatively spared in MID cases as well as AD cases.

The border zone between the middle and anterior cerebral arteries is a frequent site of cerebral infarction,[108] and there is a strong predisposition for hypertension-associated lacunar infarcts to affect the basal ganglia and thalami. Therefore, metabolic deficits that affect frontal and subcortical gray matter structures, predominantly, may be expected to be the hallmark of MID. Also, the well-known phenomenon of crossed cerebellar hypometabolism (i.e., reduced cerebellar metabolism on the side opposite predominant cortical hypometabolism) commonly reported in stroke cases may be expected to be a common phenomenon in MID cases. In a preliminary report, Kuhl and colleagues[123] found that the parietal-cerebellar ratio was significantly lower in AD than in MID cases, suggesting that parietal metabolism was relatively spared in MID. Duara and colleagues,[60] however, were unable to confirm this when they classified PET scan patterns in demented patients into those with frontal and deep gray matter deficits vs those with parietotemporal deficits. They compared these patterns of metabolic deficits to the clinical diagnosis of dementia and were unable to find a statistically significant difference in frequency of any particular pattern in AD and MID cases. Crossed cerebellar hypometabolism in demented patients,[9] however, was found to be significantly more frequent in MID cases.

SPECT STUDIES

Sharp and colleagues[195] described ^{123}I-isopropyl-amphetamine (IMP) SPECT studies in 13 patients diagnosed as MID on the basis of a Hachinski ischemic score greater than 8. No typical pattern of IMP distribution was found, and the appearances varied from a near-normal pattern to one with marked focal defects. The majority of the deficits were in posterior parietal-temporal and posterior frontal regions, which is similar to what was found in AD cases. Cohen and associates[37] reported that they correctly identified three patients with MID in their sample on the basis of SPECT findings of asymmetric defects involving the gray matter or both gray and white matter. It seems, however, unlikely that they could truly distinguish defects in the white matter using a SPECT scanner because of the poor spatial resolution of these devices and because rCBF is relatively low in normal white matter, rendering it anatomically indistinguishable from the lateral ventricles. No other SPECT studies in MID patients have been reported to date.

Regardless of the etiology of dementia, when the pathology is widespread in the brain, the metabolism or perfusion deficits are likely to be diffuse. In several PET scan studies of stroke patients, the metabolism or blood flow deficits have been found to be much more widespread than the apparent structural deficits on CT scan. Thus, multiple focal lesions on CT or MRI scans in MID cases are likely to be represented by large confluent cortical deficits on PET or SPECT scans (see Fig. 5–11C and D). This may then account for the lack of clear distinguishing factors in the PET and SPECT scan appearances of AD and MID cases.

Normal Pressure Hydrocephalus

NPH is a disorder described initially by Hakim and Adams[96] consisting of a clinical triad of signs and symptoms, namely dementia, gait disorder, and urinary incontinence. Dilatation of the ventricular system with normal CSF pressure on lumbar puncture (i.e., less than 180 mm of water) are features of the disorder. An entirely satisfactory name for this entity has not yet been found because it has been determined that intermittently CSF pressure may be raised.[202] NPH is an infrequent cause of dementia in the elderly (as described in Chapter 8), with several studies reporting incidence rates of less than 1% of all dementing diseases.

CT STUDIES

Dilatation of the ventricular system is an absolute requirement for the diagnosis of NPH. The extent of the dilatation is variable, although it has been suggested that at least a "moderate" degree of ventricular enlargement along with "rounding" of the frontal horns of the lateral ventricles be present to support the diagnosis.[207] More specifically, LeMay and Hochberg[133] report a frontal horn ratio (ratio of the maximum width of the frontal horns to the external skull diameter at the corresponding level) of 50% as being a feature indicative of NPH. In addition, they emphasize enlargement of the temporal horn tips to 2 mm or more in width. Nevertheless, Petersen and associates[176] and others could not establish any relationship of ventricular size to response to a shunting procedure, nor could they relate the degree of reduction of ventricular size after shunting to clinical response to the procedure.

Obliteration of the cerebral sulci has also been a requirement by many but not all investigators for the diagnosis of NPH. LeMay and Hochberg[133] state that "the sylvian fissures and superficial sulci could be seen, although not very wide, in 14 of the 100 patients" with NPH. Vassilouthis[207] observed that obliteration of the sulci at higher levels was sometimes observed in association with dilatation of the subarachnoid spaces, such as sylvian fissures, at lower levels, perhaps indicating obstruction of the subarachnoid space of the convexity. This author also documented the reappearance of cerebral sulci postoperatively. Parenthetically, it should be noted that the obliteration of the subarachnoid space unilaterally in experimental animals leads to ipsilateral ventricular dilatation.[91] As was the case for ventricular size, Petersen and colleagues[176] could not document any relationship of extent of sulcal enlargement (from none to moderate) to response to a shunting procedure.

The presence of periventricular low density areas may be regarded as an important feature of NPH. This finding has been considered to be a reflection of transependymal resorption of CSF, which is a phenomenon known to occur experimentally. This phenomenon may, in fact, account for the reduction of ventricular pressure to normal levels in NPH. Yamada and associates[219] have identified a specific low-density pattern that appears in NPH following subarachnoid hemorrhage, consisting of a fan-shaped irregular area of lucency extending from the anterior horns to the frontal pole, which disappears following a shunting procedure. These authors considered the possibility that the seepage of the CSF into frontal white matter may have an independent effect on mentation and also on continence and gait. However, Petersen and colleagues[176] were once again unable to document a relationship between either the presence of periventricular lucency or its disappearance after shunting and the response to the shunting procedure.

In summary, CT scan studies in NPH are important for documenting the presence of ventricular dilatation. The findings of moderate to severe enlargement of frontal horns, obliteration of sulci over the convexity, and presence of periventricular hypodensity are common in NPH cases but do not necessarily predict, by their presence, a good response to a shunting procedure. On the other hand, the coexistence of the clinical triad of symptoms and a relatively short duration of symptoms (less than 2 years) generally helps to predict good shunt responses. In general, symptoms of gait disorder and incontinence respond better to a shunt procedure than do the intellectual deficits.

MRI STUDIES

MRI has certain potential advantages over CT in the evaluation of NPH. First, because of the freedom from beam-hardening artifacts (see Chapter 1), assessment of the subarachnoid space over the convexity is much more accurate with MRI (Fig. 5–13A and B). Second, presumably because of transependymal seepage of fluid, the periventricular lucencies seen with CT can be assessed with much greater sensitivity with MRI. Distinctions may be possible between lesions that result from deep white matter infarctions versus those that are contiguous with the ependymal surface and represent fluid. Finally, the flow of CSF in the aqueduct of Sylvius would be expected to be abnormally slow in NPH and can be assessed by the CSF flow void sign (see Chapter 2). Normally, the signal from CSF in the aqueduct is reduced compared with the signal from the CSF in lateral ventricles, on T_2-weighted spin echo scans, because of the increased

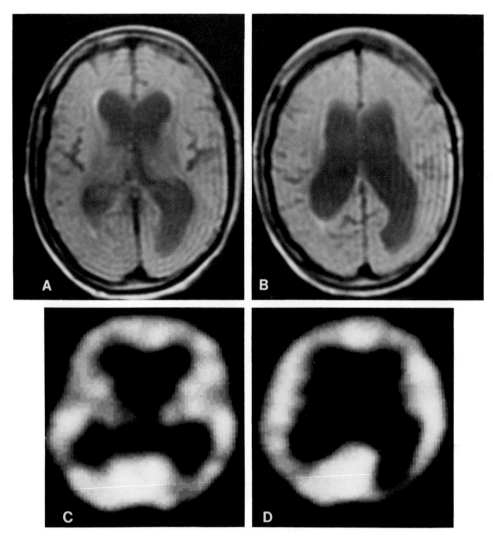

Figure 5–13. Normal pressure hydrocephalus (NPH). *A*, MRI at basal ganglia level. Note the prominent ventricular enlargement. Rounding of frontal horns is evident with surrounding cap of periventricular signal increase. *B*, MRI at midventricular level. Note the prominence of ventricles with rounding of contours. *C*, PET scan slice at basal ganglia level. Note the prominent central areas of minimal metabolic activity (representing ventricles) and normal cortical metabolism. *D*, PET scan slice at midventricular level. Note the very prominent ventricular impression centrally (minimal metabolic activity), with normal cortical metabolism.

velocity and turbulence of CSF in the aqueduct. This CSF flow void sign can best be assessed with longer TEs and thinner sections.[23] In NPH, because of the decrease in compliance of the ventricular walls, pulsatile CSF flow through the aqueduct is more turbulent and accelerated than in nonhydrocephalic cases, even though the bulk flow of CSF via the adqueduct may be re-

duced. Hence, the CSF flow void sign is likely to be more prominent in NPH.

A comprehensive evaluation of the utility of MRI in NPH and comparison to the use of MRI in other forms of dementia was done by Jack and associates.[110] They found that periventricular signal intensity was greater in NPH than in non-AD dementia (presumably MID), which in turn had greater signal intensity than did AD. Response to a shunt procedure was "slightly" better in those with a greater degree of periventricular signal intensity. The presence of deep white matter lesions was most strongly related to age. These lesions were more frequently found in demented than nondemented patients. Although NPH patients had a higher incidence of deep white matter lesions than any other diagnostic group, the response to a shunt procedure was best in those NPH cases without these lesions. This would be the expected finding, given that these deep white matter lesions may indicate ischemic changes in the brain. The CSF flow void sign was more prominent in patients with NPH than in any other dementing disorder. These authors did not comment on obliteration of the subarachnoid space of the convexity.

In summary, at this point, MRI is more likely than CT to contribute to the accuracy of the diagnosis of NPH and the prediction of shunt responsiveness in patients with this diagnosis.

PET AND SPECT STUDIES

Very few studies have been performed with these two modalities in NPH patients. This may, in fact, represent the relatively small number of patients who have this condition. Jagust and colleagues[113] reported on three patients with NPH studied with PET and [18]FDG. Glucose metabolic rates were reduced significantly compared with controls, but there was no regional deficit seen in NPH (Fig. 5–13C and D). Although no SPECT studies have been reported to date on NPH cases, the absence of regional deficits may be expected to be found in SPECT scans as well.

PET and SPECT studies may be useful for predicting shunt responsiveness in patients diagnosed as having NPH on the basis of clinical and CT or MRI findings. The presence of regional metabolic or blood flow deficits may indicate a concurrent disease such as MID or AD, and therefore a low likelihood of a clinically sustained response to a shunt procedure. It is of interest that a single patient evaluated by Friedland[76] presented with a gradually progressive dementia and on PET was found to have bilateral parietal metabolic defects. Performed because of enlarging ventricle size, gait disorder, and incontinence, a shunt procedure on this patient produced marked, sustained improvement of the dementia. It was argued that this patient did in fact have NPH rather than AD, although only long-term follow-up of the patient and pathologic examination of the brain will resolve the issue.

Differential Diagnosis of Dementia: The Use of CT, MRI, PET, and SPECT to Elucidate Pathophysiology in Dementing Conditions

Morphologic abnormalities that can cause or contribute to a dementing disorder are most amenable to definition and quantitation by CT or MRI scanning. For example, after a subarachnoid hemorrhage, hydrocephalus may develop and the size of the lateral ventricle on the CT scan may suggest why a persistent disorder of mentation is present. Reduction in size of the ventricle after a shunting procedure often coincides with rapid clearing of the cognitive deficit, in this specific situation. The same phenomenon is often observed with a subdural hematoma before and after it is evacuated, and CT or MRI scanning can demonstrate the resolution of the morphologic abnormality. Unfortunately these morphologic abnormalities that are best visualized by CT or MRI are relatively uncommon causes of dementia. On the other hand, a disease such as AD may or may not be associated with morphologic abnormalities such as cortical atrophy and ventricular enlargement, yet the functional deficits can be detected very early in the course of the disease by PET or SPECT scans. It can be seen that for the most common cause of dementia, AD, functional imaging is far more informative than morphologic imaging. Nevertheless, in all the previously mentioned disorders, a combination of morphologic and functional definition of the brain is useful for establishing the diagnosis and for understanding of the pathophysiology. An example of a situation where this combined information is very useful is MID. This condition cannot be effectively diagnosed without CT or MRI evidence of multiple infarcts. Multiple cerebral ischemic lesions, however, may be found in nondemented elderly individuals who may sometimes be asymptomatic. A PET or SPECT scan could then be used to determine whether physiologic deficits are also present, thereby suggesting that the morphologic lesions are having a major functional impact in that patient.

The pathophysiology of dementia in any given patient may be complex. Certain disorders such as a frontal meningioma may produce dementia by direct mechanical effects. These effects can be easily visualized by CT or MRI scanning, but secondary vascular effects may also play a part and only be detectable by functional imaging. Ambiguity often exists as to what factors have contributed to the dementia. Morphologic and functional imaging of the brain play very important roles in defining these contributions and thereby may help guide the management of these patients.

Neuroimaging techniques for assisting in the diagnosis of some major causes of dementia are described in Fig. 5–14. Clinical evaluation is the crucial first step and, not infrequently, the only step required to make the diagnosis (e.g., for medication effects, depression, endocrine disorders). Because of

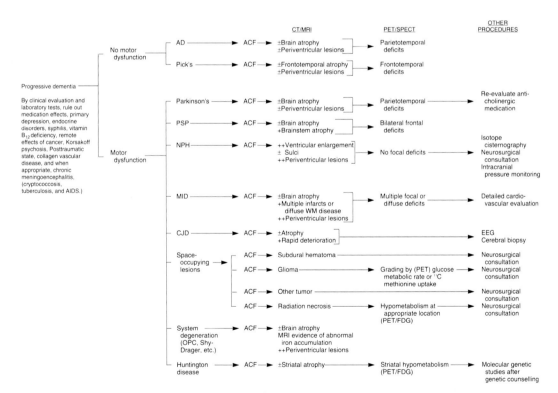

Figure 5–14. Neuroimaging methods in the differential diagnosis of dementia. Abbreviations: ACF = appropriate clinical findings; AD = Alzheimer disease; CJD = Creutzfeld Jacob disease; FDG = fluorodeoxyglucose; MID = Multi-infarct dementia; NPH = normal pressure hydrocephalus; OPC = olivopontocerebellar degeneration; PSP = progressive supranuclear palsy; WM = white matter.

the frequency with which more than one cause for a dementing syndrome may be present, however, the clinician often has to evaluate the patient further and neuroimaging methods are invariably the next step in the diagnostic process.

Once a preliminary evaluation has ruled out common and easily diagnosed conditions such as overmedication, hypothyroidism, and primary depression, appropriate clinical findings are the starting point in the evaluation of each diagnostic entity, followed by CT or MRI scans. In some instances the MRI scan provides a clear advantage over CT, as in assessing the brain stem atrophy in PSP and the extent of periventricular lesions and subarachnoid space in NPH and in obtaining evidence of iron accumulation in systems degenerations. In the case of MID, the MRI may be able to detect many more ischemic lesions than the CT scan, but the quantitative differences in these lesions in nondemented and demented subjects (if such a difference exists) is presently unclear.

PET and SPECT are particularly useful where the clinical and the CT-MRI finding are not clearly diagnostic, as is commonly the case. AD, Pick disease, and early cases of Huntington disease are such disorders where CT-MRI studies are often nonrevealing. In patients with MID and with NPH, PET and SPECT studies provide very useful additional information that may have therapeutic implications in NPH or provide evidence of the functional significance of CT-MRI lesions in MID.

CONCLUSION

This chapter has reviewed the neuroimaging features of normal aging and the major neurologic disorders that affect the elderly, namely dementia, movement disorders, and stroke. Both structural neuroimaging, using CT and MRI scans, and functional neuroimaging, using SPECT and PET scans, have been addressed. Among the various dis-

orders capable of causing dementia and movement disorders, the neuroimaging features of AD, PD, Pick disease, PSP, MID, Binswanger disease, and NPH have been described. Cerebrovascular diseases that have been addressed include lacunar stroke, TIAs, thrombotic and embolic cerebral infarction, and cerebral hemorrhage. This review of neuroimaging in geriatric neurologic conditions has emphasized the diagnostically useful radiologic features as well as the findings that illuminate aspects of pathophysiology in these various conditions.

REFERENCES

1. Adam, P, Fabre, N, Guell, A, Bessoles, G, Roulleau, J, and Bes, A: Cortical atrophy in Parkinson's disease: Correlation between clinical and CT finding with special emphasis on pre-frontal atrophy. Am J Neuroradiol 4:442–445, 1983.

2. Aharon-Peretz, L, Cummings, JL, and Hill, MA: Vascular dementia and dementia of the Alzheimer type: Cognition, ventricular size, and leuko-ariaosis. Arch Neurol 45:719–721, 1988.

3. Alavi, A, Dann, R, Chawluk, J, Alavi, J, Kushner, M, and Reivich, M: Position emission tomography imaging of regional cerebral glucose metabolism. Semin Nucl Med 16(1):2–34, 1986.

4. Albert, M, Naeser, MA, Levine, HL, and Garvey, AJ: Ventricular size in patients with presenile dementia of the Alzheimer's type. Arch Neurol 41:1258–1263, 1984.

5. Ambrosetto, P, Michelucci, R, Forti, A, and Tassinari, CA: CT findings in progressive supranuclear palsy. J Comput Assist Tomogr 8(3):406–409, 1984.

6. Awad, I, Johnson, P, Spetzler, R, and Hodak, J: Incidental subcortical lesions identified on magnetic resonance imaging in the elderly.

II. Postmortem pathological correlations. Stroke 17:1090–1097, 1986.

7. Awad, I, Spetzler, R, Hodak, J, Awad, C, and Carey, R: Incidental subcortical lesions identified on magnetic resonance imaging in the elderly. I. Correlation with age and cerebrovascular risk factors. Stroke 17:1084–1089, 1986.

8. Ball, S, Fox, P, Pardo, J, and Raichle, M: Control state stability for PET brain imaging: Rest versus task (abstr). Neurology (Suppl 1)38:362, 1988.

9. Barker, WW, Loewenstein, DA, Chang, JY, Pascal, S, Smith, D, Boothe, TE, Apicella, A, and Duara, R: FDG/PET studies of crossed cerebellar hypometabolism in dementia (abstr). Neurology (Suppl 1)38:364, 1988.

10. Baron, JC, Bousser, MG, Comar, D, Soussaline, F, and Castaigne, P: Noninvasive tomographic study of cerebral blood flow and oxygen metabolism in vivo. Eur Neurol 20:273–284, 1981.

11. Baron, JC, Bousser, MG, Rey, A, Guillard, A, Comar, D, and Castaigne, P: Reversal of focal ''misery-perfusion syndrome'' by extra-intra-cranial arterial bypass in hemodynamic cerebral ischemia. Stroke 12:454–459, 1981.

12. Baron, JC, Comar, D, Zarifian, E, Agid, Y, Crouzel, C, Loo, H, Deniker, P, and Kellershohn, C: Dopaminergic receptor sites in human brain: Positron emission tomography. Neurology 35:16–24, 1985.

13. Becker, H, Desch, H, Hacker, H, and Pencz, A: CT fogging effect with ischemic cerebral infarcts. Neuroradiology 18:185–192, 1979.

14. Benson, DF, Kuhl, DE, Hawkins, RA, Phelps, ME, Cummings, JL, and Tsai, SY: The fluorodeoxyglucose ^{18}F scan in Alzheimer's disease and multi-infarct dementia. Arch Neurol 40:711–714, 1983.

15. Berent, S, Foster, NL, Gilman, S, Hichwa, R, and Lehitnen, S: Patterns of cortical ^{18}F-FDG metabolism in Alzheimer's and progressive supranuclear palsy patients are related to the types of cognitive impairment (abstr). Neurology (Suppl)37:172, 1987.

16. Berman, KF and Weinberger, DR: Cortical physiological activation in Alzheimer's disease: rCBF studies during resting and cognitive states (abstr). Soc Neurosci Abstr 12:1160, 1986.

17. Blessed, G, Tomlinson, BE, and Roth, M: The association between quantitative measures of dementia and of senile change in the cerebral grey matter of elderly subjects. Br J Psychiatry 114:797–811, 1968.

18. Bonte, FJ, Ross, ED, Chehabi, HH, and Devous, MD, Sr: SPECT study of regional cerebral blood flow in Alzheimer disease. J Comput Assist Tomogr 10(4):579–583, 1986.

19. Botwinick, J, Storandt, M, and Berg, L: A longitudinal, behavioral study of senile dementia of the Alzheimer's type. Arch Neurol 43:1124–1127, 1986.

20. Bowen, BC, Barker, WW, Loewenstein, DA, Sheldon, J, and Duara, R: MR signal abnormalities in memory disorder and dementia. Am J Neuroradiol 11:283–290, 1990.

21. Bowen, BC, Pascal, S, Sheldon, J, Garcia, L, Gregorious, J, Norenberg, M, and Duara, R: Pathological verification of MRI-detected white matter disease in patients with Alzheimer's disease (abstr). Neurology (Suppl 1)40:176, 1990.

22. Bradac, GB and Oberson, R: CT and angiography in cases with occlusive disease of supratentorial cerebral vessels. Neuroradiology 19:193–200, 1980.

23. Bradley, WG, Jr, Kortman, KE, and Burgoyne, B: Flowing cerebrospinal fluid in normal and hydroce-

phalic states: Appearance on MR images. Radiology 159:611–616, 1986.

24. Braffman, BH, Zimmermann, R, Trojanowski, JQ, Gonatas, NK, Hickey, WF, and Shlaepfer, WW: Brain MR: Pathologic correlation with gross and histopathology. 1. Lacunar infarction and Virchow-Robin spaces. Am J Roentgenol 151:551–558, 1988.

25. Breitner, JCS and Folstein, MF: Familial Alzheimer's dementia: A prevalent disorder with specific clinical features. Psychol Med 14:63–80, 1984.

26. Brinkman, SD, Sarwar, M, Levin, HS, and Morris, HH, III: Quantitative indexes of computed tomography in dementia and normal aging. Radiology 138:89–92, 1981.

27. Brun, A and Englund, E: The pattern of degeneration in Alzheimer's disease: Neuronal loss and histopathological grading. Histopathology 5:549–564, 1981.

28. Brun, A and Englund, E: A white matter disorder in dementia of the Alzheimer type: A pathoanatomical study. Ann Neurol 19:253–262, 1986.

29. Brust, JCM: Dementia and Cerebrovascular Disease. In Mayeux, R and Rosen, WG (eds): The Dementias. Raven Press, New York, 1983, p 131.

30. Brust, JCM: Vascular dementia is overdiagnosed. Arch Neurol 45:799–801, 1988.

31. Butler, RW, Dickinson, WA, Katholi, C, and Halsey, H, Jr: The comparative effects of organic brain disease on cerebral blood flow and measured intelligence. Ann Neurol 13:155–159, 1983.

32. Cala, LA, Burns, P, Davis, R, and Jones, R: Alcohol-related brain damage—Serial studies after abstinence and recommencement of drinking. Aust Alcohol/Drug Rev 3:127–140, 1984.

33. Caplan, LR and Schoene, WC: Clinical features of subcortical arterio-

sclerotic encephalopathy (Binswanger disease). Neurology 28:1206–1215, 1978.

34. Celsis, P, Agriel, A, Puel, M, Rascol, A, and Marc-Vergnes, J-P: Focal cerebral hypoperfusion and selective cognitive deficit in dementia of the Alzheimer type. J Neurol Neurosurg Psychiatry 50;1602–1612, 1987.

35. Chase, TN, Fedio, P, Foster, NL, Brooks, R, Di Chiro, G, and Mansi, L: Wechsler adult intelligence scale performance: Cortical localization by fluorodeoxyglucose F18-positron emission tomography. Arch Neurol 41:1244–1247, 1984.

36. Chiu, HC, Teng, EL, Henderson, VW, and Moy, AC: Clinical subtypes of dementia of the Alzheimer's type. Neurology 35(11):1544–1550, 1985.

37. Cohen, MB, Graham, LS, Lake, R, Metter, EJ, Fitten, J, Kulkarni, MK, Sevrin, R, Yamada, L, Chang, CC, Woodruff, N, and Kling, AS: Diagnosis of Alzheimer's disease and multiple infarct dementia by tomographic imaging of iodine-123-IMP. J Nucl Med 27:769–774, 1986.

38. Condon, BR, Patterson, J, Wyper, D, Hadley, M, Teasdale, G, Grant, R, Jenkins, A, Macpherson, P, and Rowan, J: A quantitative index of ventricular and extraventricular intracranial CSF volumes using MR imaging. Radiology 10(5):784–792, 1986.

39. Council of Scientific Affairs, American Medical Association, Chicago: Magnetic resonance imaging of the central nervous system. JAMA 259:1211–1222, 1988.

40. Cummings, JL and Duchen, LW: Kluver-Bucy syndrome in Pick disease: Clinical and pathologic correlations. Neurology 31:1415–1422, 1981.

41. Cutler, NR, Haxby, JV, Duara, R, Grady, CL, Moore, AM, Parisi, JE, White, J, Heston, L, Margolin,

RM, and Rapoport, SI; Brain metabolism as measured with positron emission tomography: Serial assessment in a patient with familial Alzheimer's disease. Neurology 35:1556–1561, 1985.

42. D'Antona, R, Baron, JC, Samson, Y, Seraru, M, Viader, F, Agid, Y, and Cambier, J: Subcortical dementia. Frontal cortex hypometabolism detected by positron emission tomography in patients with progressive supranuclear palsy. Brain 108:785–799, 1985.

43. Dastur, DK, Lane, ML, Hansen, DB, Kety, SS, Butler, RN, Perlin, S, and Sokoloff, L: Effects of aging on cerebral circulation and metabolism in man. In Human Aging: A Biological and Behavioral Study, PHS Publication No 986. US Govt Printing Office, Washington DC, 1963, p 59.

44. DeCarli, D, Kaye, JA, Horwitz, B, and Rapoport, SI: Critical analysis of the use of computer-assisted transverse axial tomography to study human brain in aging and dementia of the Alzheimer type. Neurology 40:872–883, 1990.

45. deLeon, MJ, Ferris, SH, George, AE, Reisberg, B, Kricheff, II, and Gershon, S: Computed tomography evaluations of brain-behavior relationships in senile dementia of the Alzheimer's type. Neurobiol Aging 1:69–79, 1980.

46. deLeon, MJ, Ferris, SH, George, AE, Christman, DR, Fowler, JS, Gentes, CI, Reisberg, B, Gee, B, Kricheff, II, Emmerich, M, Yonekura, Y, Brodie, J, Kricheff, II, and Wolf, AP: Positron emission tomography studies of aging and Alzheimer disease. AJNR 4:568–571, 1983.

47. de Leon, MJ, George, AE, Ferris, SH, Christman, DR, Fowler, JS, Gentes, C, Brodie, J, Reisberg, B, and Wolf, AP: Positron emission tomography and computerized tomography of the aging brain. J Comput Tomogr 8:88–94, 1984.

48. Devous, MD, Sr, Stokely, EM, Chehabi, HH, and Bonte, FJ: Normal distribution of regional cerebral blood flow measured by dynamic single-photon emission tomography. J Cereb Blood Flow Metab 6:95–104, 1986.

49. Dolinskas, CA, Bilaniuk, LT, Zimmermann, RA, and Kuhl, DE: Computed tomography of intracerebral hematomas. I. Transmission CT observations on hematoma resolution. Am J Radiol 129:681–688, 1977.

50. Donnan, GA, Tress, BM, and Baldin, PF: A prospective study of lacunar infarction using computerized tomography. Neurology 32:49–56, 1982.

51. Dooms, GC, Hricak, H, Berthiaume, Y, Uske, A, Kucharczyk, W, Brandt-Zawadski, M, and Higgins, CB: Magnetic resonance of hemorrhagic lesions: Evolution of the intrinsic relaxation parameters from time of onset of symptoms. J Belge Radiol 69:335–343, 1986.

52. Drayer, BP, Olanow, W, Burger, P, Johnson, GA, Herfkens, R, and Reiderer, S: Parkinson plus syndrome: Diagnosis using high field MR imaging of brain iron. Radiology 159:493–498, 1986.

53. Drayer, BP: Imaging of the aging brain: Part I. Normal findings. Radiology 166:785–796, 1988.

54. Duara, R, Barker, WW, Chang, JY, Loewenstein, DA, Apicella, A, Yoshii, F, and Kothari, P: Relationship of cortical and isolated white matter MRI lesions to local cortical metabolism on FDG/PET scans (abstr). Neurology (Suppl 1)38:399, 1988.

55. Duara, R, Grady, C, Haxby, JV, Ingvar, D, Sokoloff, L, Margolin, RA, Manning, RG, Cutler, R, and Rapoport, SI: Human brain glucose utilization and cognitive function in relation to age. Ann Neurol 16:702–713, 1984.

56. Duara, R, Grady, C, Haxby, JV, Sundaram, M, Cutler, NR, Heston, L,

Moore, A, Schlageter, N, Larson, S, and Rapoport, SI: Positron emission tomography in Alzheimer's disease. Neurology 36:879–887, 1986.

57. Duara, R, Gross-Glenn, K, Barker, WW, Chang, JY, Apicella, A, Loewenstein, DA, and Boothe, T: Behavioral activation and the variability of cerebral glucose metabolic measurements. J Cereb Blood Flow Metab 7:266–271, 1987.

58. Duara, R, Gutterman, A, Loewenstein, D, Eisdorfer, C, Chang, JY, Barker, WW, and Apicella, A: The clinical and PET scan pattern of probable Pick's disease (abstr). Neurology (Suppl 1)38:415, 1988.

59. Duara, R, Yoshii, F, Barker, WW, Apicella, A, Chang, JY, and Sheldon, J: White matter (WM) and gray matter (GM) alterations in aging and dementia by magnetic resonance scanning (abstr). Neurology (Suppl):36:103, 1986.

60. Duara, R, Yoshii, F, Chang, JY, Barker, WW, Apicella, A, and Sheldon, J: PET in the differential diagnosis of dementia (abstr). Neurology (Suppl 1)37:158, 1987.

61. Dubinsky, RM and Jankovic, J: Progressive supranuclear palsy and a multi-infarct state. Neurology 37:570–576, 1987.

62. Earnest, MP, Heaton, RK, Wilkinson, WE, and Manke, WF: Cortical atrophy, ventricular enlargement and intellectual impairment in the aged. Neurology 29:1138–1143, 1979.

63. Eidelberg, D, Moeller, JR, Sidtis, JJ, Dhawan, V, Strother, DC, Ginos, JZ, Cedarbaum, J, Greene, P, Fahn, S, and Rottenberg, DA: The metabolic pathology of Parkinson's disease: Complementary ^{18}F-fluorodopa and ^{18}F-fluorodeoxyglucose PET studies (abstr). Neurology (Suppl 1)39:273, 1989.

64. Englund, E, Brun, A, and Persson, B: Correlations between histopathologic white matter changes and proton MR relaxation times in de-

mentia. Alzheimer Disease and Related Disorders 1(3):156–170, 1987.

65. Erkinjuntti, T, Ketonen, L, Sulkava, R, Sipponen, N, Vuorialho, M, and Iivanainen, M: Do white matter changes on MRI and CT differentiate vascular dementia from Alzheimer's disease? J Neurol Neurosurg Psychiatry 50:37–42, 1987.

66. Eslinger, PJ, Damasio, H, Braff-Radford, N, and Damasio, AR: Examining the relationship between computed tomography and neuropsychological measures in normal and demented elderly. J Neurol Neurosurg Psychiatry 47:1319–1325, 1984.

67. Fazekas, F, Chawluk, JB, Alavi, A, Hurtig, HI, and Zimmerman, RA: MR signal abnormalities at 1.5 T in Alzheimer's dementia and normal aging. Am J Neuroradiol 8:421–426, 1987.

68. Ferris, SH, deLeon, MJ, Wolf, AP, Farkas, T, Christman, DR, Reisberg, B, Fowler, JR, MacGregor, R, Goldman, A, George, AE, and Rampal, S: Positron emission tomography in the study of aging and senile dementia. Neurobiol Aging 1(2):127–131, 1980.

69. Foster, NL, Chase, TN, Fedio, P, Patronas, NJ, Brooks, RA, and DiChiro, G: Alzheimer's disease: Focal cortical changes shown by positron emission tomography. Neurology 33:961–965, 1983.

70. Foster, NL, Gilman, S, Berent, S, Morin, EM, Brown, MB, and Koeppe, RA: Cerebral hypometabolism in progressive supranuclear palsy studied with positron emission tomography. Ann Neurol 24:399–406, 1988.

71. Foster, NL, Hansen, MS, Siegel, GJ, and Kuhl, DE: Medial and lateral temporal glucose metabolism in aging and Alzheimer's disease studied by PET (abstr). Neurology (Suppl 1)38:133, 1988.

72. Foster, NL, Morin, EM, Kuhl, DE, and Gilman, S: Glucose metabolic ac-

tivity in the basal ganglia and thalamus differs in progressive supranuclear palsy and Alzheimer's disease (abstr). Neurology (Suppl 1)38:369, 1988.

73. Frackowiak, RSJ, Lenzi, GL, Jones, T, and Heather, JD: Quantitative measurement of regional cerebral blood flow and oxygen in man using ^{15}O and positron emission tomography: Theory, procedure, and normal values. J Comput Assist Tomogr 4(6):727–736, 1980.

74. Frackowiak, RSJ, Pozzilli, C, Legg, NJ, Du Boulay, GH, Marshall, J, Lenzi, GL, and Jones, T: Regional cerebral oxygen supply and utilization in dementia: A clinical and physiological study with oxygen-15 and positron tomography. Brain 104:753–778, 1981.

75. Frackowiak, RSJ and Wise, RJS: Positron emission tomography in ischemic cerebrovascular disease. Neurol Clin 1:183–200, 1983.

76. Friedland, RP: "Normal"-pressure hydrocephalus and the saga of the treatable dementias. JAMA 262:2577–2581, 1989.

77. Friedland, RP, Brun, A, and Budinger, TF: Pathologic and positron emission tomographic correlations in Alzheimer's disease. Lancet 1:228, 1985.

78. Friedland, RP, Budinger, TF, Brant-Zawadzki, M, and Jagust, WJ: The diagnosis of Alzheimer-type dementia. JAMA 252:2750–2752, 1984.

79. Friedland, RP, Budinger, TF, Ganz, E, Yano, Y, Mathid, CA, Koss, B, Ober, BA, Huesman, RH, and Derenzo, SE: Regional cerebral metabolic alterations in dementia of the Alzheimer type: Positron emission tomography with [^{18}F]fluorodeoxy-glucose. J Comput Assist Tomogr 7(4):590–598, 1983.

80. Friedland, RP, Yano, Y, Budinger, TF, Ganz, E, Huesman, RH, Derenzo, SE, and Knittel, B: Quantitative evaluation of blood brain barrier integrity in Alzheimer-type dementia: Positron emission tomographic studies with Rubidium-82. Eur Neurol 22(S2):19–20, 1983.

81. Gado, M, Hughes, CP, Danziger, W, Chi, D, Jost, G, and Berg, L: Volumetric measures of the cerebrospinal fluid spaces in demented subjects and controls. Radiology 144:535–538, 1982.

82. Garraway, WM, Whisnant, JP, and Drury, I: The continuing decline in the incidence of stroke. Mayo Clin Proc 58:520–523, 1983.

83. George, AE, deLeon, MJ, and Ferris, SH: Parenchymal CT correlates of senile dementia: Loss of gray-white discriminability. Am J Neuroradiol 2:205–213, 1981.

84. George, AE, deLeon, MJ, Gentes, CI, Miller, J, London, E, Budzilovich, GN, Ferris, S, and Chase, N: Leukoencephalopathy in normal and pathologic aging. 1. CT of brain lucencies. Am J Neuroradiol 7:561–566, 1986.

85. Gerard, G and Weisberg, LA: MRI periventricular lesions in adults. Neurology 36:998–1001, 1986.

86. Gibbs, JM, Wise, RJS, Leenders, K, and Jones, T: Evaluation of perfusion reserve in patients with carotid artery occlusion. Lancet 1:310–314, 1984.

87. Gilman, S, Markel, DS, Koeppe, RA, Junck, L, Kluin, KJ, Gebarski, SS, and Hichwa, RD: Cerebellar and brainstem hypometabolism in olivopontocerebellar atrophy detected with positron emission tomography. Ann Neurol 23:223–230, 1988.

88. Gomori, J, Grossman, R, Goldsberg, H, Zimmermann, R, and Bilaniuk, L: Intracranial hematomas: imaging by high-field MR. Radiology 157:87–93, 1985.

89. Goto, K, Ishii, N, and Fukasawa, H: Diffuse white-matter disease in the geriatric population. Radiology 141:687–695, 1981.

90. Groen, JJ and Hekster, REM: Computed tomography in Pick's dis-

ease: Findings in a family affected in three consecutive generations. J Comput Assist Tomogr 6(5):907–911, 1982.

91. Guinane, JE: Why does hydrocephalus progress? J Neurol Sci 32:1–8, 1977.

92. Haase, G: Diseases Presenting as Dementia. In Wells, C (ed): Dementia. FA Davis, Philadelphia, 1977, p 27.

93. Hachinski, VC, Lassen, NA, and Marshall, J: Multi-infarct dementia: A cause of mental deterioration in the elderly. Lancet July:207–210, 1974.

94. Hachinski, VC, Hiff, LD, Zilkha, E, Du Boulay, GH, McAllister, VL, Marshall, J, Russell, RWR, and Symon, L: Cerebral blood flow in dementia. Arch Neurol 32:632–637, 1975.

95. Hachinski, VC, Potter, P, and Merskey, H: Leuko-araiosis. Arch Neurol 44:21–29, 1990.

96. Hakim, S and Adams, RD: The special clinical problem of symptomatic hydrocephalus with normal cerebrospinal fluid pressure. Observations on cerebrospinal fluid hydrodynamics. J Neurol Sci 2:307–327, 1965.

97. Haldeman, S, Goldman, JW, Hyde, J, and Pribram, HFW: Progressive supranuclear palsy, computed tomography and response to antiparkinsonian drugs. Neurology 31:442–445, 1981.

98. Hawkins, RA, Mazziotta, JC, Phelps, ME, Huang, SC, Kuhl, DE, Carson, RE, Metter, RJ, and Reige WH: Cerebral glucose metabolism as a function of age in man: Influence of the rate constants in the fluorodeoxyglucose method. J Cereb Blood Flow Metab 3:250–253, 1983.

99. Haxby, JV, Duara, R, Grady, CL, Cutler, NR, and Rapoport, SI: Relations between neuropsychological and cerebral metabolic asymmetries in early Alzheimer's disease. J Cereb Blood Flow Metab 5:193–200, 1985.

100. Haxby, JV, Grady, CL, Duara, R, Schlageter, N, Berg, G, and Rapoport, SI: Neocortical metabolic abnormalities precede nonmemory cognitive defects in early Alzheimer's-type dementia. Arch Neurol 43:882–885, 1986.

101. Hellman, RS and Collier, BD: Single Photon Emission Computed Tomography: A Clinical Experience. In Freeman, LM and Weissmann, HS (eds): Nuclear Medicine Annual 1987. Raven Press, New York, 1987, p 51.

102. Herscovitch, P, Auchua, A, Gado, M, Chi, D, and Raichle, M: Correction of positron emission tomography data for cerebral atrophy. J Cereb Blood Flow Metab 6:120–124, 1986.

103. Hershey, LA, Modic, MT, Greenough, G, and Jaffee, DF: Magnetic resonance imaging in vascular dementia. Neurology 37:29–36, 1987.

104. Heston, LH and Mastri, AR: Age at onset of Pick's and Alzheimer's dementia: Implications for diagnosis and research. J Gerontol 37:422–424, 1982.

105. Huber, SJ, Paulson, GW, Shuttleworth, EC, and Chakeres, D: Magnetic resonance imaging is nonspecific to dementia in Parkinson's disease (abstr). Neurology (Suppl 1)38:329, 1988.

106. Hyman, RA and Gorey, MT: Imaging strategies for MR of the brain. Radiol Clin North Am 26:471–503, 1988.

107. Inoue, Y, Takemoto, K, Miyamoto, T, Yoshikawa, N, Taniguchi, S, Saiwai, S, Nishimura, Y, and Komatsu, T: Sequential computed tomography scans in acute cerebral infarction. Radiology 135:655–662, 1980.

108. Ishii, N, Nishihara, Y, and Imamura, T: Why do frontal lobe symptoms predominate in vascular dementia with lacunes? Neurology 36:340–345, 1986.

109. Ito, B, Hatazawa, J, Yamaura, H, and Matsuzawa, T: Age-related brain

atrophy and mental deterioration—A study with computed tomography. Br J Radiol 54:384–390, 1981.

110. Jack, CR, Jr, Mokri, B, Laws, ER, Houser, OW, Baker, HL, Jr, and Petersen C: MR findings in normal-pressure hydrocephalus: Significance and comparison with other forms of dementia. J Comput Assist Tomogr 11(6):923–931, 1987.

111. Jackson, JA, Jankovic, J, and Ford, J: Progressive supranuclear palsy: Clinical features and response to treatment in 16 patients. Ann Neurol 13:273–278, 1983.

112. Jacoby, RJ and Levy, R: Computed tomography in the elderly. 2. Senile dementia: Diagnosis and functional impairment. Br J Psychiatry 136:256–269, 1980.

113. Jagust, WJ, Friedland, RP, and Budinger, TF: Positron emission tomography differentiates normal pressure hydrocephalus from Alzheimer's disease. J Neurol Neurosurg Psychiatry 48:1091–1096, 1985.

114. Jagust, WJ, Budinger, TF, and Reed, BR: The diagnosis of dementia with single photon emission computed tomography. Arch Neurol 44:259–262, 1987.

115. Johnson, KA, Mueller, ST, Walshe, M, English, RJ, and Holman, BL: Cerebral perfusion imaging in Alzheimer's disease. Arch Neurol 44:165–168, 1987.

116. Kamo, H, McGeer, PL, Harrop, R, McGeer, EG, Calne, DB, Martin, WRW, and Pate, BD: Positron emission tomography and histopathology in Pick's disease. Neurology 37:439–445, 1987.

117. Kendall, BE and Radue, EW: Computed tomography in spontaneous intracerebal hematoma. Br J Radiol 51:563–573, 1978.

118. Kingsley, DPE, Radue, EN, and Du Boulay, EPGH: Evaluation of computed tomography in vascular lesions of the vertebrobasilar ter-

ritory. J Neurol Neurosurg Psychiatry 43:193–197, 1980.

119. Kinkel, WR, Jacobs, L, and Kinkel, PR: Gray matter enhancement: A computerized tomographic sign of cerebral hypoxia. Neurology 30:810–819, 1980.

120. Kinkel, WR, Jacobs, L, Polachini, I, Bates, V, and Heffner, RR: Subcortical arteriosclerotic encephalopathy (Binswanger's disease). Arch Neurol 42:951–959, 1985.

121. Kinkel, PR, Kinkel, WR, and Jacobs, L: Nuclear magnetic resonance imaging in patients with stroke. Semin Neurol 6:43–52, 1986.

122. Knopman, DS, Christensen, KJ, Schut, LS, and Ngo, T: Neuropsychometric and computed tomographic findings in Pick's disease (abstr). Neurology (Suppl 1)38:228, 1988.

123. Kuhl DE, Metter EJ, Benson F, Ashford JW, Riege WH, Fujikawa DG, Markham CH, Mazziotta JC, Maltese A, and Dorsey DA: Similarities of cerebral glucose metabolism in Alzheimer's and Parkinson's dementia. J Cereb Blood Flow Metab (Suppl 1)5:S169–170, 1985.

124. Kuhl, DE, Metter, EJ, and Riege, WH: Patterns of local cerebral glucose utilization determined in Parkinson's disease by the [^{18}F]fluorodeoxyglucose method. Ann Neurol 15:419–424, 1984.

125. Kuhl, DE, Metter, EJ, Riege, WH, and Phelps, ME: Effects of human aging on patterns of local cerebral glucose utilization determined by the [^{18}F]fluorodeoxyglucose method. J Cereb Blood Flow Metab 2:163–171, 1982.

126. Kuhl, DE, Small, GW, Riege, WH, Fujikawa, EJ, Metter, EJ, Benson, DF, Ashford, JW, Mazziotta, JC, Maltese, A, and Dorsey, DA: Cerebral metabolic patterns before the diagnosis of probable Alzheimer's disease (abstr). J Cereb Blood Flow Metab (Suppl)7:S406, 1987.

127. Kunitz, S, Gross, CR, Heyman, A, Kase, CS, Mohr, JP, Price, TR, and Wolf, PA: The pilot stroke data bank: Definition, design, data. Stroke 15:740–746, 1984.

128. Ladurner, G, Sager, WD, Iliff, LD, and Lechner, H: A correlation of clinical findings and CT in ischemic cerebrovascular disease. Eur Neurol 18:281–288, 1979.

129. Lassen, NA: The luxury-perfusion syndrome and its possible relation to acute metabolic acidosis localized within the brain. Lancet 2:1113–1115, 1966.

130. Lebrun-Grandie, P, Baron, J, Soussaline, F, Loch, H, Sastre, J, and Bousser, M: Coupling between regional blood flow and oxygen utilization in the normal human brain. Arch Neurol 40:230–236, 1983.

131. Leifer, D, Buonanno, FS, and Richardson, EP, Jr: Clinicopathologic correlations of cranial magnetic resonance imaging of periventricular white matter. Neurology 40:911–198, 1990.

132. LeMay, M: CT changes in dementing diseases: A review. Am J Neuroradiol 7:841–853, 1986.

133. LeMay, M and Hochberg, FH: Ventricular differences between hydrostatic hydrocephalus and hydrocephalus ex vacuo by computed tomography. Neuroradiology 17:191–195, 1979.

134. LeMay, M, Stafford, JL, Sandor, T, Albert, M, Haykal, H, and Samani, A: Statistical assessment of perceptual CT scan ratings in patients with Alzheimer type dementia. J Comput Assist Tomogr 10(5):802–809, 1986.

135. Lenzi, GL, Frackowiak, RS, and Jones, T: Cerebral oxygen metabolism and blood flow in human cerebral infarction. J Cereb Blood Flow Metab 2:321–335, 1982.

136. Lenzi, GL, Frackowiak, RS, Jones, T, Heather, JD, Lammertsma, AA, Rhodes, CG, and Pozzilli, C: $CMRO_2$ and CBF by the oxygen-15 inhalation technique. Results in normal volunteers and cerebrovascular patients. Eur Neurol 20:285–290, 1981.

137. Levasseur, M, Setter, G, Pappata, S, Laplane, D, Tran, Dubois, B, Baulac, M, and Baron, JC: Abnormal frontal cortex glucose utilization (CMRglu) in behaviorally impaired subjects with bilateral pallidal lesions (BPL): A PET study (abstr). Neurology (Suppl 1)38:397, 1988.

138. Ley, D, Soetaert, G, Petit, H, Fauquette, A, Pruvo, J-P, and Steinling, M: Periventricular and white matter magnetic resonance imaging hyperintensities do not differ between Alzheimer's disease and normal aging. Arch Neurol 47:534–537, 1990.

139. Liston, EH and La Rue, A: Clinical differentiation of primary degenerative and multi-infarct dementia: A critical review of the evidence. II. Pathological studies. Biol Psychiatry 18(12):1467–1484, 1983.

140. Loeb, C and Gandolfo, C: Diagnostic evaluation of degenerative and vascular dementia. Stroke 14(3):399–401, 1983.

141. Loewenstein, D, Yoshii, F, Barker, WW, Apicella, A, Emran, A, Chang, JY, and Duara, R: Predominant left hemisphere metabolic dysfunction in dementia. Arch Neurol 46:146–152, 1989.

142. Lotz, PR, Ballinger, WE, Jr, and Quisling, RG: Subcortical arteriosclerotic encephalopathy: CT spectrum and pathologic correlation. Am J Neuroradiol 7:817–822, 1986.

143. Maher, ER and Lees, AJ: The clinical features and natural history of the Steele-Richardson-Olszewski syndrome (progressive supranuclear palsy). Neurology 36:1005–1008, 1986.

144. Manon-Espaillat, R, Lanska, D, Ruff, RL, and Marsaryk, T: Magnetic resonance imaging in progressive supranuclear palsy: Decreased

signal intensity in the basal ganglia (abstr). Neurology (Suppl 1)38:192, 1988.

145. Marshall, VG, Bradley, WG, Jr, Marshall, CE, Bhoopat, T, and Rhodes, RH: Deep white matter infarction: Correlation of MR imaging and histopathologic findings. Radiology 167:517–522, 1988.

146. Martin, WRW, Palmer, MR, Peppard, RF, and Caine, DB: Quantitation of presynaptic dopaminergic function with positron emission tomography (abstr). Neurology (Suppl 1)39:163, 1989.

147. Mayeaux, R, Stern Y, and Spanton, S: Heterogeneity in dementia of the Alzheimer type: Evidence of subgroups. Neurology 35:453–461, 1985.

148. McGeachie, RE, Fleming, JO, Sharer, LR, and Hyman, RA: Diagnosis of Pick's disease by computed tomography. J Comput Assist Tomogr 3(1):113–115, 1979.

149. McGeer, PL, Kamo, H, Harrop, R, Li, DKB, Tuokko, H, McGeer, EG, Adam, MJ, Ammann, W, Beattie, BL, Cane, DB, Martin, WRW, Pate, BD, Rogers, JG, Ruth, TJ, Sayre, CI, and Stoessel, AJ: Positron emission tomography in patients with clinically diagnosed Alzheimer's disease. Can Med Assoc J 134:597–607, 1986.

150. McGeer, PL, Kamo, H, McGeer, EG, Martin, WRW, Pate, BD, and Li, DKB: Comparison of PET, MRI and CT with pathology in a proven case of Alzheimer's disease. Neurology 36:1569–1574, 1986.

151. McKhann, G, Drachman, D, Folstein, M, Katzman, R, Price, D, and Stadlan, EM: Clinical diagnosis of Alzheimer's disease: Report of the NINCDS-ADRDA work group under the auspices of department of health and human services task force on Alzheimer's disease. Neurology 34:939–944, 1984.

152. Melamed, E, Lavy, S, Bentin, S, Cooper, G, and Rinot, Y: Reduction in regional cerebral blood flow during normal aging in man. Stroke 11:31–35, 1980.

153. Messina, AV and Chernick, NL: Computed tomography: The "resolving" intracerebral hemorrhage. Radiology 118:609–613, 1976.

154. Meyer, JS, Sakai, F, Naritomi, H, and Grant, P: Normal and abnormal patterns of cerebrovascular reserve tested by ^{133}Xe inhalation. Arch Neurol 35:350–359, 1978.

155. Miller, JD, deLeon, MJ, Ferris, SH, Kluger, A, George, AE, Reisberg, B, Sachs, SJ, and Wolf, AP: Abnormal temporal lobe response in Alzheimer's disease during cognitive processing as measured by ^{11}C-2 deoxy-d-glucose and PET. J Cereb Blood Flow Metab 7:248–251, 1987.

156. Miyashita, K, Naritomi, H, Sawada, T, Nakamura, M, Kuriyama, Y, Ogawa, M, and Imakita, S: Identification of recent lacunar lesions in cases of multiple small infarctions by magnetic resonance imaging. Stroke 19:834–839, 1988.

157. Mohr, JP: Lacunes. Stroke 13:3–11, 1982.

158. Mohr, JP and Barnett, HJM: Classification of Ischemic Stroke. In Barnett, HJM, Stein, BM, Mohr, JP, and Yatsu, FM (eds): Stroke— Pathophysiology, Diagnosis, Management. Churchill Livingstone, New York, 1986, p 281.

159. Molsa, PK, Paljärvi, L, Rinne JO, Rinne, UK, and Sako, E: Validity of clinical diagnosis in dementia: A prospective clinicopathological study. J Neurol Neurosurg Psychiatry 48:1085–1090, 1985.

160. Morris, JC, Cole, M, Banker, BQ, and Wright, D: Hereditary dysphasic dementia and the Pick-Alzheimer spectrum. Ann Neurol 16:455–466, 1984.

161. Moseley, IF and Olney, J: Intracranial Hemorrhage in the Elderly: Neuroradiology. In Cecchini, A, Nappi, G, and Arrigo, A, (eds): Cerebral Pathology in Old Age: Neu-

roradiological and Neurophysiological Correlations. Emiras, Pavia, 1982, p 215.

162. Moss, MB, Albert, MS, Butters, N, and Payne, M: Differential patterns of memory loss among patients with Alzheimer's disease, Huntington's disease, and alcoholic Korsakoff's syndrome. Arch Neurol 43:239–246, 1983.

163. Munoz-Garcia, D and Ludwin, K: Classic and generalized variations of Pick's disease: A clinicopathological, ultrastructural, and immunocytochemical comparative study. Ann Neurol 16:467–480, 1984.

164. Naritomi, H, Meyer, JS, Sakai, F, Yamaguchi, F, and Shaw, T: Effects of advancing age on regional cerebral blood flow: Studies in normal subjects and subjects with risk factors for atherothrombotic stroke. Arch Neurol 36:410–416, 1979.

165. Neary, D, Snowden, JS, Shields, RA, Burjan, AWI, Northen, B, MacDermott, N, Prescott, MC, and Testa, HJ: Single photon emission tomography using ^{99m}Tc-HM-PAO in the investigation of dementia. J Neurol Neurosurg Psychiatry 50:1101–1109, 1987.

166. O'Brien, MD: Vascular dementia is underdiagnosed. Arch Neurol 45:797–798, 1988.

167. Pantano, P, Baron, J, Lebrun-Grandie, P, Duqesnoy, N, Bousser, M, and Comar, D: Regional cerebral blood flow and oxygen consumption in human aging. Stroke 15:635–641, 1984.

168. Pastakia, B, Polinsky, R, Di Chiro, G, Simmons, JT, Brown, R, and Wener, L: Multiple system atrophy (Shy-Drager syndrome): MR imaging. Radiology 159:499–502, 1986.

169. Pawlik, G, Heiss, WD, Beil, C, Wienhard, K, Herholz, K, and Wagner, R: PET demonstrates differential age dependence, asymmetry and response to various stimuli of regional brain glucose metabolism in healthy volunteers (abstr). J Cereb Blood Flow Metab (Suppl 1)7:S376, 1987.

170. Perani, D, DiPiero, V, Lucignani, G, Gilardi, MC, Pantano, P, Rosetti, C, Pozzilli, C, Gerundini, P, Fazio, F, and Lenzi, GL: Remote effects of subcortical cerebrovascular lesions: A SPECT cerebral perfusion study. J Cereb Blood Flow Metab 8:560–567, 1988.

171. Perani, D, Di Piero, V, Vallar, G, Cappa, S, Messa, C, Bottini, G, Berti, A, Passafiume, D, Scarlato, G, Gerundini, P, Lenzi, GL, and Fazio, F: Technetium-99m HM-PAO-SPECT study of regional cerebral perfusion in early Alzheimer's disease. J Nucl Med 29:1507–1514, 1988.

172. Perlmutter, JS and Raichle, ME: Regional blood flow in hemiparkinsonism. Neurology 35:1127–1134, 1985.

173. Perlmutter, JS, Kilbourn, MR, Raichle, ME, and Welch, MJ: Positron emission tomographic demonstration of upregulation of radioligand-receptor binding in human MPTP-induced parkinsonism (abstr). J Cereb Blood Flow Metab (Suppl 1)7:S371, 1987.

174. Perlmutter, JS, Powers, WJ, Herscovitch, P, Fox, PT, and Raichle, ME: Regional asymmetries of cerebral blood flow, blood volume, and oxygen utilization and extraction in normal subjects. J Cereb Blood Flow Metab 7:64–67, 1987.

175. Perrone, P, Candelise, L, Scotti, G, De Grandi, D, and Scialfa, G: CT evaluation in patients with transient ischemic attack: Correlation with clinical and angiographic findings. Eur Neurol 18:217–221, 1979.

176. Petersen, RC, Mokri, B, and Laws, R, Jr: Surgical treatment of idiopathic hydrocephalus in elderly patients. Neurology 35:307–311, 1985.

177. Podreka, I, Suess, E, Goldenberg, G, Steiner, M, Brucke, T, Muller, C, Lang, W, Neirinckx, RD, and Deecke, L: Initial experience with Technetium-99m HM-PAO brain SPECT. J Nucl Med 28:1657–1666, 1987.

178. Powers, WJ, Martin, WRW, Herscovitch, P, Raichle, ME, Grubbs, RL Jr: Extracranial-intracranial bypass surgery: Hemodynamic and metabolic results. Neurology 34:1168–1174, 1984.

179. Quinn, NP, Rossor, MN, and Marsden, CD: Dementia and Parkinson's disease—Pathological and neurochemical considerations. Br Med Bull 42(1):86–90, 1986.

180. Radue, EW, du Boulay, GH, Harrison, MJG, and Thomas, DJ: Comparison of angiographic and CT findings between patients with multi-infarct dementia and those with dementia due to primary neuronal degeneration. Neuroradiology 16:113–115, 1978.

181. Raynaud, C, Rancurel, G, Samson, Y, Baron, JC, Soucy, JP, Kieffer, E, Cabanis, E, Majdalani, A, Ricard, D, Bardy, A, Bourguignon, M, Syrota, A, and Lassen, N: Pathophysiologic study of chronic infarcts with I-123 isopropyl iodoamphetamine (IMP): The importance of peri-infarct stroke. Stroke 18:21–29, 1987.

182. Rinne, UK, Laihinen, A, Rinne, JO, Nagren, K, Bergman, J, and Ruotsalainen, U: Positron emission tomography (PET) demonstrates dopamine receptor supersensitivity in the striatum of patients with early Parkinson's disease (abstr). Neurology (Suppl 1)39:273, 1989.

183. Risberg, J: Regional Cerebral Blood Flow Measurements by ^{133}Xe-Inhalation: Methodology and applications in neuropsychology and psychiatry. Brain Lang 9:9–34, 1980.

184. Roberts, MA and Caird, FI: Computerized tomography and intellectual impairment in the elderly. J

Neurol Neurosurg Psychiatry 39:986–989, 1976.

185. Roman, GC: Senile dementia of the Binswanger type. A vascular form of dementia in the elderly. JAMA 258(13):1782–1788, 1987.

186. Rosenberg, GA, Kornfeld, M, Stovring, J, and Bicknell, JM: Subcortical arteriosclerotic encephalopathy (Binswanger): Computerized tomography. Neurology 29:1102–1106, 1979.

187. Sage, MR: Blood-brain barrier: Phenomenon of increasing importance to the imaging clinician. Am J Radiol 138:887–898, 1982.

188. Savoiarado, M: CT Scanning. In Barnet, HJM, Stein, BM, Mohr, JP, and Yatsu, FM, (eds): Stroke—Pathophysiology, Diagnosis, Management. Churchill Livingstone, New York, 1986, p 189.

189. Schapiro, MB, Ball, MJ, Grady, CL, Haxby, JV, Kaye, JA, and Rapoport, SI: Dementia in Down's syndrome: Cerebral glucose utilization, neuropsychological assessment, and neuropathology. Neurology 38:938–942 1988.

190. Schapiro, MB, Grady, C, Ball, MI, DeCarli, C, and Rapoport, SI: Reductions in parietal/temporal cerebral glucose metabolism are not specific for Alzheimer's disease (abstr). Neurology (Suppl 1)40:152, 1990.

191. Schlageter NL, Carson, RE, and Rapoport, SI: Examination of blood-brain barrier permeability in dementia of the Alzheimer type with [^{68}Ga]EDTA and positron emission tomography. J Cereb Blood Flow Metab 67:1–8, 1987.

192. Schlageter, NL, Horwitz, B, Creasey, H, Carson, R, Duara, R, Berg, GW, and Rapoport, SI: Relation of measured brain glucose utilization and cerebral atrophy in man. J Neurol Neurosurg Psychiatry 50:779–785, 1987.

193. Schneider, E, Fisher, PA, Jacobi, P, Becker, H, and Hacker, H: The sig-

nificance of cerebral atrophy for the symptomatology of Parkinson's disease. J Neurol Sci 42:187–197, 1979.

194. Schwartz, M, Creasey, H, Grady, CL, DeLeo, JM, Frederickson, HA, Cutler, NR, and Rapoport, SL: Computed tomographic analysis of brain morphometrics in 30 healthy men aged 21 to 81 years. Ann Neurol 17:146–157, 1985.

195. Sharp, P, Gemmell, H, Cherryman, G, Besson, J, Crawford, J, and Smith, F: Application of iodine-123-labeled Isopropylamphetamine imaging to the study of dementia. J Nucl Med 27:761–768, 1986.

196. Shibayama, H, Kitoh, J, Marui, Y, Kobayashi, H, Iwase, S, and Kayukawa, Y: An unusual case of Pick's disease. Acta Neuropathol 59:79–87, 1983.

197. Sjogren, T, Sjogren, H, and Lindgren, A: Morbus Alzheimer and morbus Pick: Genetic, clinical and pathoanatomic study. Acta Psychiatr Scand (Suppl)82:1–152, 1952.

198. Soininen, H, Puranen, M, and Riekkinen, PJ: Computed tomography findings in senile dementia and normal aging. J Neurol Neurosurg Psychiatry 45:50–54, 1982.

199. Sroka, H, Elizan, TS, Yahr, MD, Burger, A, and Mendoza, MR: Organic mental syndrome and confusion states in Parkinson's disease. Relationship to computerized tomographic signs of cerebral atrophy. Arch Neurol 28:339–342, 1981.

200. Steiner, A, Gomori, JM, and Melamed, E: Features of brain atrophy in Parkinson's disease. Neuroradiology 27:158–160, 1985.

201. Steingart, A, Hachinski, V, Lau, C, Fox, A, Diaz, F, Cape, R, Lee, D, Initari, D, and Merskey, H: Cognitive and neurologic findings in subjects with diffuse white matter lucencies on computed tomographic scan (leuko-araiosis). Arch Neurol 44:32–35, 1987.

202. Symon, L, and Dorsch, NWC: Use of long-term intracranial pressure measurement to assess hydrocephalic patients prior to shunt surgery. J Neurosurg 42:258–273, 1975.

203. Sze, G, DeArmand, SJ, Brant-Zawadzki, M, Davis, RL, Norman, D, and Newton, TH: Foci of MRI signal (pseudolesions) anterior to the frontal horns: Histological correlations of normal findings. Am J Radiol 147:331–337, 1986.

204. Tomlinson, RB, Blessed, G, and Roth, M: Observations on brains of demented old people. J Neurol Sci 53:413–421, 1970.

205. Unger, EC, Gado, MH, Fulling, KF, and Littlefield, JL: Acute cerebral infarction in monkeys: An experimental study using MR imaging. Radiology 162:789–795, 1987.

206. Valentine, AR, Moseley, IF, and Kendall, BE: White matter abnormalities in cerebral atrophy: Clinicoradiological correlations. J Neurol Neurosurg Psychiatry 43:139–142, 1980.

207. Vassilouthis, J: The syndrome of normal-pressure hydrocephalus. J Neurosurg 61:1501–1509, 1984.

208. Vonofakos, D and Artmann, H: CT findings in hemorrhagic cerebral infarct. Comput Radiol 7:75–83, 1983.

209. Wade, JPH, Mirsen, TR, Hachinski, VC, Fisman, M, Lau, C, and Merskey, H: The clinical diagnosis of Alzheimer's disease. Arch Neurol 44:24–29, 1987.

210. Wechsler, AF, Verity, MA, Rosenschein, S, Fried, I, and Scheibel, AB: Pick's disease: A clinical, computed tomographic, and histologic study with Golgi impregnation observations. Arch Neurol 39:287–290, 1982.

211. Weinberger, DR, Gibson, RE, Coppola, R, Jones, DE, Berman, KF, Braun, AR, Zeeberg, B, Sunderland, T, and Reba, RC: ^{123}IodoQNB SPECT in Alzheimer's and Pick's disease (abstr). Neurology (Suppl 1)39:165, 1989.

212. Wilson, RS, Fox, JH, Huckman, MS, Bacon, LD, and Lobick, JJ: Computed tomography in dementia. Neurology 32:1054–1057, 1982.

213. Wing, SD, Norman, D, Pollock, JA, and Newton, TH: Contrast enhancement of cerebral infarcts in computed tomography. Radiology 121:89–92, 1976.

214. Wise, RJ, Bernardi, S, Frackowiak, RS, Legg NJ, and Jones T: Serial observations on the pathophysiology of acute stroke. The transition from ischaemia to infarction as reflected in regional oxygen extraction. Brain 106:197–222, 1983.

215. Wolf, PA, Kannel WB, and McGee, LD: Epidemiology of strokes in North America. In Barrett, HJM, Stein, BM, Mohr, JP, and Yatsu, FM, (eds): Stroke—Pathophysiology, Diagnosis, Management. Churchill Livingstone, New York, 1986, pp 19–29.

216. Wolfson, LI, Leenders, KL, Brown, LL, and Jones, T: Alterations of regional cerebral blood flow and oxygen metabolism in Parkinson's disease. Neurology 35:1399–1405, 1985.

217. Wong, DF, Wagner, HN, Jr, Dannals, RF, Links, JM, Frost, JJ, Ravert, HT, Wilson, AA, Rosenbaum, AE, Gjedde, A, Douglass, KH, Petronis, JD, Folstein, MF, Toung, JKT, Burns, D, and Kuhar, MJ: Effects of age on dopamine and serotonin receptors measured by positron emission tomography in the living human brain. Science 226:1393–1396, 1984.

218. Wu, S, Schenkenbert, T, Wing, SD, and Osborn AG: Cognitive correlates of diffuse cerebral atrophy determined by computed tomography. Neurology 31:1180–1184, 1981.

219. Yamada, F, Fukuda, S, Samejima, H, Yoshii, N, and Kudo, T: Significance of pathognomonic features of normal-pressure hydrocephalus. Neuroradiology 16:212–213, 1978.

220. Yerby, MS, Sundsten, JW, Larson, EB, Wu, SA, and Sumi, SM: A new method of measuring brain atrophy: The effect of aging in its application for diagnosing dementia. Neurology 35:1316–1320, 1985.

221. Yoshii, F, Barker, WW, Chang, JY, Loewenstein, D, Apicella, A, Smith, D, Boothe, T, Ginsberg, MD, Pascal, S, and Duara, R: Sensitivity of cerebral glucose metabolism to age, gender, brain volume, brain atrophy, and cerebrovascular risk factors. J Cereb Blood Flow Metab 8:654–661, 1988.

222. Zatz, LM, Jernigan, TL, and Ahumada, AJ: Changes on computed cranial tomography with aging: Intracranial fluid volume. Am J Neuroradiol 3:1–11, 1982a.

223. Zatz, LM, Jernigan, TL, and Ahumada, AJ: White matter changes in cerebral computed tomography related to aging. J Comput Assist Tomogr 6(1):19–23, 1982b.

224. Zilkha, A: Intraparenchymal fluid-blood level: A CT sign of recent intracerebral hemorrage. J Comput Assist Tomogr 7:301–305, 1983.

225. Zimmerman, RD, Fleming, CA, Lee, BCP, Saint-Louis, LA, and Deck, MDF: Periventricular hyperintensity as seen by magnetic resonance. Am J Radiol 146:443–450, 1986.

Chapter 6

NEUROPSYCHOLOGIC ASSESSMENT OF DEMENTIA IN THE ELDERLY

David P. Salmon, Ph.D., and
Nelson M. Butters, Ph.D.

**COMPOSITION OF THE UCSD-ADRC
  NEUROPSYCHOLOGIC TEST
  BATTERY
DIFFERENTIATING DEMENTIAS
  WITH EXPLICIT AND IMPLICIT
  MEMORY TESTS**

In view of the prevalence of dementia among the elderly, systematic neuropsychologic evaluations serve several important diagnostic functions. First, the cognitive deficits associated with the early stages of dementia can be differentiated from the mild changes that are a normal consequence of aging. Second, a comprehensive neuropsychologic examination allows the global cognitive impairment of dementia to be distinguished from selective deficits that may occur as a result of focal brain dysfunction, metabolic factors, and psychiatric disorders. Third, identifying the patterns of neuropsychologic deficits produced by patients with dementias of various etiologies may be useful for differential diagnosis.

The initial section of this chapter will describe the neuropsychologic tests comprising the assessment battery used at the University of California, San Diego Alzheimer's Disease Research Center (UCSD-ADRC). The test battery includes measures of those cognitive functions that are most often compromised in various forms of dementia; attention, memory, language, abstraction and cognitive flexibiltiy, and constructional and visuospatial abilities. We have found that this 4-hour test battery provides sufficient detailed information to determine whether a patient has the deficits in two or more areas of cognition required to diagnose dementia, and more specifically, dementia of the Alzheimer type (DAT, or simply Alzheimer disease [AD]) according to the National Institute of Neurological and Communicative Disorders and Stroke-Alzheimer Disease and Related Disorders Association (NINCDS-ADRDA) criteria.[39]

The second section of the chapter will discuss the patterns of performance seen on some of these neuropsychologic tests by patients with dementias arising from different etiologies (e.g., AD or Huntington disease [HD]). Because most of these tests involve memory, our descriptions will concentrate on this function.

COMPOSITION OF THE UCSD-ADRC NEUROPSYCHOLOGIC TEST BATTERY

The following test battery is intended to serve as an example of the kinds of tasks that should be employed for the diagnosis of dementia (Table 6–1). Since there are numerous tests that adequately evaluate the critical cognitive functions, our specific choices should not be considered a testimonial for any particular measure. Rather, we only wish to emphasize that the diagnosis of dementia requires the assessment of a wide range of cognitive abilities, with special emphasis placed on memory.

Table 6–1 UCSD-ADRC NEUROPSYCHOLOGIC TEST BATTERY

I. Attention
   A. Digit Span Test
   B. Visual Span Test
II. Memory
   A. Explicit memory tests
     1. Rey Auditory Verbal Learning Test
     2. Moss Recognition Span Test
     3. Buschke-Fuld Selective Reminding Test
     4. Logical Memory Test
     5. Visual Reproduction Test
     6. Number Information Test
     7. Remote Memory Battery
   B. Implicit memory tests
     1. Pursuit Rotor Task
     2. Lexical Priming Test
     3. Semantic Priming Test
III. Abstraction and problem solving
   A. Modified Wisconsin Card Sorting Test
   B. Similarities Test
   C. Trail-Making Test: Parts A and B
IV. Language
   A. Boston Naming Test
   B. Letter and Category Fluency Tests
   C. Token Test
   D. Vocabulary Test
V. Constructional and visuospatial abilities
   A. Block Design Test
   B. Digit-Symbol Substitution Test
   C. Clock Drawing Test
   D. Clock Setting Test
   E. Copy a Cube Test
VI. Mental status examinations
   A. Mini-Mental State Examination
   B. Information-Memory-Concentration Test
   C. Dementia Rating Scale

The chosen tasks must be reliable and valid and have available norms for healthy elderly individuals.

Attention

An important component of the neuropsychologic examination is the assessment of attention. Impaired attention can detrimentally affect performance on all other neuropsychologic tests. Because verbal and nonverbal attention mechanisms can be selectively impaired, they should be evaluated independently. The Digit Span and Visual Memory Span Tests of the Wechsler Memory Scale-Revised (WMS-R)[56] are comparable tests of attention for verbal and nonverbal information, respectively.

DIGIT SPAN TEST (WMS-R)

This task requires the subject to repeat a sequence of single-digit numbers read aloud by the examiner. In the first condition, the subject must repeat the digits in the same order (i.e., digits forward); in the second condition, the digits must be repeated in reverse order (i.e., digits backward). In both the forward and backward conditions, the lengths of the sequences increase progressively from as few as three digits to a maximum of nine (two to eight digits in the backward condition).

VISUAL MEMORY SPAN TEST (WMS-R)

On this nonverbal span task, subjects watch the examiner touch a series of colored squares distributed on a white card and then immediately attempt to repeat the sequence in either the same (forward) or reversed (backward) order. The forward condition is always administered before the backward condition. The lengths of the sequences increase progressively from two to eight items (two to seven items in the backward condition).

Memory

Memory impairment is a cardinal feature of dementia. In the usual case, declines in the ability to remember simple information such as the location of a parked car, a short shopping list, and names of acquaintances are the most prominent patient complaints in the initial stages of the disorder. The ubiquitous presence of memory dysfunction in all forms of dementia is reflected by its inclusion as a necessary component of the diagnostic criteria for dementia established in the American Psychiatric Association's most recent edition of the *Diagnostic and Statistical Manual of Mental Disorders.*[3]

The prevalence and significance of memory impairments in dementia require that its assessment be a major focus of the neuropsychologic evaluation of the elderly patient. Since various types of dementia are associated with specific patterns of impairment on *explicit, implicit,* and *remote* memory tests,[4,11] it is important to emphasize these in the assessment process.

EXPLICIT MEMORY TESTS

Explicit memory tests are those that require the conscious recollection of information. The tests can employ either a recall or recognition format and can assess either semantic or episodic* memory.[52] The explicit memory tests employed by our center in the neuropsychologic assessment of elderly patients include the Rey Auditory Verbal

---

*Following Tulving's distinction,[52] semantic memory refers to the store of general knowledge, rules, and procedures that are highly overlearned and context free (e.g., rules of grammar, geographic facts, multiplication tables). In contrast, episodic memory refers to memory for information that is closely associated with the particular spatial and temporal context in which it was originally acquired (e.g., a particular list of words; yesterday's breakfast). Although semantic memory, like episodic memory, is impaired in most forms of dementia, the processes underlying the impairments differ depending on the nature of the disorder.[9]

Learning Test (RAVLT), the Moss Recognition Span Test, the Buschke-Fuld Selective Reminding Test, the Logical Memory and Visual Reproduction Tests from the original Wechsler Memory Scale (WMS)[53], and the Number Information Test.

Rey Auditory Verbal Learning Test.[36] This test assesses learning and retention of a list of words. On each of five trials, a list of 15 common words is presented orally, and the subject is immediately asked to recall as many words as possible. Following a 20-mintue delay filled with unrelated psychometric testing, the subject is asked to recall (i.e., delayed recall) as many words as possible from the list.

Our modified recognition form of the RAVLT[14] consists of five trials in which a list of 15 to-be-remembered (target) words is presented orally to the subject. Immediately following each presentation of the list, a yes-no recognition test consisting of 30 words (15 targets and 15 distractor words) is administered. Delayed recognition is assessed 20 minutes after the fifth recognition trial.

Moss Recognition Span Test.[41] This test, adapted from the spatial delayed nonmatching-to-sample task originally employed with nonhuman primates, measures a subject's ability to retain increasingly longer strings of information in memory. Recognition spans are determined for spatial, verbal (i.e., words), and complex visual (i.e., faces) information. For each stimulus condition, recognition span should be measured at least twice.

Recognition span for spatial information is determined by placing identical disks, one at a time, in various locations on a test board and having the subject point to the added "new" disk on each trial. Since a disk placed on the board always remains in the same position, the subject has to retain the position of an additional disk with each successive trial. Recognition span is the number of new disks correctly identified prior to the first error.

In the verbal condition, each of the 14 disks has a unique five-letter word mounted on the top, and the subject must identify the new word on each trial. The previously exposed disks are moved randomly around the board on each trial to eliminate spatial cues. A new word is added to the board, even if the previous response was incorrect, until all 14 words are presented. Free recall of the words is assessed 15 seconds (i.e., immediate recall), and again 2 minutes (i.e., delayed recall) after completion of the last recognition test series.

On the face recognition form, 14 photographs of faces from a military academy yearbook are mounted on the disks. This form is administered in the same manner as the verbal one except that each test series is terminated after the first error and no recall attempt is required.

Buschke-Fuld Selective Reminding Test.[8] This verbal list learning task provides information on storage, retention, and retrieval. Subjects are read 10 unrelated words at a rate of one word every 2 seconds and then asked for immediate recall of the entire list. On the second trial the subjects are read only those words they failed to recall on the first list and again asked for recall of the entire list. This procedure of presenting only those words they failed to recall on the preceding trial is followed for six trials. With this test procedure, and the scoring methods described by Buschke and Fuld,[8] it is possible to derive measures of the number of items in short- and long-term storage, random retrieval, consistent retrieval, and the total number of items recalled during testing. In addition, the subject's performance may be analyzed for intrusion errors. Several reports have indicated that the number of intrusion errors correlates significantly with both neuropathologic and neurochemical abnormalities in AD.[23,33]

Logical Memory Test (WMS). This test assesses memory for short prose passages. The examiner reads aloud a short story consisting of several lines and then immediately asks the subject to recall as much of the story as possible. The procedure is repeated with a second, different story. Each story contains 23 memory units or "ideas." The subject receives one point for each idea recalled. Thirty minutes after the first recall attempt, the subject is again asked to recall each story. The difference between immediate and delayed recall provides a measure of forgetting.

Russell's Adaptation of the Visual Reproduction Test[44] **(WMS).** This test assesses memory for geometric forms. On each of three trials, the subject must reproduce a complex geometric figure from memory immediately following a 10-second study period. Three increasingly complex stimuli containing from 4 to 10 components are presented on successive trials. As a measure of long-term retention (i.e., delayed recall), the subject is asked again after 30 minutes of unrelated testing to reproduce the figures. Finally, the subject is asked to simply copy the stimulus figures to assess any visuospatial dysfunction that may be contaminating visual memory performance. The subject's reproductions are scored for the number of accurately drawn components from the original stimulus materials.

Although memory for these geometric patterns correlates highly with performance on other visuospatial and so-called "right hemisphere" tasks, the figural stimuli comprising this test can be easily given verbal labels and remembered employing this mnemonic ability of the left hemisphere.

Number Information Test.[25] This test consists of 24 general knowledge questions, each of which has a number for an answer. For example, "How many minutes are in an hour?" and "At what temperature does water freeze?" The Number Information Test differs from the other tests of explicit memory described above in that it assesses semantic rather than episodic memory.

IMPLICIT MEMORY TESTS

A number of recent investigations have indicated that the ability to acquire and retain certain kinds of information is preserved in amnesic patients with severe anterograde and retrograde amnesias. These patients show normal classical conditioning of the eyeblink response, psychophysical biasing, acquisition of motor and visuoperceptual skills, and lexical and semantic priming (for review, see references 48 and 51.) A common thread connecting these diverse tasks is their implicit nature.[48] That is, none of the tasks requires the conscious recollection of information; rather, they allow knowledge to be expressed through the performance of the specific operations comprising the task. In many forms of implicit memory, the subject's performance is unconsciously facilitated by the presentation of previous stimulus materials.

As will be described in a later section of this chapter, some implicit memory tests can be used to distinguish different forms of dementia. For this reason, the Pursuit Rotor Task and the Lexical and Semantic Priming Tests are included in our neuropsychologic test battery. However, it should be emphasized that the implicit memory tests described in this chapter are still experimental in nature and have not been extensively standardized with an elderly control population.

Pursuit Rotor Task.[35] This motor skill learning task requires subjects to try to maintain contact between a stylus held in their preferred hand and a small metallic disk on a rotating turntable (15, 30, 45, or 60 rpm). Subjects are tested on six four-trial (20 seconds per trial) blocks. The total time on target is recorded for each trial.

To equate the initial level of performance of all subjects, the first test series is preceded by a block of practice trials in which the speed of the turntable is increased on successive trials. The turntable is then set for the remainder of a subject's testing to that speed which was associated with a score closest to 5 seconds (i.e., on target 25% of the time).

Lexical Priming Test.[27] Subjects are first exposed to a list of 10 target words (e.g., motel, abstain) and asked to rate each word in terms of its "likeability." Following two presentations and ratings of the entire list, the subjects are shown three-letter stems (e.g., mot, abs) of words that were or were not on the presentation list and asked to complete the stems with "the first word that comes to mind." Half of the stems can be completed with previously presented words, whereas the other half are used to assess baseline guessing rates. Several studies have shown that amnesic patients who are unable to intentionally recall the rated words will produce these words, rather than more probable associates (e.g., motor, absent), when given these "free association" instructions.[27]

Semantic Priming Test.[47] The subjects are first exposed to a list of 10 target word pairs (e.g, bird-robin) and asked to rate the degree of association between the words. After two ratings of the word pairs, subjects are asked to "free associate" to the first words of previously presented (and rated) word pairs (to assess priming) and to words that were not previously presented (to assess baseline guessing rates). An increased propensity to produce the second word of the previously presented semantically related pair is indicative of semantic priming. Amnesic patients show this propensity despite their inability to intentionally recall the specific words associated with the first word of each pair.[24,50]

REMOTE MEMORY TESTS

Impairment of remote memory is characteristic of many forms of dementia.[1,4,20,57] Furthermore, different patterns of remote memory deficits are exhibited by patients with dementias of different etiologies. The Remote Memory Battery, originally developed by Albert and colleagues,[2] and recently updated by Beatty and colleagues,[4] has been administered to patients with AD, HD, and Parkinson disease (PD). Although this battery appears to provide a valid measure of retrograde amnesia, it may be susceptible to cultural and geographic differences in patient populations. Normative data collected from elderly subjects in one locale or from one cultural background may not be applicable to all subjects. Individuals growing up and living in different parts of the United States do not have the same exposure to the same public events and famous people. Thus, it is suggested that investigators in different geographic locales develop and norm their own versions of remote memory tests.

The revised version of the Remote Memory Test used at the UCSD-ADRC consists of 75 photographs of famous individuals (i.e., Marilyn Monroe) and 75 public events questions from the 1940s to the 1980s. For each of the five decades (1940s, 1950s, 1960s, 1970s, 1980s) there are 30 items (i.e., 15 faces, 15 public event questions). The items are presented, one at a time, and if the subject cannot name the person or identify the public event, a standard set of semantic cues is read (e.g., actress, World War II pinup girl, starred in "The Outlaw" for Jane Russell) and the subject is allowed to respond again. Each subject receives a score for *with* and *without* cues.

Abstraction and Problem Solving

An impairment of abstract thinking and problem solving, and deficient ability to shift or maintain set, are prominent features of dementia.[16] Although the emergence of these deficits may occur at different stages in the various dementias, they are invariably present by the middle stages of the disorders.

The specific tests of abstraction and cognitive flexibility included in the UCSD-ADRC battery are the Wisconsin Card Sorting Test (WCST), Similarities Test, and the Trail-Making Test.

MODIFIED WISCONSIN CARD SORTING TEST[28]

The WCST is widely accepted as a measure of abstracting ability that is sensitive to frontal lobe pathology.[40] In Nelson's [42] modified version of the test, subjects must sort 48 response cards on which are printed one to four symbols (triangle, star, cross, or circle) in one of four colors (red, green, yellow, or blue). Four stimulus cards containing one red triangle, two green stars, three yellow crosses, and four blue circles, respectively, are arranged in a row in front of the subject. Each response card matches three of the stimulus cards in terms of one, and only one, attribute (either number, symbol, or color) and has no attribute in common with the fourth stimulus card. The subject must place the response cards, one by one, below the stimulus cards according to a principle (number, symbol, or color) that the subject must deduce from the pattern of the examiner's responses to the subject's placement of the cards. Each principle remains in effect until the subject achieves six correct placements in a row, at which point the subject is told that a new principle is now in effect. The test continues until six sorts (principles) are achieved or until all 48 response cards have been sorted.

A subject's performance is assessed by the number of sorts achieved, the total number of correct card placements, the number of perservative errors (i.e., persisting with a category despite negative feedback) and the number of nonperseverative errors.

SIMILARITIES TEST (WAIS-R)

The Similarities Test requires the subject to describe how two items or concepts (e.g., dog-lion, praise-punishment) are alike (e.g., both animals, both ways of controlling behavior). Fourteen stimulus pairs are presented, and the subject's responses are scored according to their correctness and degree of abstraction.

TRAIL-MAKING TEST: PARTS A AND B

The Trail-Making Test (from the Halstead-Reitan Neuropsychological Test Battery)[43] requires immediate recognition of overlearned symbols, an ability to scan a page continuously to identify the next number or letter in a sequence, and flexibility in shifting from number to letter sets. Part A consists of 25 circles, numbered 1 through 25, which the subject must connect with a pencil line as quickly as possible in ascending numerical order. Part B also consists of 25 circles, but these circles are either numbered (1 through 13) or contain letters (A through L). Now the subject must connect the circles while alternating between numbers and letters in an ascending order (e.g., 1 to A; A to 2; 2 to B; B to 3). A subject's performance is judged in terms of the time (in seconds) required to complete each trial and by the number of errors of commission and omission.

Language

The assessment of language in the elderly patient should minimally include measures of confrontation naming, fluency, and comprehension. Of these three language functions, confrontation naming and fluency have been most thoroughly studied in the demented patient. Confrontation naming deficits are evident relatively early in the course of AD,[16] but they develop only in the latter stages of other dementing disorders such as HD.[12] In contrast, fluency deficits occur relatively early in almost all dementing disorders.[9] As will be discussed later in this chapter, these different patterns of impairment on naming and fluency tests

may be indicative of different underlying linguistic and memory deficits.

The widely employed tests of language described below include an evaluation of confrontation naming (Boston Naming Test), two tests of verbal fluency (letter fluency and category fluency tests), a verbal comprehension test (Token Test), and the Vocabulary test from the WAIS-R.

BOSTON NAMING TEST[32]

The test requires subjects to name 60 objects (e.g., tree, pretzel) depicted in outline drawings. The drawings are graded in difficulty, with the easiest drawings always presented first. If a subject encounters difficulty in naming an object, a stimulus or phonemic cue is provided. A subject's performance is evaluated by the number of spontaneous and cued correct responses, perceptual errors, circumlocutions, paraphasias, and perseverations.

LETTER AND CATEGORY FLUENCY TESTS[6,9]

On the letter fluency test the subject is asked to generate orally as many words as possible that begin with the letters "F," "A," and "S," excluding proper names and different forms of the same word. For each letter, the subject is allowed 1 minute to generate words. Performance is measured by the total number of correct words produced for the three letters. Perseverations (i.e., repetitions of a correct word) and intrusions are also recorded.

On the category fluency test the subject is asked to generate orally as many different kinds of animals, fruits, and vegetables as possible in 1 minute. For each category, the subject is allowed 1 minute to generate items. The subject's score is the total number of items correctly named during the 1-minute time period.

Although fluency tests are sensitive to language dysfunctions, they also reflect an individual's capacity to retrieve information from semantic memory. If other language abilities, such as confrontation naming and comprehension, are intact, impaired fluency may be due to an inability to initiate systematic retrieval of information in semantic storage.[13]

TOKEN TEST[17]

This test of comprehension consists of a series of 62 oral commands involving "tokens" that vary in shape (circles, rectangles), size, and color (red, yellow, blue, green, or white). The commands issued in the test range from simple (i.e., "Touch the red circle") to complex (i.e., "Before touching the yellow circle, pick up the red rectangle"). This task is highly sensitive to linguistic functions in general and verbal comprehension specifically.

VOCABULARY TEST (WAIS-R)

The Vocabulary Test correlates highly with overall verbal IQ and is considered a measure of "crystallized" intelligence that can act as an indicator of premorbid intellectual abilities. The subjects are required to define 35 words, the frequency of which range from very common to moderately uncommon. The subject's definitions are scored according to the criteria described by Wechsler.[55]

Constructional and Visuospatial Abilities

Impairment of constructional and visuospatial abilities occurs in varying degrees in most forms of dementia.[16] Although they are often not prominent in the early stages of AD, constructional and visuospatial problems are evident by the middle stages of the disease.[16] There is also evidence that a small percentage of AD patients may present initially with deficits in these cognitive spheres.[15,37]

For purposes of assessing constructional and visuospatial problems among the elderly, the Block Design test from the Wechsler Intelligence Scale for Children-Revised (WISC-R),[54] Digit-Symbol Subsitutiton, Clock Drawing, Clock Setting, and Copy-a-Cube Tests have proved useful at our center.

BLOCK DESIGN TEST (WISC-R)

For this constructional task, the subject is presented with four or nine red-and-white blocks and asked to construct replicas of 11 designs. Eight of the designs require four blocks; three need all nine blocks. All blocks are red on two sides, white on two sides, and half white–half red on two sides. The four-block designs have either 60- or 75-second limits; the nine-block designs 2-minute limits. The subject's score depends on both accuracy and speed. For the first two block designs, the subject copies the examiner's block constructions; for the remaining nine designs, he or she copies two-dimensional pictures of the designs.

DIGIT-SYMBOL SUBSTITUTION TEST (WAIS-R)

This visuoperceptual task requires the subject to associate single digit numbers with unfamiliar symbols. A stimulus set of nine printed digit-symbol pairs is presented above rows of numbers without the appropriate symbols. The subject is instructed to draw the correct symbol below each of the numbers using the digit-symbol code presented above. After four practice items, the subject completes as many substitutions as possible in 90 seconds.

Memory for the digit-symbol associations is assessed 1 minute after completion of the substitution task. The numbers one through nine are presented without the associated symbols and the subject is instructed to draw the correct symbol below each number without using the digit-symbol code.

CLOCK DRAWING TEST[26]

In the first part of this task, the subject is asked to draw a clock with numbers indicating the hours and then to draw the two hands to show "ten past eleven." In the second part of the test, the subject attempts to copy a picture of a clock with the hands set at ten past eleven. The subject's drawings are scored on a three-point scale that stresses circularity of the clock's face, correctness and symmetry of number placement, and accuracy in placement of the hour and minute hands.

CLOCK SETTING TEST[26]

The subject is asked to draw the hour and minute hands on four clocks that have 12 indistinguishable slashes (instead of numbers) positioned symmetrically around the inner contour of their faces. The desired settings of the hands are presented numerically (e.g., 3:15, 7:30) below each clock. The subject's score on this task depends on the accuracy of the placement of the hands.

COPY A CUBE TEST[26]

The subject is required to copy a two-dimensional drawing of a three-dimensinal cube. The drawing is scored for the correct number of lines, the presence and correctness of all angles, and the three-dimensionality of the drawing.

Mental Status Examinations

Several standardized mental status examinations have been developed that assess multiple areas of cognition in the potentially demented elderly patient. Although these relatively brief examinations are not adequate for detecting the subtle cognitive impairments that are often present in the earliest stages of dementia, recent evidence suggests that they are useful for tracking the progression of dementia[34] and may supply some clues for differentiating etiologically distinct forms of dementia.[7] The Mini-Mental State Examination,[19] Fuld's adaptation[21] of the Blessed Information–Memory-Concentration Test,[5] and the Dementia Rating Scale[38] are three commonly used, brief instruments that have proved useful for screening and follow-up evaluations.

Scores on the Mini-Mental State Examination range from a low of 0 to a maximum of 30 correct. Demented individuals generally score 23 or below on this test. The Information-Memory-Concentration Test is scored in terms of errors, which may range from 0 to 33. A score of six or more errors is usually indicative of dementia on the Blessed test. The Dementia Rating Scale scores range from 0 to 144 points for correct responses. A score of 133 or less on this rating scale is usually indicative of dementia or some other neurologic dysfunction.

Summary of Clinical Findings

The battery of neuropsychologic tests described above has proved useful for differentiating early AD from the benign cognitive changes associated with normal aging. Our experience suggests that deficits in memory and problem solving abilities are usually the initial cognitive dysfunctions apparent in AD. Patients in the early stages of AD can be differentiated from normal elderly individuals by their severe impairments on all of the explicit memory and verbal priming tests described previously.[9,22,47] On several of the memory (e.g., Logical Memory, Visual Reproduction) and problem solving tests, the early AD patients' impaired performances are also characterized by numerous perseverative tendencies and intrusion errors (for review, see reference 11).

As AD progresses to the middle and advanced stages, impairment of attention and language and visuospatial abilities also become prominent. The language dysfunctions are characterized by both naming and comprehension deficits. In terms of visuospatial and constructional impairments, performances on the Block Design and all of the drawing tasks are severely affected.

In addition to this modal pattern of progression, a small percentage of early AD patients have presented initially with language (i.e., aphasic) and visuospatial-constructional deficits. For these patients, many memory functions remain relatively spared until the later stages of the disease. These different patterns of early impairments are consistent with the heterogeneous nature of initial presentation reported by other investigators.[37]

DIFFERENTIATING DEMENTIAS WITH EXPLICIT AND IMPLICIT MEMORY TESTS

Of all the neuropsychologic tests, those assessing memory functions have proved the most useful in differentiating various forms of dementia. Although all demented patients will evidence significant deficiencies on numerous memory tests, they may be distinguished by their patterns of intact and impaired performances and by the processes (e.g., storage, retrieval) underlying their deficiencies. To exemplify this point, the pattern of memory deficits that differentiate AD patients from normal elderly individuals and from patients with other forms of progressive dementias (e.g., HD, PD) will be stressed in this section. Special emphasis will be placed on the specific memory tests described in the previous section of this chapter.

In comparison to normal elderly and to demented patients with HD, early AD patients are highly sensitive to proactive interference. That is, previously learned information will often hinder the AD patients' attempts to acquire and retrieve new materials. Fuld[22] has noted that this sensitivity to interference often results in the production of the numerous *intrusion* errors that characterize AD patients' memory performances and that correlate with specific neuropathologic and neurochemical markers of this disease.[23] In a recent study from our laboratory, intrusion errors were found to be diagnostically important on a memory task involving the recall of short passages (i.e., stories).[9] AD patients, HD patients, alcoholics with Korsakoff syndrome (AK), and normal controls were read aloud sequentially a series of four short passages similar to those comprising the Logical Memory Test. Thirty seconds after the presentation of each story the subjects were asked to recall as much of the story as possible. The subjects' performances were scored for the number of correctly recalled ideas (i.e., total of 23 for each story) and for the number of prior-story (i.e., a correctly recalled item from one story that is recalled as part of a subsequent story) and extra-story (i.e., ideas recalled by the subject that were never presented in any of the four stories) intrusion errors.

Figures 6–1 and 6–2 show that all three patient groups were severely impaired compared with their age-matched controls in the number of ideas they correctly recalled. The major differences among the three patient groups become apparent when the numbers of prior-story and extra-story intrusion errors are examined. Both the patients with AD and the amnesic alcoholics made more intrusion errors than did their age-matched controls and the HD patients. When the performances of the subject groups are evaluated in terms of proportions (percentage) of the total responses that are correct (Fig. 6–2), the differences among the three patient groups are even more apparent. Although the HD patients did not recall many phrases from the four stories, what little they did recall was usually correct (78%). In contrast, less than 50% of the impaired

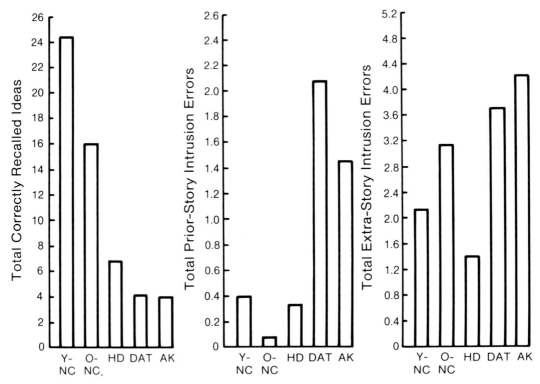

Figure 6–1. Performance of young normal control (Y-NC) and old normal control (O-NC) subjects and patients with Huntington disease (HD), Alzheimer disease (AD)—dementia of the Alzheimer type (DAT), and alcoholic Korsakoff (AK) syndrome on the story recall test. (Adapted from Butters et al,[9] p 485.)

recall of the AD and Korsakoff patients was correct. Most of the AD and AK patients' recall represented a combination of intra-story and extra-story intrusion errors.

Evidence that AD patients' tendencies to generate intrusion errors is not limited to verbal memory tests has been presented by Jacobs and colleagues.[31] These investigators assessed the performance of mildly and moderately demented AD and HD patients on the Visual Reproduction Test described in the previous section. In addition to scoring the accuracy of the patients' immediate recall of the four geometric patterns, intrusions of parts of one figure into the attempted recall of another were also tallied. The results showed that although both AD and HD patients were severely impaired in their recall of the designs, these two patient groups could be distinguished by the occurrence of

prior-figure intrusion errors. Patients with AD made numerous intrusions from one figure into another, whereas HD patients produced only slightly more of these errors than did intact middle-aged subjects (Fig. 6–3). The findings also demonstrated that the diagnostic utility of intrusion errors may be limited to the early stages of dementia. Mildly demented AD and HD patients differed in their production of intrusion errors, but moderately demented patients with these two disorders made similar numbers of these errors. This loss of clinical utility was due to a marked increase in intrusion errors as the dementia of HD progressed.

A second feature of AD patients, even in the early stages of the disorder, is a very rapid rate of forgetting of what little verbal and figural material they can initially acquire. Moss and colleagues[41] compared AD, HD, AK, and intact el-

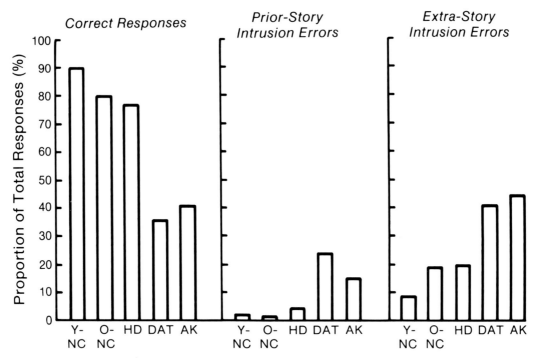

Figure 6–2. Story recall performance is presented as a proportion of the total number of story recall test responses for Y-NC and O-NC subjects and for patients with HD, AD (DAT), and AK syndrome. Abbreviations: See legend to Figure 6–1. (Adapted from Butters et al,[9] p 486.)

derly controls on the Recognition Span Test described previously. Although all three patient groups had very limited recognition spans for verbal, spatial, and figural materials, they differed in terms of their immediate (15-second) and delayed (2-minute) recall of the words used on the verbal form of the test. All three patient groups were impaired on both recall attempts, but the AD patients showed the least amount of savings (i.e., the most rapid forgetting) between immediate and delayed recall (Fig. 6–4). The HD patients, amnesic alcoholics, and intact controls exhibited almost perfect retention over the 2-minute delay period. Salmon and co-workers[46] have replicated this difference between AD and HD patients with an abbreviated form of the Moss and colleagues test.

In a recent study concerned with the validation of the WMS-R, Butters and colleagues[10] compared AD, HD, and AK patients' performances on immediate and delayed recall of the Visual Reproduction and Logical Memory Tests. As anticipated on the basis of the findings of Moss and colleagues, the AD patients demonstrated less savings than did the HD and normal control subjects (Visual Reproduction: AD = 20%; HD = 43%; NC = 88%; Logical Memory: AD = 15%; HD = 63%; NC = 85%). In contrast to their relatively normal savings scores on the Recognition Span Test,[41] the AK patients also exhibited rapid forgetting on both the Visual Reproduction (13%) and Logical Memory (9%) tests.

A third feature of AD patients' memory problems involves a disruption of the linguistic structure underlying semantic knowledge. Although both AD and HD patients often fail tests involving semantic memory (e.g., Number Information Test, Vocabulary), the processes underlying these deficits are separable. Patients with HD perform poorly on all explicit memory tests (both episodic and semantic) due to an inabil-

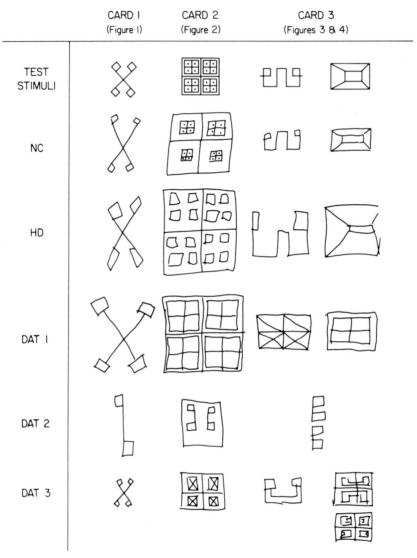

Figure 6–3. Performance of five subjects on the Visual Reproduction Test. Abbreviations: See legend to Figure 6–1. (Adapted from Jacobs et al,[31] p 53.)

ity to initiate systematic retrieval strategies,[13] whereas, the AD patients' source of impairment seems to be rooted in a disruption or actual loss of semantic knowledge. In the Butters and colleagues study,[9] semantic memory was evaluated in AD and HD patients with letter and category fluency tests. If searching for exemplars of an abstract concept (i.e., animals) demands that the hierarchic organization of semantic knowledge be relatively intact,[37] AD pa-

tients should be more impaired on category than on letter fluency tests, especially in the early stages of the disease. On the other hand, given HD patients' profound problems with initiating cognitive strategies, retrieval using phonologic (i.e., letter fluency) and semantic (i.e., category fluency) cues should be equally impaired.

The results for the two fluency tests were consistent with these expectations (Fig. 6–5). The HD patients were

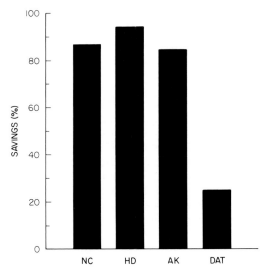

Figure 6–4. Difference between number of words recalled at 15-second and 2-minute delay intervals. Abbreviations: See legend to Figure 6–1. (Adapted from Moss et al,[41] p 243.)

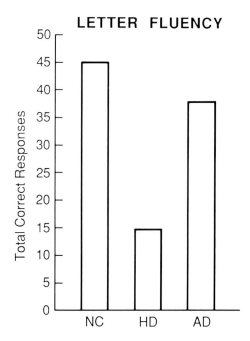

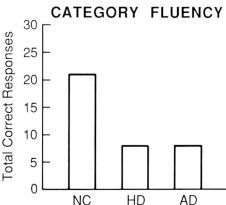

Figure 6–5. Performance of AD (DAT) patients, HD patients, and NC subjects on letter and category fluency tests. Abbreviations: See legend to Figure 6–1.

severely impaired on both letter and category fluency tests, but the performance of the AD patients was directly related to the linguistic demands of the two fluency tasks. On the letter fluency test, the patients with AD generated almost as many correct words as did the control subjects and actually produced more correct words than did the HD patients. However, on the category fluency task, the performance of the AD patients was severely impaired. They generated significantly fewer correct animal names than did the controls, and their scores were indistinguishable from those of the severely impaired HD patients. Clearly, the greater the linguistic demands of the task, the greater the AD patients' impairments on this type of semantic memory test.

Further evidence that AD patients endure significant disruption of semantic knowledge can be found in studies of implicit memory systems. Salmon and colleagues[47] administered the previously described semantic priming test to elderly AD, HD, and intact (elderly and middle-aged) control subjects. Briefly, the subjects were asked to judge categorically or function-ally related word pairs (e.g., bird-robin, needle-thread) and later to say the first word that came to mind (i.e., "free associate") when presented with the first word (e.g., bird, needle) of a pair. Semantic priming, as well as an intact organization of semantic memory, is indicated by the subjects' tendency to produce the second word of the related word pairs. Amnesic patients, who are unable to intentionally recall the words presented with the first word, will usually exhibit normal priming when this free association format is followed.[50] It is such performances by amnesic patients that serve as the most compelling evidence for the existence of an unconscious implicit memory system.

Figure 6–6 shows the percentage of previously presented words generated on the semantic priming task by each group in the Salmon and colleagues[47]

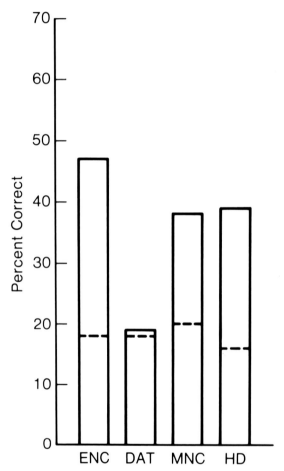

Figure 6–6. The percentage of previously presented words correctly produced in the free association task by patients with AD (DAT), patients with HD, elderly normal control subjects (ENC), and middle-aged normal control subjects (MNC). The baseline guessing rate of each group is indicated by the broken line. Abbreviations: See legend to Figure 6–1. (Adapted from Salmon et al,[47] p 487.)

study. The HD patients showed normal semantic priming on this task and performed significantly better than did the AD patients. The AD group not only was impaired compared with their age-matched control group but also was the only group that did not prime above baseline guessing rates.

These results support the notion that AD patients, but not HD patients and elderly controls, experience a breakdown in the hierarchic-associative structure of their semantic memories. The categorical and functional cues may have failed to activate traces of previously presented stimuli due to the dissolution of the semantic network governing verbal materials. For example, the cue bird may not have evoked an unconscious activation of the categorical associate robin because the association between the two words has been greatly weakened. Such a disruption of the organization of semantic memory would also account for the AD patients' reported deficiences on lexical priming tests.[49] That is, the associaton in semantic memory between a word stem such as mot and the word motel may be sufficiently disrupted to negate the facilitating effect of the word's presentation.

A fourth characteristic of AD patients is their intact ability to acquire motor skills, another type of implicit memory. Eslinger and Damasio[18] have reported that elderly AD patients can acquire in normal fashion the motor skills underlying the pursuit rotor task. Heindel and co-workers[29] extended this assessment of motor skill learning to include HD and amnesic patients as well as patients with AD and normal controls. The results (Fig. 6–7) showed that three of the four groups evidenced systematic learning of the pursuit rotor task over six blocks (four 20-second test trials comprised each block) of training. Specifically, the AD and amnesic patients and normal controls all improved their performance to approximately 52% time on target on Block 6, whereas HD patients maintained contact between the stylus and the disk for

PURSUIT ROTOR PERFORMANCE

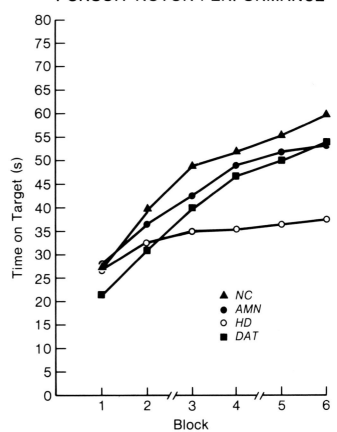

Figure 6–7. Performance of NC subjects, amnesic (AMN), HD patients, and patients with AD (DAT) on the pursuit rotor task. Abbreviations: See legend to Figure 6–1. (Adapted from Heindel et al,[29] p 143.)

only 36% of the time on this last test block. In this and a more recent investigation[30] no correlations were found between the HD patients' deficits on the skill learning task and the severity of their motor symptoms, a finding that suggests that failures on this implicit memory task cannot be reduced to deficiencies in motor performance per se.

The nature and severity of the Alzheimer patients' remote memory deficits provide a fifth differentiating characteristic. Like some forms of amnesia, AD patients often have a very severe and extensive loss of remote autobiographic and public events.[4,45,57] In the early stages of the disorder, the loss is temporally "graded," with memories from the patients' childhood and early adulthood relatively preserved.[4] When

AD patients progress to the middle stages (i.e., moderately demented) of the disorder, all periods of their lives appear to be equally affected.[57]

In comparison with AD, HD is associated with a somewhat milder and temporally "flat" retrograde amnesia. That is, when tested with public events questionnaires and photographs of famous people, HD patients in the early and middle stages of the disease exhibit a moderate and equivalent deficit for all periods of their lives.[1] As shown by Beatty and colleagues,[4] when AD and HD patients' correct responses on the Remote Memory Test are plotted according to the decade from which they emanate, the differences between temporally "graded" and "flat" retrograde amnesias are quite apparent (Fig. 6–8).

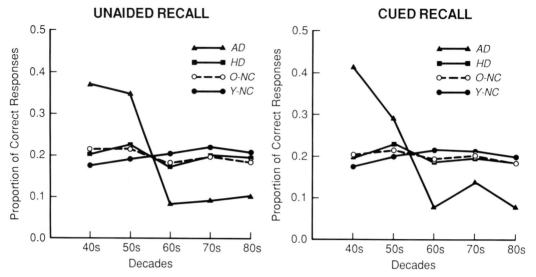

Figure 6–8. Mean proportion of memories recalled by AD and HD disease patients and by Y-NC and O-NC subjects for each of the five decades sampled with the remote memory battery. Performance for both unaided recall (*left panel*) and cued recall (*right panel*) are shown. Abbreviations: See legend to Figure 6–1. (Adapted from Beatty et al,[4] p 184.)

CONCLUSION

This description of the major features of AD patients' explicit and implicit memory disorders provides abundant rationale for the administration of extensive neuropsychologic examinations when evaluating elderly individuals for dementia. Neuropsychologic assessment of the major cognitive functions not only can distinguish dementia from normal aging and track the progression of intellectual loss, but also can play a prominent role in determining the etiology of patients' cognitive decline. Also, if pharmacologic therapies for dementia ever become a reality, the ability of neuropsychologic tests to dissect the processes underlying impaired performance will be critical in evaluating both short- and long-term effects of such treatments.

ACKNOWLEDGMENTS

The research reported in this chapter was supported by funds from the Medical Research Service of the Veterans Administration, by NIAAA grant AA-00187 to Boston University, and by NIA grant AG-05131 to the University of California, San Diego.

REFERENCES

1. Albert, MS, Butters, N, and Brandt, J: Patterns of remote memory in amnesic and demented patients. Arch Neurol 38:495–500, 1981.
2. Albert, MS, Butters, N, and Levin, J: Temporal gradients in the retrograde amnesia of patients with alcoholic Korsakoff's disease. Arch Neurol 36:211–216, 1979.
3. American Psychiatric Association: Diagnostic and Statistical Manual of Mental Disorders, ed 3. American Psychiatric Association, Washington, DC, 1980.
4. Beatty, WW, Salmon, DP, Butters, N, Heindel, WC, and Granholm, EL: Retrograde amnesia in patients with Alzheimer's disease or Huntington's disease. Neurobiol Aging 9:181–186, 1988.
5. Blessed, G, Tomlinson, BE, and Roth, M: The association between quantitative measures of dementia and

of senile change in the cerebral grey matter of elderly subjects. Br J Psychiatry 114:797–811, 1968.

6. Borkowski, JG, Benton, AL, and Spreen, O: Word fluency and brain damage. Neuropsychologia 5:135–140, 1967.

7. Brandt, J, Folstein, SE, and Folstein, MF: Differential cognitive impairment in Alzheimer's disease and Huntington's disease. Ann Neurol 23:555–561, 1988.

8. Buschke, H and Fuld, PA: Evaluating storage, retention, and retrieval in disordered memory and learning. Neurology 24:1019–1025, 1974.

9. Butters, N, Granholm, E, Salmon, DP, Grant, I, and Wolfe, J: Episodic and semantic memory: A comparison of amnesic and demented patients. J Clin Exp Neuropsychol 9:479–497, 1987.

10. Butters, N, Salmon, DP, Cullum, CM, Cairns, P, Troster, AI, Jacobs, D, Moss, M, and Cermak, LS: Differentiation of amnesic and demented patients with the Wechsler Memory Scale-Revised. Clin Neuropsychologist 2:133–148, 1988.

11. Butters, N, Salmon, DP, Heindel, W, and Granholm, EL: Episodic, Semantic and Procedural Memory: Some Comparisons of Alzheimer's and Huntington's Disease Patients. In Terry, RD (ed): Aging and the Brain. Raven Press, New York, 1988, p 63.

12. Butters, N, Sax, DS, Montgomery, K, and Tarlow, S: Comparison of the neuropsychological deficits associated with early and advanced Huntington's disease. Arch Neurol 35:585–589, 1978.

13. Butters, N, Wolfe, J, Granholm, E, and Martone, M: An assessment of verbal recall, recognition, and fluency abilities in patients with Huntington's disease. Cortex 22:11–32, 1986.

14. Butters, N, Wolfe, J, Martone, M, Graholm, E, and Cermak, LS: Memory disorders associated with Huntington's disease: Verbal recall, verbal recognition and procedural mem-

ory. Neuropsychologia 23:729–744, 1985.

15. Crystal, HA, Horoupian, DS, Katzman, R, and Jotkowitz, S: Biopsy-proven Alzheimer disease presenting as a right parietal lobe syndrome. Ann Neurol 12:186–188, 1982.

16. Cummings, JL and Benson, DF: Dementia; A Clinical Approach. Buttersworths, Boston, 1983.

17. De Renzi, E and Vignolo, LA: The Token Test: A sensitive test to detect disturbances in aphasics. Brain 85:665–678, 1962.

18. Eslinger, PJ and Damasio, AR: Preserved motor learning in Alzheimer's disease: Implications for anatomy and behavior. J Neurosci 6:3006–3009, 1986.

19. Folstein, MF, Folstein, SE, and McHugh, PR: "Mini-Mental State": A practical method for grading the cognitive state of patients for the clinician. J Psychiatr Res 12:189–198, 1975.

20. Freedman, M, Rivoira, P, Butters, N, Sax, DS, and Feldman, RS: Retrograde amnesia in Parkinson's disease. Can J Neurol Sci 11:297–301, 1984.

21. Fuld, PA: Psychological Testing in the Differential Diagnosis of Dementias. In Katzman, R, Terry, RD, and Bick, KL (eds): Alzheimer's Disease: Senile Dementias and Related Disorders. Aging Series, Vol 7. Raven Press, New York, 1978, p 185.

22. Fuld, PA: Word intrusion as a diagnostic sign in Alzheimer's disease. Geriatr Med Today 2:33–41, 1983.

23. Fuld, PA, Katzman, R, Davies, P, and Terry, RD: Intrusions as a sign of Alzheimer dementia: Chemical and pathological verification. Ann Neurol 11:155–159, 1982.

24. Gardner, H, Boller, F, Moreines, J, and Butters, N: Retrieving information from Korsakoff patients: Effects of categorical cues and reference to the task. Cortex 9:165–175, 1973.

25. Goodglass, H, Biber, C, and Freedman, M: Memory factors in naming disorders in aphasics and Alzheimer

patients. Paper presented at the meeting of the International Neuropsychological Society, Houston, Texas, February, 1984.

26. Goodglass, H and Kaplan, E: The Assessment of Aphasia and Related Disorders. Lea & Febiger, Philadelphia, 1972.

27. Graf, P, Squire, LR, and Mandler, G: The information that amnesic patients do not forget. J Exp Psychol [Learn Mem Cogn] 10:164–178, 1984.

28. Grant, DA and Berg, EA: A behavioral analysis of degree of reinforcement and ease of shifting to new responses in a Weigl-type card-sorting problem. J Exp Psychol 38:404–411, 1948.

29. Heindel, WC, Butters, N, and Salmon, DP: Impaired learning of a motor skill in patients with Huntington's disease. Behav Neurosci 102:141–147, 1988.

30. Heindel, WC, Salmon, DP, Shults, CW, Walicke, PA, and Butters, N: Neuropsychological evidence for multiple implicit memory systems: A comparison of Alzheimer's, Huntington's and Parkinson's disease patients. J Neurosci 9:582–587, 1989.

31. Jacobs, D, Salmon, DP, Troster, AI, and Butters, N: Figural intrusion errors in early and advanced Alzheimer's and Huntington's disease. Arch Clin Neuropsychol 5:49–57, 1990.

32. Kaplan, E, Goodglass, H, and Weintraub, S: The Boston Naming Test. Lea & Febiger, Philadelphia, 1983.

33. Katzman, R, Brown, T, Fuld, PA, Thal, L, Davies, P, and Terry, RD: Significance of Neurotransmitter Abnormalities in Alzheimer's Disease. In Martin, J and Barchas, J (eds): Neuropeptides in Neurologic and Psychiatric Disease. Raven Press, New York, 1986, p 279.

34. Katzman, R, Brown, T, Thal, LJ, Fuld, PA, Aronson, M, Butters, N, Klauber, MR, Wiederholt, W, Pay, M, Renbing, X, Ooi, WL, Hofstetter, R, and Terry, RD: Comparison of rate of annual change of mental status score in four independent studies of patients with Alzheimer's disease. Ann Neurol 24:384–389, 1988.

35. Koerth, W: A pursuit apparatus: Eye-hand coordination. Psychol Monogr 31:288–292, 1922.

36. Lezak, MD: Neuropsychological Assessment. Oxford University Press, New York, 1983.

37. Martin, A: Representation of semantic and spatial knowledge in Alzheimer's patients: Implications for models of preserved learning in amnesia. J Clin Exp Neuropsychol 9:191–224, 1987.

38. Mattis, S: Mental Status Examination for Organic Mental Syndrome in the Elderly Patient. In Bellack, L and Karasu, TB (eds): Geriatric Psychiatry. Grune & Stratton, New York, 1976, p 77.

39. McKhann, G, Drachman, D, Folstein, M, Katzman, R, Price, D, and Stadlan, EM: Clinical diagnosis of Alzheimer's disease: Report of the NINCDS-ADRDA Work Group under the auspices of Department of Health and Human Services Task Force on Alzheimer's disease. Neurology 34:939–944, 1984.

40. Milner, B: Some Effects of Frontal Lobectomy in Man. In Warren, JM and Akert, K (eds): The Frontal Granular Cortex and Behavior. McGraw-Hill, New York, 1964, p 313.

41. Moss, MB, Albert, MS, Butters, N, and Payne, M: Differential patterns of memory loss among patients with Alzheimer's disease, Huntington's disease and alcoholic Korsakoff's syndrome. Arch Neurol 43:239–246, 1986.

42. Nelson, HE: A modified sorting test sensitive to frontal lobe deficits. Cortex 12:313–324, 1976.

43. Reitan, R: Validity of the trail making test as an indicator of organic brain disease. Percept Mot Skills 8:271–276, 1958.

44. Russell, EW: A multiple scoring method for the assessment of complex memory functions. J Consult Clin Psychol 43:800–809, 1975.

45. Sagar, HJ, Cohen, NJ, Sullivan, EV, Corkin, S, and Growdon, JH: Remote memory function in Alzheimer's disease and Parkinson's disease. Brain 111:185–206, 1988.

46. Salmon, DP, Granholm, E, McCullough, D, Butters, N, and Grant, I: Recognition memory span in mild and moderately demented patients with Alzheimer's disease. J Clin Exp Neuropsychol 11:429–443, 1989.

47. Salmon, DP, Shimamura, AP, Butters, N, and Smith, S: Lexical and semantic priming deficits in patients with Alzheimer's disease. J Clin Exp Neuropsychol 10:477–494, 1988.

48. Schacter, DL: Implicit memory: History and current status. J Exp Psychol [Learn Mem Cogn] 13:501–517, 1987.

49. Shimamura, AP, Salmon, DP, Squire, LR, and Butters, N: Memory dysfunction and word priming in dementia and amnesia. Behav Neurosci 101:347–351, 1987.

50. Shimamura, AP and Squire, LR: Paired-associate learning and priming effects in amnesia: A neuropsychological study. J Exp Psychol [Gen] 113:556–570, 1984.

51. Squire, LR: Memory and Brain. Oxford University Press, New York, 1987.

52. Tulving, E: Elements of Episodic Memory. Oxford University Press, New York, 1983.

53. Wechsler, D: A standardized memory scale for clinical use. J Psychol 19:87–95, 1945.

54. Wechsler, D: WISC-R Manual. Wechsler Intelligence Scale for Children—Revised. Psychological Corp, New York, 1974.

55. Wechsler, D: WAIS-R Manual. Wechsler Adult Intelligence Scale—Revised. Psychological Corp, New York, 1981.

56. Wechsler, D: Wechsler Memory Scale—Revised. Psychological Corp, New York, 1987.

57. Wilson, R, Kaszniak, AW, and Fox, JH: Remote memory in senile dementia. Cortex 17:41–48, 1981.

Part III
SPECIAL ISSUES

Chapter 7

DIAGNOSIS AND MANAGEMENT OF DEMENTIA

Robert Katzman, M.D.

DEMENTIA AS A CLINICAL
  SYNDROME
ALZHEIMER DISEASE
DEMENTIA AND PARKINSON
  DISEASE
PROGRESSIVE SUPRANUCLEAR
  PALSY
MULTI-INFARCT DEMENTIA
THE ROLE OF THE PHYSICIAN IN
  THE MANAGEMENT AND
  TREATMENT OF THE PATIENT
  WITH A PROGRESSIVE DEMENTIA

DEMENTIA AS A CLINICAL SYNDROME

One of the major responsibilities of the geriatrician and neurologist is to recognize the presence of dementia. Dementia is a clinical syndrome that can be caused by many disorders; it is most often due to Alzheimer disease (AD)—(see also Chapter 8) but may be caused by or occur in the context of more than 70 conditions, some progressive and ultimately fatal, a number treatable, a few actually reversible.

The past decade has been marked by a major advance in the accuracy of clinical diagnosis of dementia, AD, and other dementing illnesses. Retrospective studies in the late 1970s found error rates of 30% to 50% that occurred in regard to the diagnosis of dementia generally, and AD specifically. In more recent series using newly developed clinical criteria, the accuracy of the diagnosis of "dementia" is reported to exceed 95%, and the accuracy of the diagnosis of "probable" AD to exceed 85%, the latter based on pathologic verification[113,115,126,177,181,189,199] (Table 7–1).

This advance in diagnostic accuracy has occurred because of the evolving recognition of the components of the syndrome or symptom complex denoted by the term *dementia* and the evolving recognition of the features specific to AD. The consensus that developed in regard to dementia as a syndrome or symptom complex caused by many disorders was formalized in the 1980 revision of the *Diagnostic and Statistical Manual of Mental Disorders* (DSM-III) of the American Psychiatric Association (APA).[5] The criteria for the clinical diagnosis of AD were formalized by the National Institute of Neurological and Communicative Disorders and Stroke/Alzheimer's Disease and Related Disorders Association (NINCDS/ADRDA) workshop,[140] and the criteria for the pathologic diagnosis by the National Institute on Aging/American Association of Retired Persons (NIA/AARP) workshop.[116]

The DSM-III criteria for the diagnosis of dementia syndrome, summarized in Table 7–2, have proved to be extremely useful. The criteria depend upon phe-

Table 7–1 DIAGNOSIS OF DEMENTIA SYNDROME: MISCLASSIFICATION BASED ON FOLLOW-UP STUDIES

Study	Original Diagnosis		Outcome Diagnosis		Misclassification		
	Total N	Demented	Nondemented	Demented	Nondemented	N	%
Kendell, 1974[115]	98	98	0	75	23	16	23
Ron et al, 1979[189]	51	51	0	35	16	16	31
Smith and Kiloh, 1981[199]	200	200	0	164	36	36	18
Rabins, 1981[177]	41	41	0	37	4	4	10
Reding et al, 1984[181]	56	56	0	55	1	1	<2
Larson et al, 1985[126]	200	200	0	198	2	2	1

Source: Adapted from Katzman et al, [113] p 17.

nomena that the clinician can readily ascertain by proper history and mental status examination. Dementia is characterized by deterioration in intellectual functioning of sufficient severity to interfere with occupational or social performance, or both. The cognitive defect involves memory and other areas of cognition such as impairment of abstract thinking, learning new skills, problem solving, language, praxis, constructional abilities, and orientation in space; there is often a change in personality. Most important, until the late stages of dementia there is a normal state of alertness and awareness, a feature of dementia that differentiates it from delirium.

This late development of criteria for the diagnosis of dementia had its roots in the historic fact that except for general paresis, dementia held little interest for physicians, including neurologists, during the first half of this century.[112] The 1888 edition of Gowers' classic text *A Manual of Diseases of the Nervous System*, a text over 1300 pages long, spent only 16 lines on "senile dementia."[71] Even in the 1951 edition of Walshe's text *Diseases of the Nervous System*,[213] there was no description of the differential diagnosis of dementia, no description of dementia as associated with subacute combined degeneration, no description of AD, and only three pages on general paresis. However, the term dementia had been used by physicians for many decades. In 1952, the APA, in its first *Diagnostic and Statistical Manual of Mental Disorders* (DSM-I), did not include the term dementia, but instead introduced a new term, *chronic organic brain syndrome*.[4] Neurologists found this new terminology cumbersome and poorly conceived. The definition of chronic organic brain syndrome included the requirement that the condition be progressive and irreversible, a feature that was not true of many disorders that produce chronic intellectual deterioration, for example, normal-pressure hydrocephalus (NPH). A clinician is often uncertain about the reversibility of a condition at the time of the initial patient evaluation. The use of a phenomenologic definition and the restoration of the term dementia by the APA in 1980 was most welcome.

The two disorders that caused the greatest difficulty in differential diagnosis of the dementia syndrome in the 1970s were delirium and depression. A major feature differentiating delirium from dementia is that the dementia patient is alert and aware, whereas the

Table 7–2 DIAGNOSTIC CRITERIA FOR DEMENTIA

A loss of intellectual abilities of sufficient severity to interfere with social or occupational functioning.
Cognitive deficit always involves memory: usually impairment of abstract thinking, problem solving, impaired judgment, aphasia, apraxia, agnosia, "constructional difficulty," personality change.
Alert and awake until late stages.

Source: Adapted from DSM-III,[5] p 107.

patient with delirium presents with a fluctuating level of awareness or clouding of consciousness. This is discussed in detail in Chapter 9.

The misinterpretation of depression as dementia was apparently common prior to DSM-III. For example, in 1979 Ron and colleagues[189] reported the results of a 4-year follow-up of a group of patients who had been diagnosed as having presenile dementia of the Alzheimer type at the Maudsely Hospital, a leading psychiatric referral hospital in London. Thirty percent were found to have been misdiagnosed, the most common error occurring in patients in whom depression was misinterpreted as dementia. Kiloh[117] had introduced the term *pseudodementia* to describe patients who presented with memory problems or psychomotor retardation associated with a depressive episode rather than a dementing condition. Wells[216] identified a group of individuals with complaints of memory loss but inconsistent findings on neuropsychologic tests who often had depression or other psychiatric conditions, rather than dementia. Wells noted that in the majority of cases careful evaluation of symptoms and the use of a mental status examination will distinguish between individuals with "pseudodementia" due to depression and true dementia. Indeed, inconsistencies on neuropsychological testing are sometimes diagnostic of "pseudodementia." Yet there is a group of patients with a history of recurrent depression who on aging have depressive symptoms associated with true memory problems.[50] Typically, there is a past history of recurrent depressions and of psychiatric treatment for depression, a subacute onset of the cognitive impairment, and a tendency for the cognitive impairment to plateau.[139] Neuropsychologic testing confirms the memory loss, but there is no evidence of language disturbances or other "cortical" signs. These patients usually respond to vigorous antidepressant drug treatment, but sometimes electroconvulsive therapy is needed. Folstein and McHugh[50] demonstrated that such patients may show marked improvement in cognition following treatment of the depression, a finding that led them to suggest that the term *dementia in depression* is more appropriate than the term *pseudodementia* for such patients.

Depression and dementia often coexist.[21,139,143,180,182,183,197] A trial of therapy for depression may be needed to determine what role the depressive state plays in the etiology of cognitive impairment in these patients.[183] This is more a complex management issue than a problem in initial diagnosis because a high proportion of AD patients show symptoms of depression, usually without fulfilling the full DSM-III criteria for depression. Depression in patients with AD may occur at any stage of severity of cognitive impairment.[197]

Although the diagnosis of dementia is now made with much greater accuracy, the underdiagnosis of dementia remains a serious problem as indicated by hospital and nursing home surveys.[41,65,119,187] In studies in general hospitals, it has been found that cognitive deficits caused by either mild delirium or dementia are often ignored by physicians when the patient has been admitted for another condition. This occurs particularly in persons with early symptomatology who are able to maintain some conversation and who do not complain of memory loss or cognitive impairment. These patients may show no abnormality unless specifically tested for mental status and memory. Early in the course of dementia, a person may have a normal verbal IQ and be fluent at a time when ability to recall a memory phrase or the date is already impaired. For this reason a mental status examination should be a routine part of the examination of every older individual seeking medical attention.

In a small number of patients, the differentiation of dementia from the mild memory loss characteristic of normal aging (see Chapter 2) continues to present a problem. As public awareness of AD has focused attention on memory deficits in dementia, physicians are in-

Table 7–3 DISEASES PRESENTING AS DEMENTIA

ALZHEIMER DISEASE

With or without vascular disease
With or without Parkinson disease
With or without other dementing diseases

OTHER PROGRESSIVE DEMENTIAS

DEGENERATIVE DISEASES
Pick disease
Huntington disease
Progressive supranuclear palsy
Parkinson disease
Diffuse Lewy body disease
Cerebellar degenerations
Amyotrophic lateral sclerosis (ALS)
Parkinson-ALS-dementia complex of Guam
and New Guinea
Rare genetic and metabolic diseases
(Hallervorden-Spatz, Kuf's, Wilson, late-
onset metachromatic leukodystrophy,
adrenoleukodystrophy)

VASCULAR DEMENTIAS
Multi-infarct dementia
Cortical microinfarcts
Lacunar dementia
Binswanger disease
Cerebral embolism by fat or air

ANOXIC DEMENTIA
Cardiac arrest
Cardiac failure (severe)
Carbon monoxide

TRAUMATIC
Dementia pugilistica (boxer's dementia)
Head injuries (open or closed)

INFECTIONS
Acquired immunodeficiency syndrome (AIDS)
Primary AIDS encephalopathy
Opportunistic infections
Creutzfeldt-Jakob disease (subacute
spongiform encephalopathy)
Progressive multifocal leukoencephalopathy
Postencephalitic dementia
Behçet syndrome

TREATABLE DEMENTIAS

INFECTIONS
Herpes encephalitis
Fungal meningitis or encephalitis
Bacterial meningitis or encephalitis
Parasitic encephalitis
Brain abscess
Neurosyphillis (general paresis)

**NORMAL PRESSURE HYDROCEPHALUS
(COMMUNICATING HYDROCEPHALUS OF
ADULTS)**

SPACE-OCCUPYING LESIONS
Chronic or acute subdural hematoma
Primary brain tumor
Metastatic tumors (carcinoma, leukemia,
lymphoma, sarcoma)

MULTIPLE SCLEROSIS (SOME CASES)

AUTOIMMUNE DISORDERS:
Disseminated lupus erythematosus
Vasculitis

TOXIC DEMENTIA
Alcoholic dementia
Metallic poisons (e.g., lead, mercury, arsenic,
manganese)
Organic poisons (e.g., solvents, some
insecticides)

OTHER DISORDERS
Concentration camp syndrome
Whipple disease
Heat stroke

REVERSIBLE CAUSES OF DEMENTIA

PSYCHIATRIC DISORDERS
Depression
Sensory deprivation
Other psychoses

DRUGS
Sedatives
Hypnotics
Antianxiety agents
Antidepressants
Antiarrhythmics
Antihypertensives
Anticonvulsants
Digitalis and derivatives
Drugs with anticholinergic side effects
Others (mechanism unknown)

NUTRITIONAL DISORDERS
Pellagra (vitamin B_6 deficiency)
Thiamine deficiency (Wernicke syndrome,
acute phase treatable)
Cobalamin deficiency (vitamin B_{12}) or
pernicious anemia
Folate deficiency
Marchiafava-Bignami disease

METABOLIC DISORDERS
Hyper- and hypothyroidism (thyroid
hormones)
Hypercalcemia (calcium)
Hyper- and hyponatremia (sodium)
Hypoglycemia (glucose)
Hyperlipidemia (lipids)
Hypercapnia (carbon dioxide)
Kidney failure
Liver failure
Cushing syndrome
Addison disease
Hypopituitarism
Remote effect of carcinoma

Note: Most of these disorders in the treatable-
reversible categories produce dementia in only a
small percentage of patients.
Source: Adapted from Katzman et al,[113] pp
18–19.

creasingly asked to evaluate symptoms such as forgetfulness of details that might represent the earliest stages of a dementing process. In many of these patients, administration of a standardized mental status examination with which the physician is comfortable will serve to establish the diagnosis. Even so, there will be individuals in whom diagnosis will be uncertain. Detailed neuropsychologic evaluation is very helpful at this juncture, especially if the patient is anxious about the diagnosis. The normal elderly patient who does well on such examinations is reassured. In a few cases, one may have to repeat the neuropsychologic examination after 6 to 9 months to determine if a progressive process is indeed present.

Disorders That Produce the Dementia Syndrome

It is recognized that dementia may be produced by a wide variety of diseases. In 1977, Haase[76] noted more than 50 disorders that may cause dementia. The list has increased to approximately 70 disorders, as shown on Table 7–3.[113]

An important autopsy series with over 1000 patients with a diagnosis of dementia during life was reported in 1976 by Jellinger.[95] This series is most interesting in that it preceded computed tomography (CT) and magnetic resonance imaging (MRI) and, as shown in Table 7–4, about 7% of the series had such structural causes of dementia as brain tumors in silent areas, hydrocephalus, or subdural hematomas.[95] Clinical series of diseases that produce the dementia syndrome are also shown in Table 7–5.[33,39,55,113,126,144,177,199] In these clinical series, conditions that produce the dementia syndrome include not only the conditions found at postmortem examination but also depression, drug toxicity, dehydration, water intoxication, electrolyte imbalances, pernicious anemia, and other vitamin deficiencies. All of these conditions are treatable and sometimes reversible and therefore must be considered in the workup. In one series, adverse drug reactions caused cognitive impairment in 35 of 300 patients evaluated for cognitive function, with long-acting sedative hypnotic agents and antihypertensive drugs primarily implicated. The risk of

Table 7–4 PATHOLOGIC DIAGNOSES IN DEMENTIA

	<70 Years of Age		>70 Years of Age	
	N	%	N	%
Alzheimer atrophy	73	44.8	502	52.7
Vascular	25	15.4	214	22.5
Mixed vascular–Alzheimer	1	0.6	148	15.2
Pick	15	9.2	8	0.8
Parkinson	3	1.8	10	10
Olivo-ponto-cerebellar	3	1.8	1	0.1
Wernicke encephalopathy	6	3.7	6	0.6
Postanoxic	—		2	0.2
Posttraumatic	—		5	0.5
Hydrocephalus	9	5.5	5	0.5
Tumor	14	8.6	34	3.5
Creutzfeldt-Jakob	5	3.1	4	0.4
Inflammatory (MS–general paresis)	9	5.5	6	0.6
Unclassified or normal	—		8	0,8
Total N	163		953	

Source: From Jellinger;[95] Tomlinson;[209] and Terry (personal communication, 1985); and adapted from Katzman et al,[113] p 33.

Table 7–5 DISORDERS PRODUCING DEMENTIA: DIAGNOSES IN NINE CLINICAL SERIES

Diagnosis	N	%
ALZHEIMER	499	
+ Parkinson	10	
+ Vascular	8	
Total	517	65.9
OTHER PROGRESSIVE DEMENTIAS		
Vascular MID	85	
Parkinson	10	
Huntington	15	
PSP	3	
ALS	1	
Kuf	1	
Postanoxic-CO	5	
Posttraumatic	8	
Postencephalitic	3	
Creutzfeldt-Jakob	3	
Total	134	17.1
TREATABLE DEMENTIAS		
Neurosyphilis	2	
Fungal infections	2	
Tumor	22	
Alcohol	22	
Subdural	4	
Hydrocephalus	27	
Epilepsy	3	
Total	82	10.5
REVERSIBLE DEMENTIAS		
Drug toxicity	21	
Metabolic	16	
Hepatic	1	
Hyponatremia	1	
Calcium-PTH	4	
Vitamin B_{12}	2	
Thyroid	7	
Hypoglycemia	1	
Total	37	4.7
CAUSE UNCERTAIN	14	1.8
Total N	784	100

Note: Series include Marsden and Harrison,[144] Freeman and Rudd,[55] Coblentz et al,[33] Smith and Kiloh,[199] Rabins,[177] Delaney,[39] Garcia et al,[65] Larson et al,[126] and Katzman et al (unpublished).
Source: Adapted from Katzman et al,[113] p 32.

an adverse reaction increased as the number of prescription drugs taken by an individual patient increased.[125]

MULTI-INFARCT DEMENTIA

Because AD is the most common cause of dementia in the western world, accounting for 50% to 70% of cases, and since as yet there is no effective treatment for AD, it has often been believed in the past—and this belief has recently resurfaced—that dementia as a whole is untreatable. Multi-infarct dementia (MID) is the second most common cause of dementia in most countries; in Finland and Japan where there is very high incidence of hypertension, MID may be more common than AD. Although it is certainly true that advanced cases of MID do not respond to treatment and are generally as progressive and fatal as AD, MID is largely a preventable disorder and if caught in its earliest stages may be stabilized. Clearly, in the United States the occurrence of MID has been declining *pari passu* with the decline in occurrence of large thromboembolic strokes during the last 20 years and now constitutes less than 10% of dementia cases in most current practices.[181,215] It is likely that even in countries such as Finland and Japan, where stroke is a predominant cause of death and MID is more common, the effective treatment of hypertension and the prevention of atherosclerosis will reverse the situation.

AIDS DEMENTIA

In large metropolitan areas of the United States, particularly on the east and west coasts, acquired immunodeficiency syndrome (AIDS) dementia has a growing importance and in some centers has now assumed the role of the second most common cause of dementia. Dementia can present in AIDS patients either as a result of opportunistic infections, lymphomas, or other malignancies, or due to direct infection of the brain by the AIDS virus. In AIDS encephalopathy, a mild to moderate degree of cognitive impairment occurs, usually presenting as a *subcortical* dementia as defined below.[87,174] For the most part, the demography of AIDS patients and the presentation of symptoms are so different from that of AD that misdiagnosis is rare, but as the number of middle-aged and elderly AIDS patients increases and as seropositive individuals with early AIDS encephalopathy begin to seek medical attention, the differential diagnosis may become medically important. This is especially likely because current studies suggest that AZT and other drugs may be useful in treatment of AIDS encephalopathy.

CORTICAL AND SUBCORTICAL DEMENTIA

The concept of cortical and subcortical dementia was introduced some years ago by Albert[3] who described progressive supranuclear palsy (PSP) as a *subcortical dementia* characterized by marked retardation of psychomotor processes. Individuals with this disorder may be exceedingly slow in responding to a question and yet give the right answer after an abnormally long period of attempted retrieval. In addition to slowness of thought processes, there is forgetfulness and the impaired ability to manipulate acquired knowledge. Apathy or depression may also be present.[37] Other conditions producing subcortical dementia include chronic communicating hydrocephalus and Huntington diseaseHD). In contrast, in a cortical dementia such as AD, evidence of cortical dysfunction (e.g., primary language disturbances) usually develops. Some neurologists have doubted whether dementia occurs as a result of involvement of subcortical structures other than the hippocampus and thalamus; in disorders such as hydrocephalus and HD, it is assumed that there is secondary involvement of the cerebral cortex. However, recent data obtained with positron emission tomography (PET) have shown that cortical metabolism is regularly impaired in AD, whereas metabolism of subcortical structures is reduced in HD and hydrocephalus.[15,121] Patients with MID show spotty areas of depressed cerebral metabolism consistent with the multifocal nature of this condition.

REVERSIBLE OR TREATABLE DEMENTIAS

The reversible conditions that can produce dementia account for only a small percentage of cases. Clarfield[32] reviewed 32 published studies (2889 subjects) to investigate the question of "The Reversible Dementias: Do They Reverse?" In the overall series, AD accounted for 56.8%, MID 13.3%, depression 4.5%, alcohol abuse 4.2%, and drug abuse 1.5%. Potentially reversible causes made up 13.2% of all cases. In only one third of cases was follow-up provided; in these cases 11% of dementias resolved either partially (8%) or fully (3%). The most common reversible causes were drugs (28.2%), depression (26.2%), and metabolic conditions (15.5%). In our experience, infectious processes, specifically chronic fungal meningitides, also need to be considered here, the latter requiring cerebral spinal fluid (CSF) examination for diagnosis. Another recently reported reversible dementia was that of hyperlipidemic dementia: the case described occurred in a 60-year-old with a 10-fold increase in serum triglycerides and impairment of recent and remote memory, calculation, and reasoning power without aphasia or apraxia; the condition reversed with treatment of the hyperlipidemia.[147] Larson and associates[126] noted that in a diagnostic evaluation of 200 elderly outpatients with dementia (70% of whom had a clinical diagnosis of AD) 31% had more than one illness contributing to the dementia state; the most prominent of these coexistent conditions was drug toxicity. Improvement occurred in 55 patients on treatment and persisted for at least 1 year in 28 (14%). This series was notable in that only 1% had MID, whereas 1.5% had myxedema.

Several of the treatable or reversible dementias are controversial. Lindenbaum and co-workers[131] reported that below-normal serum vitamin B_{12} levels occurred in 1.5% of the patients in the Larson series.[126] In our experience, in the majority of instances vitamin B_{12}

deficiency is found unrelated to an anemia, and administration of vitamin B_{12} corrects the biochemistry without affecting the cognitive deficit. However, there are occasional cases in which vitamin B_{12} deficiency is truly the cause of a dementia, and the search for this benign cause of a disastrous disorder is worthwhile.

Perhaps the most controversial "treatable" dementing illness has been NPH. It is predominantly a disorder of late middle age.[103] In the Jellinger series, hydrocephalus constituted 5% of the dementia cases in those who died under age 70 but only 0.2% in those over age 70. Thus, NPH appears to be an age-related rather than an age-dependent disorder. We have estimated that the total number of cases in the United States is 10,000 ± 5000, about one per neurologist. Nevertheless, cases do occur in the senium and need to be identified as a treatable form of dementia. In the case of hydrocephalus, although response to shunt is disappointing in some patients, it is remarkable in others as we have been reminded recently by Robert Friedland,[57] who reported a patient in her late 70s with a progressive dementia, moderate to severe in degree, diagnosed at one time as "probable Alzheimer's disease," who, 2 years following ventriculoperitoneal shunt, is approaching normality in her cognition. In regard to stroke, although we do not have an effective way of increasing the rate of recovery following a stroke, we are now learning effective methods of preventing additional strokes by use of drugs that act on platelet adhesiveness and calcium channels; the availability of recombinant tissue plasminogen activator (TPA) and streptokinase means that treating acute stroke is now possible for the first time. The most important risk factor for stroke is a prior stroke, and families of individuals at very high risk of stroke should be taught to recognize the symptoms of an oncoming stroke within the first few minutes as part of preventive medicine today.

Initially described by Adams and colleagues[2] in 1965 as a "treatable" syndrome and referred to by them as symptomatic occult hydrocephalus with "normal" CSF pressure, this condition occurs secondary to overt causes, such as subarachnoid hemorrhage, trauma, or meningeal infection, but frequently has no obvious cause. More than 600 adults with secondary hydrocephalus had been reported in the literature by 1977,[103] with 60% showing definite improvement after shunting. It is the idiopathic form that is controversial. Following the initial description of the syndrome in the middle 1960s, there was great excitement, the hope being that demented individuals with large ventricles would benefit from a shunting procedure. In fact, most large ventricles are *ex vacuo,* that is, they occur due to atrophy, loss of white matter, and are found in about 20% of cases of AD[95] and in many with MID, including most cases of Binswanger disease and related cerebrovascular disorders. Shunting of patients with AD does not lead to improvement of dementia and may in fact shorten the life span.[91] Thus, there has been great interest in the accurate diagnosis of idiopathic NPH. Evidence of enlarged ventricles with minimal cortical atrophy on CT, and radioisotope cisternograms have proved of limited accuracy in predicting who will benefit from shunting.[26]

Patients with NPH, in fact, have periods of elevated intracranial pressure. Monitoring intracranial pressure for periods up to 24 hours has shown that these patients invariably have elevations of intracranial pressure identical to the B-type plateau waves observed in the presence of frankly elevated intracranial pressure.[207] In a follow-up of patients with "normal pressure" hydrocephalus it was found that if B waves occupied less than 5% of the recording time, shunting failed to improve symptoms; if B waves occupied more than 50% of the recording time, shunting was almost always successful; but if, as in many cases, B waves occupied 5% to 50% of the recording time, the outcome of shunting could not be predicted.[26] On the assumption that patients with NPH suffer intermittently from a problem with CSF outflow, we introduced an infusion-manometric test.[2,111] This test also proved to be only partially predictive of improvement after shunting, even when modified as described by Nelson and Goodman.[162] Børgesen and Gjerris[27] reported that a direct measure of CSF conductance to outflow, utilizing a ventricular catheter, does predict outcome with quite good accuracy. However, the fact that this method requires intraventricular catheterization has limited its applicability. The picture has been further clouded by the discovery that some cases presenting as typical NPH with excellent initial improvement after ventricular shunting turned out to have multiple lacunes at autopsy.[44,120]

In the experience of many neurologists, the best predictor of response to shunting is the clinical presentation. Although the clinical picture can include a variety of symptoms, including behavioral ones,[136] the typical presentation of NPH has been best described by C. M. Fisher.[48] He recounts the first patient treated by Dr. Adams and himself, a woman aged 63 with a 6-month history of insidiously progressing, wobbling gait, 3 months of forgetfulness, slowness in verbal response, difficulty concentrating, and several weeks of urinary incontinence. This classic triad of gait disturbance, mild dementia (usually memory deficit and psychomotor retardation), and urinary incontinence together with the demonstration of enlarged ventricular system forms the typical picture. Fisher states that his own initial concern over whether the enlarged ventricles represented an atrophic process was overcome when the improvement in such patients became apparent. In regard to the intellectual deficit, Fisher noted that the rule was that verbal performance is preserved while nonverbal performance is more impaired, consistent with a *subcortical* dementia. Dyscalculia does occur, but speaking, reading, and writing are usually preserved.

Sometimes an abulic state with marked psychomotor retardation and akinetic mutism occurred if there were rapid decompensation as would sometimes occur in the 1960s after a pneumoencephalogram; this abulic state needed to be differentiated from the usual presentation. Thus the patient who needs to be investigated is the patient with gait difficulty, associated with, or preferably preceding, a mild to moderate *subcortical* dementia syndrome,[72] sometimes with urinary incontinence. In addition, some patients show improvement, especially of gait, after withdrawal of CSF, a finding that indicates the likelihood of further improvement after shunting. It has recently been reported that measurement of regional cerebral blood flow using tomographic methods to distinguish the AD type of cortical changes from those of NPH is helpful in the diagnosis,[73] but this finding needs to be replicated.

One of the most interesting aspects of NPH from a neurologic perspective has been the gait disturbance. Many observers have felt that there is a stereotyped pattern of gait abnormality, sometimes termed a "magnetic" gait (with apparent difficulty in lifting the foot off the ground), sometimes as an apractic gait. However, the findings in different patients are not consistent, and Adams has described the gait disturbance simply as "unsteady," as nonspecific a term as can be applied.[1] Sudarsky and Simon[204] carried out a detailed analysis of the gait disturbance and concluded that the gait is not apractic and not due simply to stretching of descending frontal motor fibers by the expanding ventricles as many of us have assumed, but instead represents a loss of subcortical control of gait patterning.

The finding that truly reversible dementias are infrequent in the elderly has led to the suggestion by several authors that the workup by primary care physicians be brief, a conclusion motivated in part by a cost-effectiveness argument. Clarfield summarizes, "A critical review of the literature does not support . . . the need for clinicians at the primary and secondary level to subject all demented patients to . . . an exhaustive workup."[32] Larson[123] suggests utilizing selective test-ordering strategies (specifically omitting the CT or MRI in many cases), stating that it in most cases it would be unlikely that a reversible case of dementia would be found by use of the complete workup. Larson's argument is based on a series of 200 patients (described earlier) each of whom had a CT scan, which, however, did not detect any illnesses that led to treatment changes. However, this was an unusually selected series, the patients having been referred to a geriatric program by a department of psychiatry known for its interest in AD. The fact that there were no cases of NPH and only 1 patient among the 200 had MID attests to the possibility of a high degree of physician-selection or self-selection bias that led to these referrals. Based in part on Larson's reports, a "consensus" conference published in *JAMA* in 1987[40] recommended CT only if the history suggested a mass or if there were focal neurologic signs or dementia of brief duration; however, they then stated that "unless . . . diagnosis is obvious on first contact, computed tomography should be performed." One could not argue that numerous patients with truly reversible conditions would be missed if the comprehensive workup were discarded. It is our belief, however, that the individual disasters that occur when a reversible case is missed, together with the potential cost to society of providing custodial care for an individual who could be restored to function, justifies the comprehensive workup.

Treatable, if not reversible, conditions are frequently encountered that depend on CT for diagnosis. The most important examples are structural brain lesions, such as tumors, subdural hematomas, and hydrocephalus. Prior to CT technology, Jellinger found that over 7% of his sample of 1000 autopsies on dementia patients had such lesions (see Table 7–4). *Thus, omitting CT*

scans may cause the physician to miss strokes and brain tumors, including meningiomas; it will also miss NPH and chronic subdural hematomas in subjects who do not present with a specific clinical picture.[108a,124] Although neurosurgical treatment of such conditions does not always reverse existing cognitive impairment if there has been permanent brain damage, it successfully reverses the cognitive impairment in some instances and prevents progression in others. It must be emphasized that the brain tumors or other structural lesions we are concerned with here are not those in locations that produce early focal lesions. Because they are located in so-called silent areas, the neurologic examination may show only nonspecific changes and thus cannot be used as the basis of the decision to carry out a CT. Similarly, the use of CT or MRI greatly improves the identification of vascular lesions located in the thalamus, prefrontal, or other areas where such lesions may produce the dementia syndrome without focal neurologic signs. The identification of vascular lesions is important not only for prognosis but also to alert the physician to undertake more vigorous steps to prevent further strokes and to determine the nature of the vascular lesions; for example, the pattern of lesions on CT might suggest a cerebral vasculitis, an important treatable condition. For these reasons we are strong advocates of the view that every patient presenting with a dementing illness is entitled to a CT or MRI.

The Workup for the Differential Diagnosis of Dementia

The comprehensive workup of subjects with dementia[104,160,214] is outlined in Table 7–6. This workup should follow the same plan whether the patients are in their 40s or 80s and should include history, physical, neurologic, and mental status examinations; CT scan

Table 7–6 WORKUP FOR THE DIFFERENTIAL DIAGNOSIS OF DEMENTIA

BY THE EXAMINER
History
Mental status examination
Physical examination
Neurologic examination

BY SPECIAL TESTS
CT or MRI
EEG
Blood: metabolic screen; thyroid profile; vitamin B_{12} level serology; AIDS
Neuropsychologic evaluation
Lumbar puncture in selected cases

Source: Adapted from Katzman,[104] p 344.

or MRI; blood workup with a chemical screen; thyroid function tests; vitamin B_{12} and folate levels; serologic test for syphilis; and if indicated and permitted, a test for AIDS.[104,105,108,214] In addition, neuropsychologic evaluation assists in establishing the presence of dementia, depression, or both, determining whether the dementia is a cortical, subcortical, or multifocal dementia, and in assessing level of functioning[217] (see Chapter 6). The EEG can contribute both to confirming the presence of an organic process and to ruling out seizure activity as a cause of the dementia. The utility of the P300 and other event-related potentials is still a matter of clinical investigation.[68,168] The use of PET, single-photon emission computed tomography (SPECT), or xenon CBF may assist in the differential diagnosis in a limited number of cases.

CLINICAL EVALUATION

The most critical aspects of the workup are the history, the mental status examination, and the neurologic examination. Essential to the diagnosis of dementia is a history of deterioration of performance on the job or the home or in the social sphere. To evaluate deterioration of function, the patient's education level, occupational history, and, if retired, social functioning, and activities prior to the development of

symptoms must be detailed. Usually there is no difficulty obtaining a history of deterioration of function, but it is of fundamental importance that the physician try to obtain information from more than one informant. The patient's report may not be as reliable as that of relatives or friends who have known the patient for some period of time.

The functional disturbances commonly associated with dementia, such as incontinence or the need for assistance in dressing, eating, and other activities of daily living, represent end-stage changes. Conversely, changes in higher level functioning occur early in the course of a dementing illness. The ability to handle finances is one of the most demanding tasks in our society, and the loss of the ability to prepare one's income tax return or balance a checking account statement are significant early signs. The Pfeffer functional scale addresses these areas of dysfunction.[171]

The usual symptoms of dementia are forgetfulness, memory loss, exaggerated repetitiveness, difficulty finding words, getting lost, difficulty in carrying out routine calculations, loss of interest or ability at work, confusion, behavioral disturbances, and personality change. With regard to the history, the nature of the onset is critical in differential diagnosis. The clinical hallmark of AD is an insidious onset, by which is meant that it is literally impossible to pinpoint the time of occurrence; typically one member of a family remembers some problem that the proband had with memory 6 months earlier, whereas another family member remembers an incident that occurred perhaps a year before. On the other hand, one is sometimes faced with a story agreed on by family members, that the patient was in good health until an operation, hospitalization, or death in the family, following which there was a marked decline in memory. This is an especially difficult story for a clinician to deal with, because, for example, asystole during anesthesia could be responsible for the onset of memory loss.

In such instances it may not be possible to establish whether the onset was indeed acute or, instead, acutely recognized.

It is important to ask about changes in affect; in appetite or sleep, symptoms that might represent vegetative signs of depression; the occurrence of gait difficulty, falls, or incontinence, symptoms that suggest hydrocephalus or brainstem and deep white matter involvement as in lacunar state. Changes in language, vision, and hearing should be documented. Also, whether there have been seizures, myoclonus, tremor, or abnormal movements (such as are in HD or in Parkinson disease [PD]). The presence or absence of paranoid ideation and hallucinations must be determined. In regard to past history, it is critical to know if the patient has had one or more strokes or transient ischemic attacks (TIAs); if there has been hypertension, diabetes, or cardiac problems; if the patient has been hospitalized in the past decade; if cancer has been present; the patient's alcohol history and medication and drug history; if there has been a serious head injury leading to unconsciousness; if the patient has engaged in amateur or professional boxing, an enterprise that can lead directly to dementia pugilistica or increase the risk for AD.

Once the history is obtained, as much from the patient as possible and the remainder from a relative or friend, the clinician possesses considerable information about the cognitive state of the patient. At this point the physician should know a great deal about the patient's past and current memory, fluency, and state of awareness. Nevertheless, it is critical to carry out a mental status examination on a formal basis (see also Chapter 6).

In our experience a variety of approaches to the formal mental status examination can be legitimately used. It should be noted that at least two of the mental status examinations sometimes used[100,172] fail to identify individuals with early dementia[46] because of the absence of specific tests of recent memory and concentration. If time or circumstances dictate the briefest possible test, the short six-item version of the information-memory-concentration (IMC) test[110] is sensitive, reliable, and validated; if possible, it should be used with at least one construction test such as drawing a clock ("with the numbers on it; and set the hands to 3:30") and a verbal fluency test ("please name as many animals as you can think of in the next minute"), a three-step command requiring the subject to cross the midline (e.g., "touch your right ear with your left thumb and close your eye"); and confrontation naming of simple objects and parts of objects (e.g., watch and watch strap). Whenever possible, we recommend the IMC test of Blessed and associates[18] as adapted by Fuld[63] or the Mini-Mental State Examination (MMSE) of Folstein and colleagues.[49] Both instruments have had extensive clinical and pathologic validation, and it does not take long to give them both together since there are many overlapping items. The Mattis Dementia Rating Scale (DRS)[33,149] is a more comprehensive mental status test but is too long to include in an ordinary neurologic or geriatric consultation. It is an excellent instrument for following changes in cognition in demented individuals over time, because it has a wide range of scores useful in the moderately to severely demented individual. All of the foregoing tests can be administered by a nurse after adequate training.

The mental status examination is based on the recognition that dementing illnesses impair not only memory but also intellectual functions considered to represent general, rather than focal, cerebral symptoms.[150,192,221] Among these other functions, the most useful in diagnosing dementia are loss of orientation to time (e.g., current date) and loss of ability to do serial reversals (e.g., spell a five-letter word backward or name the months in reverse order).[13,18,208] Demented patients sometimes give inappropriate responses to test questions ("intrusions"), another generalized symptom that is perhaps related to the diffusely projecting cholinergic system.[62] In addition, patients with disease processes such as AD that involve cerebral cortical association areas may show word-finding difficulties,[8] difficulty in calculating, visual spatial apraxia, and agnosias.

The degree of cognitive impairment can be conveniently specified in terms of these standardized and validated mental status tests. Thus, on the Mattis DRS, with a maximum of 144 points, a score below 124 in indicative of mild dementia, a score below 109 of moderate dementia, and a score below 90 of severe dementia. The most difficult decisions concern scores between 124 and 140; the question is whether they represent past educational deficiencies, age-associated memory impairment, or early dementia. If there is a serious question, full psychometric evaluation (see Chapter 6) is needed.

Global ratings of dementia are also useful. The most widely used are the Global DRS of Reisberg[184] and the Clinical DRS of Hughes and colleagues.[90]

The history is important in determining etiology. Whereas, as noted above, patients with AD usually have an insidious onset, patients with vascular dementia due to multiple infarcts more often have abrupt onset and stepwise progression with focal neurologic signs and symptoms. These differences were formalized in the Hachinski Ischemic Score,[77,78] later modified by Rosen and colleagues,[190] both scales validated in autopsy series. These scales fail, however, to distinguish between patients with primary vascular dementia and those with a mixture of AD and cerebral infarcts.

LABORATORY EVALUATION IN THE DIFFERENTIAL DIAGNOSIS OF DEMENTIA

The CT scan has revolutionized the diagnosis of dementia. In the largest pre-CT autopsy series,[95] 7% of persons seen for the diagnosis of dementia were found to have silent brain tumors (4.7%), intracranial masses such as subdural hematomas (1%), or hydrocephalus (1%). The advent of the CT scan has made it possible to readily diagnose these structural disorders that can produce dementia during life. In some instances, patterns of cortical atrophy are diagnostic, as in cases with marked frontal-temporal atrophy suggesting Pick disease, or in cases with caudate atrophy, diagnostic of HD. With high-resolution CT scanners it is now possible to diagnose MID in an increasing number of individuals who show evidence of areas of focal attenuation on a CT scan consistent with the scars of old cerebral infarcts. These scanners make possible the objective diagnosis in some cases of lacunar state. Binswanger disease had been found to present a characteristic picture of focal attenuation in white matter, particularly in periventricular areas[191] (see Chapter 5).

In contrast to the demonstrated utility of the CT scan in diagnosing these disorders, CT evidence of cerebral atrophy in the diagnosis of AD has been less satisfactory (see Chapter 5). Atrophy of the brain is part of the normal aging process, and although as a group AD patients show greater atrophy, this finding is not diagnostic in an individual patient.

MRI is now available at many hospitals. MRI is an alternative imaging procedure that is more expensive than CT but more sensitive. MRI will identify the major structural lesions visualized on CT and will provide additional information in that smaller infarcts in the brain can be identified. The downside of MRI as currently used is that it is so sensitive that white matter lesions originally considered to be indications of vascular change—but now known to occur in both normal aging and in AD as well as in vascular dementia—have misled many physicians to overdiagnose vascular dementia. The situation may change radically, however, in the next several years as sophistication in the use of MRI improves. Specifically, regions of the brain that are first to atrophy in AD, such as the hippocampus, can now be visualized quite specifically. Early indications are that visualizations of the structures may provide a more specific radiologic diagnosis of AD and other neurodegenerative disorders than has been available in the past.

The problem of diagnosing patients with vascular dementia has been both aided and hindered by the availability of CT and MRI. On the one hand, high-resolution images make it possible to unequivocally identify large infarcts and lacunes, including infarcts that may occur in so-called silent areas such as the right frontotemporal lobes, infarcts that may not be diagnosable on neurologic examination. On the other hand, a plethora of white matter changes are seen on CT scans and especially T_2 images on MRI which have been incorrectly assumed by some radiologists to be diagnostic of subacute arteriosclerotic encephalopathy, or Binswanger disease.

The electroencephalogram (EEG) can also contribute to differential diagnosis. Focal processes may be revealed by focal findings on the EEG. In AD there is a characteristic slowing of the EEG to the extent that the usual alpha activity at a given age shows further slowing; also the relative amount of theta and delta activity is increased.* As AD progresses, there is on average a decrease in absolute alpha power and an increase in absolute delta power, with theta power remaining unchanged.[200] These EEG changes are found in a high percentage of individuals with AD and help differentiate such persons from age-matched normal subjects. However, there is considerable heterogeneity in regard to EEG patients among AD patients, and some do not show significant changes over several years of follow-up.[178] In both the Ron and colleagues series[189] and in one of our early follow-up series,[130] the EEG proved, in retrospect, to be one of the more useful

tests in differentiating the AD patients who did show abnormalities from patients with Korsakoff psychosis or depression misdiagnosed as AD, who, on initial examination, had had normal EEGs. One of these patients was later found to have Korsakoff psychosis and improved on therapy; a second patient, known to be depressed, showed an improvement in cognitive function following antidepressive treatment.[130] In our series, these were the only persons with normal EEGs. It must be emphasized that the EEG is not always as diagnostic as it was in these series, but it remains a very useful test.

When event-related potentials were first studied in AD patients, they appeared to offer a promise of a new diagnostic tool.[69] It has now become apparent that the most commonly studied of the event-related potentials, the P300 component, which is generated in response to irregular and infrequent stimuli—the so-called odd-ball event—separates normal aging, AD patients, and depression but is not sufficiently discriminating "to be used in differentiating demented persons on an individual basis for clinical diagnosis."[194] Still, there may be some diagnostic utility if one utilizes earlier (N1 and P2) and later (N2 and P3) phases of the auditory evoked responses; these are reported to allow separation of AD, HD, and PD from each other and from normal subjects, the P2 latency being exceptionally long in PD as compared to AD and normal subjects, the P2 being prolonged in HD, and prolonged latency of the N2 and P3 separating AD from normal.[67,168]

Both PET and SPECT are markers of regional metabolism and blood flow. In cases that meet the clinical criteria for probable AD,[38,51,54,58,59] these studies often show a typical biparietal and temporal pattern of reduced metabolism and blood flow. Regional CBF measured by the noninvasive [133] xenon inhalation method also clearly differentiates clinically diagnosed AD patients with mild to moderate dementia from control subjects.[56,89,92,94,175] The ability of these im-

*References 9, 22, 70, 98, 101, 137, 158, 164, 165, 169, 178, 186, 200.

aging techniques to identify atypical cases of AD or to identify AD in the presence of other disorders such as PD, MID, or NPH has not been demonstrated yet.

With the discovery of marked pathologic changes in olfactory epithelium, olfactory bulb, and olfactory cortex in AD, a number of investigators are attempting to determine whether tests of olfactory recognition or memory might specifically diagnose AD in persons who have intact olfaction.[155,159] The loss of ganglion cells in the retina in AD is correlated with a decrease in amplitude of the electroretinogram[102]; whether this is a useful diagnostic marker in early or complicated cases is under investigation.

ALZHEIMER DISEASE

Diagnostic Criteria

In the diagnosis of AD, as in the diagnosis of the dementia syndrome, specific criteria have contributed to an improvement in diagnostic accuracy. The DSM-III included criteria for the diagnosis of *primary degenerative dementia*, a term meant to include AD, Pick disease, and other unspecified degenerative disorders.[5] In part, this term was developed in the belief that these various disorders could not be distinguished one from another on purely clinical grounds. However, increasing experience and attention paid to symptoms and course have led to an improvement in diagnostic capabilities. A special task force jointly convened by the NINCDS and the ADRDA[140] classified the diagnosis of AD as *definite, probable*, and *possible*. To be *definite*, one had to have a biopsy or autopsy confirmation of the neuropathologic findings diagnostic of AD. The clinical diagnosis of probable AD, however, has been correct about 90% of the time as discussed below. This level of accuracy is quite comparable to that found acceptable for other clinically diagnosed medical disorders.

The diagnosis of *probable* AD, the highest level of certainty currently possible without histologic confirmation, requires a workup to rule out other intracerebral or systemic diseases that could produce dementia. The patient must present with the clinical features typical of AD, that is, an insidious onset, a progressive course, cognitive deficits in two or more areas of cognition, including memory, and an alert and aware state. The diagnosis of *possible* AD was proposed for patients with either atypical courses, for example, with unusual clinical presentations, or for the group of individuals who have coexistent intracerebral or systemic disease that, however, the physician does not consider to be a significant cause of the dementia. Approximately one third of AD patients do not meet the criteria for probable AD, but meet the criteria for possible AD. As shown in Table 7–7 these can be separated into

Table 7–7 CRITERIA FOR THE CLINICAL DIAGNOSIS OF ALZHEIMER DISEASE

CRITERIA FOR THE CLINICAL DIAGNOSIS OF *PROBABLE* ALZHEIMER DISEASE:

- Dementia established by clinical examination and documented by mental status test and confirmed by neuropsychologic tests
- Deficits in two or more areas of cognition
- Progressive worsening of memory and other cognitive functions
- No disturbance of consciousness
- Absence of systemic disorders or other brain diseases that in and of themselves could account for the progressive deficits in memory and cognition

CRITERIA FOR THE CLINICAL DIAGNOSIS OF *POSSIBLE* ALZHEIMER DISEASE:

- May be made on the basis of the dementia syndrome, in the absence of other neurologic, psychiatric, or systemic disorders sufficent to cause dementia, and in the presence of variations in the onset, in the presentation, or in the clinical course
- May be made in the presence of a second systemic or brain disorder sufficient to produce dementia, which is not considered to be *the* cause of the dementia

Source: Adapted from McKhann et al,[140] p 940.

two groups, those with coexistent cerebral systemic disease and those with atypical presentations. As individuals age, the likelihood of a coexistent disease that could produce dementia greatly increases. For example, many older individuals, either because of changes in their ability to absorb vitamin B_{12} from the gastrointestinal tract or because of dietary changes leading to deficient intake of vitamin B_{12}, are found to have serum levels of B_{12} below normal limits. It has been established in a small number of patients that vitamin B_{12}, deficiency can produce dementia without signs of pernicious anemia, a dementia that can be reversed with appropriate therapy.[131] However, in most individuals with low serum vitamin B_{12}, administering sufficient vitamin B_{12} to correct the deficit does not alter the progression of the dementing syndrome. In these individuals a diagnosis of possible AD can appropriately be made if the clinical history and findings are typical of AD. This is similarly true for many individuals who are on thyroid therapy. Both hypothyroidism and hyperthyroidism can lead to cognitive impairment, but for most patients being treated with thyroid medication, this is a coincident disorder rather than a cause of dementia. A similar group includes those who have had a single stroke yet clearly do not have MID; rather, during the course of an AD process, they have had a coincident stroke. For all of these patients the diagnosis of possible AD can be used.

Atypical presentations are not only a diagnostic challenge, but they also highlight the problem of the relationship of pathology to cognitive symptoms.[35,107,196] In the majority of patients with AD, there is quite early (usually at the time of the first examination) evidence on clinical mental status or on neuropsychologic testing of deficiencies in several areas of cognition. In a small subset of patients, however, a deficit in one area of cognition dominates the clinical condition early in the course of the disease, leading to initial presentations of syndromes of progressive aphasia, progressive constructional apraxia, progressive visual agnosia, isolated behavioral changes, or pure memory loss. Although in most of these AD patients the focal presentation lasts for only months to a year or two, in some patients it predominates for longer periods of time. For example, in the patient reported by Crystal and co-workers[35] a 57-year-old woman developed astereognosis and pseudoathetosis in her left hand, a tendency to ignore space on the left side of her body, and constructional apraxia, findings characteristic of a right parietal lobe syndrome. On an imaging study, her right cerebral ventricle was larger than her left ventricle, consistent with specific atrophy of her right parietal lobe. On neuropsychologic examination, there was only the most minor memory deficit in addition to evidence of the right parietal deficits. Because of the focal nature of her deficit, which progressed over a period of 3.5 years, a cortical biopsy was carried out. The biopsy of the right frontal lobe showed numerous neuritic plaques (NP) and neurofibrillary tangles (NFT), indicating that there was not only an AD process but that it involved the cortex diffusely. Five years later the patient had deteriorated, showing evidence of cognitive impairment in every sphere, thus becoming a typical AD patient. Why had this individual presented with such focal signs? We do not understand the focal functional vulnerability of specific areas of cerebral cortex in these subsets of AD patients.

Language disturbance is an almost universal feature of AD in its moderately severe to severe states[8,10,11,36,151] (see Chapter 6). Language deficits may also occur as an early symptom in many patients, and in a few are the dominant symptoms. Although there have been reports that aphasic symptoms occur more often in patients with onset below age 70, this has not held up in other series. Left temporal lobe atrophy on CT or MRI is often seen in patients in whom progressive language difficulty is the predominant clinical feature. Not all such patients end up with a pathologic diagnosis of AD at autopsy,[152] but a number do. It should be noted that if such patients are followed for several years, then more typical, generalized cognitive deficits usually arise if the condition is caused by AD.

The existence of a memory deficit as the primary cognitive change creates a problem in distinguishing AD from the amnestic syndrome (DSM-III). The latter, in the absence of focal temporal lobe lesions, is usually due to Korsakoff syndrome. In our society, Korsakoff syndrome is commonly associated with alcoholism, although it can occur because of thiamine (vitamin B_1) deficiencies in other circumstances, for example, prisoners of war. As described in Chapter 6, however, neuropsychologic studies have shown that the nature of the memory loss is quite different in AD patients compared to Korsakoff patients so that neuropsychologic testing is diagnostic in such situations. With a few exceptions to be noted later, AD patients show progression and Korsakoff patients do not on yearly neuropsychologic evaluations.

The typical AD patient who meets the diagnosis of probable AD shows biparietal temporal deficits, sometimes greater on one side than on the other on PET.[60,179] In these studies, greater reduction of cerebral metabolism on one side of the brain is often associated with corresponding cognitive asymmetry, again showing how variable the onset of the disease may be when one begins to look at specific regions of the brain, even in patients who meet the criteria for probable AD.

A very difficult group to diagnose includes those in whom personality and behavioral changes occur early. These changes may not necessarily be isolated but may occur together with memory deficits so that one anticipates that indeed there is an AD process. Here, the differential diagnosis of Pick disease becomes very important. These patients often present on neuropsychologic tests with involvement considered to indicate frontal lobe dysfunction, and this combination of neuropsychologic evidence of frontal lobe dysfunction and behavioral change has been described as a frontal lobe type of dementia. This presentation occurs in Pick disease. In some patients with ALS, a frontal lobe type of dementia with personality and behavioral changes antedates amyotrophy by several years.[88,154,219] But a similar frontal lobe type of presentation may occur in AD patients, leading to a potential problem in diagnosis. Early in their course, Pick and ALS patients do not show involvement of parietal lobe function, so that if there is coincident involvement of parietal lobe function with the personality changes, the diagnosis of probable AD can safely be made. The personality changes here often include agitation, irritability, episodic evidence of temper, and occasionally violent actions. The physician often needs to protect the patient and caregiver from injury due to behavioral aberrations and at times needs to commit the patient.

Pick disease is a neurodegenerative disorder characterized by the loss of neurons and cortical atrophy that is most prominent in the frontal and temporal lobes, with sparing of the posterior portion of the superior temporal gyrus, so that the diagnosis can sometimes be made by the pathologist at brain cutting; the characteristic focal atrophic pattern can occasionally be seen on CT scan.[138] Histologically, on silver stain, there are neuronal inclusions termed *Pick bodies* (PB) that stain positively with antibodies to tau, A-68, and ubiquitin but do not show the paired helical filament (PHF) morphology observed in the NFT; the pathogenetic relationship to AD is unknown at this time.[83,134] Pick disease is usually sporadic, but about 15% of the relatives of Pick disease probands develop the disorder[84] and occasional families with apparent autosomal dominant inheritance have been reported.[74] At times, Pick and AD changes may coexist pathologically[17]; both were present in a remarkable family with hereditary dysphasic dementia with onset in the late fifties.[156] Pick disease is an "age-associated" rather than an "age-dependent" disorder as defined in Chapter 1, because most cases begin at ages between 40 and 70 years, and the incidence does not rise in later years as it does in AD. As a consequence, the percentage of dementia patients in any series with Pick disease will depend upon the age distribution of the patients. In autopsy series involving older nursing home subjects, Pick disease is rarely reported or is absent; in the Heston Minnesota autopsy series from state hospitals where the patients tended to be under age 70 at onset of illness, 5% of the cases regarded as progressive dementia during life had Pick disease. On the basis of reported series and our own experience, it is likely that overall there is about 1 Pick case for every 50 AD cases in the United States.

The accuracy of the diagnosis of probable AD has now been well established. Autopsy series have shown that the accuracy of ADRDA-NINCDS diagnosis of probable AD usually exceeds 85%.[52,157,161,205] However, the accuracy of the diagnosis of possible AD has not yet been reported in published autopsy series. In our own limited experience in this regard, the diagnosis is almost as accurate as probable AD. In one series in which autopsies verified the clinical diagnosis of AD in 26 of 26 cases, an accurate diagnosis had been made in 17 cases while the patients had a mild dementia (CDR1 according to classification of Hughes[90]).[157]

Joachim and associates[97] reported on the autopsy results in 150 cases in which brains of patients diagnosed as AD by a number of community physicians were sent to a research center; utilizing the NIA-AARP workshop criteria for pathologic diagnosis,[116] AD was present in 131 cases, an accuracy rate of 87%, although 35 of these cases had other finding such as contributing strokes (11/150), PD (14/150), incidental Lewy bodies (LBs) (9/150), and spongiform encephalopathy (1/150). Among the misdiagnoses, there was one case of Pick disease, one of PSP, nine cases of PD or nigral degeneration, three of vascular dementia, and one of chronic meningoencephalitis (no organisms); two had no specific abnormality. Thus, even in the general community without specified use of diagnostic criteria, a high degree of accuracy is now being achieved.

Despite the marked improvement in diagnosis of AD that has resulted from use of the NINCDS-ADRDA criteria, these criteria are not adequate to permit the diagnosis of AD coexisting with such dementing disorders as NPH, multiple strokes, or PD; in many of these instances, the coincident AD plays a major and often determining role in regard to the presence or severity of the dementia. Further improvement in clinical criteria is unlikely to eliminate such diagnostic problems; objective diagnostic markers of AD are needed.

At present, a clinically and autopsy-proven objective diagnostic marker for AD does not exist, but research holds promise. A number of investigators are currently seeking a biochemical marker for AD, either in CSF or in peripheral tissue, such as skin, fibroblasts, platelets, or lymphocytes.[19,195] Although a number of biochemical markers can distinguish *groups* of AD subjects from controls or those with other neurologic disorders, no existing marker has been shown to be effective in individual cases. Often, in such studies, differences in group means are significant statistically but considerable overlap exists for individual values. Among the most promising markers are those for the abnormal proteins (amyloid precursor fragments, PHF, tau, A-68) that accumulate in AD brain; in addition, a number of metabolic markers have been reported in peripheral tissue, none wholly specific.

The insidious onset of progressive course so typical of AD has been verified in prospective studies. In a prospective study of a cohort of more than 400 apparently nondemented 75- to 84-year-old volunteers, a cohort that developed DSM-III dementia at a rate of about 3% per year,[109] the majority of those developing AD had mental status examination scores at the upper limits of "normal" in the year prior to recognition of the dementia, at a time when they were considered to be symptomatically and functionally normal. Their initial scores may have represented the onset of a dementing process unrecognized by patient, family, or doctor, truly insidious in onset. But other patients show a marked change in cognition as measured by mental status and neuropsychologic tests, with no functional change noted by the family. In this latter situation, the patient under the stress of an event may become overtly confused, for example, during a trip, after an operation, or following the death of a spouse. The experienced clinician may easily understand the circumstances that led to the behavior that appears to the family as an abrupt onset. Under the initial DSM-III criteria, such cases could not be classified. The category of possible AD, as specified in the NINCDS-ADRDA criteria, provides such leeway.

The original DSM-III criteria included a "uniformly progressive course" as a feature of AD. This is frequently not the case. Among autopsy-confirmed AD cases, we have had patients who showed no change on mental status scores over a 2-year period, and clinically diagnosed patients whose mental status has remained on a plateau for 3 years before progression resumed. In other cases there has been abrupt worsening. The most dramatic in our own experience was a 65-year-old retired elementary school teacher who had begun to have problems during the year prior to evaluation. According to her history, she had lost her way while driving, increasingly misplaced objects, and had difficulty filling out her retirement papers.[6] A detailed evaluation showed the presence of a mild dementia with scores of 7/33 errors on the IMC, 26/30 on the MMSE, and 122/144 on the Mattis DRS. There were masked facies, but she was ambulatory, partially independent, and did not show other neurologic signs. Over a 3-month pe-

riod after this examination, her condition worsened so that when evaluated in the hospital for a possible intercurrent condition she could no longer perform the activities of daily living without help and she had error scores of 16/33 on the IMC, 9/30 on the MMSE, and 39/144 on the DRS. She died a month later, and the only intracranial process was an advanced AD with coexistent LB, an example of the LB variant (LBV) of AD to be discussed later. This extraordinarily rapid worsening of an AD dementia was not associated with any evident change in her living status, nutrition, or intercurrent infection. Conversely, studies of demented patients with plateaus have not yielded any clue as to factors that might influence the rate of decline.

Extrapyramidal Findings in Alzheimer Disease

Extrapyramidal findings often develop in the course of AD. Chui and colleagues[31] reported extrapyramidal findings in 43 of 146 AD patients (29%), and Mayeux and co-workers[151] reported extrapyramidal findings in 34 of 121 AD patients (28%), the AD diagnoses in both series based on criteria that excluded patients with clinical evidence of PD before the onset of intellectual decline as well as those with an elevated Hachinski ischemic score. The extrapyramidal signs were unrelated to psychotropic drugs. Patients with extrapyramidal signs did not differ from other AD patients in regard to age, but their performance on mental status examinations and their functional capacity were significantly poorer. In the Mayeux series, there was greater occurrence of organic psychosis with hallucinations and delusions, and a family history of dementia was more prevalent in the patients with extrapyramidal signs. Rigidity and bradykinesia were the most frequent extrapyramidal signs, tremor was rare.

The problem of the dementia patient with a history and cognitive changes suggestive of cortical involvement, who has coexistent extrapyramidal features, has turned out to be more complicated than was initally envisioned. In most patients under consideration, the extrapyramidal features do not meet the current criteria for parkinsonism. In particular, this group of patients does not show resting tremor,[42] and seldom parkinsonian gait; rigidity and bradykinesia being the most common findings. Also, the response to L-dopa is usually disappointing. Leverenz and Sumi[128] found that the clinical extrapyramidal findings are 2.5 to 3.5 times greater in prevalence than expected for age and gender. In one autopsy series, the presence of LB in the SN (substantia nigra) was 3.8 times that expected in nonparkinsonian subjects of similar age. The highest percentage of PD findings in AD is the series of Larson[126]; in 17 autopsies, AD was confirmed in 15, AD with coexistent PD in 2, AD, Pick, and PD combined in 1, and PD without AD findings in 1.

LBs, one of the hallmarks of PD, have traditionally been identified in the SN and nucleus basalis of Meynert (nbM) by the presence of a halo highlighting the eosinophilic neuronal inclusions. As noted in Chapter 8, LBs in cerebral neocortex that are not surrounded by a halo are often difficult to identify. Even so, there has been recent identification of a small number of dementia cases in which the major pathologic feature has been LBs present throughout neocortex, as well as in brain stem, so-called diffuse LB disease. The immunohistochemical identification of LBs, made possible by the availability of antiubiquitin antibody,[148] has permitted further exploration of LBs.[82]

Hansen and associates[82] found that as many as one third of subjects diagnosed as AD with autopsy findings of NP and NFT distribution typical of AD, also had diffuse neocortical and subcortical LBs. The patients with AD pathology plus diffuse neocortical LBs appear to constitute a distinct neuropathologic and clinical subset of AD,

the *Lewy body variant* (LBV). The LBV group shows gross pallor of the SN, greater neuron loss in the locus cerulens (LC), SN, and substantia innominata (SI), lower neocortical choline acetyl-transferase (ChAT) levels, and fewer midfrontal NFT than pure AD, along with the frequent occurrence of medial temporal spongiform vacuolization. We compared findings in nine subjects with autopsy-proved LBV and nine with pure AD, subjects matched on age and initial mental status test scores (mean IMC score was 17.5 errors), who had been selected on the basis of their ability during life to cooperate with an extensive neuropsychologic test battery on initial examination. The LBV subset had similar brain weights, numbers of NP and NFT, and neuronal cell counts to the AD subset, but a greater reduction in ChAT. Clinically, the majority of the LBV patients had masked facies, and a number had an action (not a typical parkinsonian) tremor, mild nuchal rigidity, and slowing of rapid alternating movements, but did not show gait impairment, rest tremor, or cogwheel rigidity. Although closely matched on mental status test scores with patients with pure AD, their neuropsychologic tests showed greater deficiencies in attention, fluency, and visuospatial processing. However, in terms of dementia symptomatology, history, and other neuropsychologic tests, the LBV patients were identical to the typical AD patients. Hence, we believe that these subjects represent a clinically and pathologically defined subtype of AD, the LBV of AD. It may be possible to diagnose these cases prospectively, although this has not yet been proved.

Myoclonus and Epilepsy in Alzheimer Disease

Myoclonus and epilepsy occur in some AD patients. Generalized seizures occur in 5% to 10% of AD patients. Usually, myoclonus tends to occur after several years of progression, as dementia becomes severe.[31] However, Mayeux and co-workers[151] reported that myoclonus was present in 11 of 121 patients on first evaluation, 5 of these patients also showing extrapyramidal findings. They also reported that patients with myoclonus tended to be younger, but that late-onset cases, in which myoclonus is a prominent early feature, do occur.[45] The myoclonus in AD has been reported to be distinguishable electrophysiologically from the myoclonus of Creutzfeldt-Jakob (CJ) disease.[220] AD patients with myoclonus do not show the periodic spike or wave discharge characteristic of CJ disease but rather diffuse bursts of high-amplitude sharp waves.

DEMENTIA AND PARKINSON DISEASE

Just as PD findings occur with increased frequency in AD, dementia both with and without concurrent AD pathology occurs in patients who present clinically with initial symptoms of typical PD. Widespread recognition of the importance of dementia in parkinsonism is a relatively recent phenomenon. In his initial description of the "shaking palsy" in 1817, James Parkinson specified that "the senses and intellects being uninjured."[167] At the turn of the century, a small group of writers called attention to the presence of dementia,[173] yet as late as 1967 the classic paper of Hoehn and Yahr,[86] which reviewed the clinical findings in 801 PD patients examined between 1949 and 1964, did not describe dementia as a symptom. Although this paper established the most widely used of the clinical scales for rating the severity of PD, the scale does not include cognitive deficit as a component.

In the late 1960s, several observers began to study cognitive deficit in PD. A particularly instructive study was a 1973 report in which Martin and colleagues[145] described the symptomatology in 100 patients who sought treatment with L-dopa, a drug that had just been released. These investigators noted frequent occurrence of intellectual impairment and frontal release signs in their patients. On a mental status test with 28 items, 25% made 8 or more errors. Subsequently, a number of observers have reported that 20% to 40% of their PD patients were demented,* although one series reported only 10%.[151] It should be noted that several of these series were collected prior to L-dopa therapy so that prolongation of life by L-dopa is not the explanation, although an overall increase in life expectancy and hence an increase in the very elderly in PD series might play a role. Hietanen and Teravainen[85] reported that only 1 of 108 with onset before age 60 was demented according to DSM-III criteria, but that in patients over the age of 60 at onset, 25% were demented. Others, however, have not found such a significant change in the proportion of PD patients with dementia during aging.[28]

PD patients without dementia do not perform as well as age-matched controls in a number of neuropsychologic tests such as block design and picture completion subtests from the Wechsler Adult Intelligence Scale (WAIS); the logical, associate, and visual memory subtests from the Wechsler Memory Scale; and in the trail making and reaction time tasks. It has been assumed that these neuropsychologic changes result from the loss of dopaminergic neurons.

As might be anticipated, the presence of clinically diagnosed dementia in PD is somewhat greater in series based on autopsy cases. In a study of 300 PD patients who had come to autopsy, Jellinger[96] found evidence of AD in 16.9% of those who died under age 70 and in 32.6% in older subjects. Yoshimura[223] reported that 37 of 56 cases of PD who came to autopsy had been demented during life; two thirds of the brains of

---

*References 14, 24, 28, 30, 129, 132, 146, 153, 173, 206.

these demented cases showed changes typical of AD. These investigators also noted that cortical LBs were more frequent in demented than in nondemented PD patients and tended to vary in parallel with the frequency of senile changes and degree of dementia. Similar findings were reported by Boller and associates.[20] In our series of 137 consecutive nursing home autopsies,[114] there were 4 demented patients who had PD plus AD and 5 who were demented without coincident AD. It must be concluded that AD is much more common than chance in PD and that some PD patients develop a mild to moderate dementia on the basis of the PD alone, showing changes in frontal lobe and nbM, in addition to the typical midbrain and LC involvement. Whether these patients also had diffuse LB disease is unknown because antiubiquitin staining was not available at the time this series was studied.

In PD cases without numerous NP or NFT, there is often a significant deficit in frontal, and sometimes temporal lobe, ChAT[114,170] and a 50% to 75% loss of neurons in the nbM,[218] which has been postulated to be related to the intellectual impairment.

Because the coincidence of PD and AD findings are significantly above chance, in terms of existing prevalence figures, one might speculate that the diseases are in some way etiologically related or that one disease process triggers the other. Quinn and colleagues[176] argued that the high percentage of dementia in PD is due to the occurrence of PD with subclinical AD, superimposing pathologic and biochemical changes, leading to clinical expression of the dementia at a time when the AD changes would not ordinarily be expressed clinically. This argument supposes a high incidence, in normal aging, of hippocampal NFT and other AD changes as reported by Tomlinson and others[209,211] based on autopsy series primarily from chronic hospitals. It should be noted that this hypothesis is not consistent with the findings of Hakim and Mathie-

son,[81] who reported that in 18 autopsied cases of dementia in patients who had been clinically diagnosed as having PD, only 2 lacked typical AD changes, whereas even very mild AD changes occurred in less than 20% of age-matched control brains of persons dying of trauma and stroke.

From the clinical point of view, the patient who initially presents with the typical features of AD and then develops mild extrapyramidal features is most likely to have the LBV of AD. The patient who initially presents with tremor, postural and gait changes, rigidity, and bradykinesia is diagnosed as having PD. Mild cognitive changes probably occur in the majority of PD patients, perhaps attributable to involvement of the nbM. In the 20% to 40% of the PD patients who develop frank dementia, about half will be found at autopsy to have AD. There is not yet a firm basis, however, on which to make the differential diagnosis, to predict clinically which demented PD patients also have AD.

PROGRESSIVE SUPRANUCLEAR PALSY

PSP, also termed the *Steele, Richardson, Olzsewski syndrome*,[202] is an important dementing disorder that is often misdiagnosed. It is still often omitted from clinical and neuropathologic series, and it is not understood why this disorder was not described prior to 1964. In our experience, this disorder is at least as common as Pick disease, it is almost always sporadic, and we have not observed any familial cases. Pathologically, there are tangles containing aggregates of 15-nm straight filaments rather than the 10-nm helical filaments found in NFT of AD, nevertheless reacting with antibodies to ubiquitin, tau phosphorylated neurofilaments, and tubulin.[134] These tangles are present particularly in basal ganglia, brain stem, and deep cerebellar nuclei.[64] Clinically, this disorder is characterized by the impairment of extraocular movements, particularly vertical gaze, occasional association with photophobia, slowing of motor processes, memory and visual spatial disturbance,[3,37] variable extrapyramidal features (not including tremor), clumsiness, dysarthria and other pseudobulbar features, poor postural stability, and gait disturbance. As discussed earlier, Albert[3] considered the psychomotor retardation of PSP patients to be the prototype of subcortical dementia. Dubois and colleagues[43] found that central processing time was increased in patients with PSP as compared with both PD and control subjects. The increase was associated with impairment in frontal lobe test performance, suggesting that this slowing may be related to striatofrontal dysfunction. Language, however, is spared. The patient may be dysarthric and say few words, but the words are informative; questions are answered appropriately; comprehension and repetition are retained.

We have seen PSP patients misdiagnosed as AD, PD, MID, and dementia of unknown etiology. In some cases, missed diagnoses occur because the eye movement abnormalities may not occur for months or even a year or two after other symptoms, but more often eye movements are not carefully examined or abnormalities are misinterpreted. Thus, the gait difficulty and dysarthria may be misinterpreted as evidence of a lacunar state, particularly if there are a few bright intensity spots in subcortical regions on an MRI.

Other neurodegenerative disorders important in the neurologic evaluation of dementia include HD, olivo-ponto-cerebellar degeneration, Kuf disease (juvenile-onset form of hexosaminidase deficiency), and the adult form of metachromatic leukodystrophy. The onset of symptoms of these inherited disorders may occur during early adult life (olivo-ponto-cerebellar degeneration, Kufs' disease, metachromatic leukodystrophy) or in the age range of 40 to 60 years (HD), but these disorders are not normally seen in a geriatric practice.

MULTI-INFARCT DEMENTIA

Not many years ago, physicians often labeled any elderly person with mental deterioration as a case of cerebral atherosclerosis. Indeed, when one looks at the arteries of individuals of advanced age, one frequently finds atherosclerosis, but this clearly is not correlated with the presence or absence of dementia.[34] Persons with advanced AD often have minimal atheromatous change in their intracranial vessels.

The clinical-pathologic correlations of Tomlinson and associates[209–212] provided the critical evidence that dementia during life was correlated with overt pathologic changes in brain parenchyma—the number of plaques per unit area in cerebral cortex in AD, the volume of cerebral hemisphere infarcted in vascular dementia—rather than the degree of atherosclerosis in cerebral arteries, or any presumed chronic cerebral ischemia. These findings were in accord with the clinical experience of C. M. Fisher, who stated that "cerebrovascular dementia is a matter of strokes large and small."[47]

These concepts have been further strengthened by studies of cerebral metabolism and blood flow in dementia. Dementia is regularly accompanied by a decrease in both CBF and cerebral oxygen metabolism as measured in vivo by the Kety nitrous oxide technique.[56,89,127,201] However, this decrease is secondary to the decrease in neuronal activity and is not a consequence of ischemia because the arteriovenous oxygen difference is the same in persons with dementia and normal persons acting as controls. These somewhat indirect measures have been dramatically confirmed by PET with ^{15}O.[53,54] PET shows no change in oxygen extraction by cerebral cortex in AD, but a change in oxygen extraction in a multifocal pattern in vascular dementia. A similar pattern covering glucose metabolism is seen with 2-[^{18}f]fluoro-2-deoxy-D-glucose in these disorders.

On the other hand, multiple strokes are correlated with dementia, forming a distinct group of patients with senile dementia. Two forms of vascular disease most commonly produce dementia.[106] The first is multiple strokes or MID, and the second is the lacunar state. The latter is a condition in which there are multiple small lacunes, or cavities, usually in the basal ganglia and other periventricular areas, which are associated with hypertension in a very high percentage of cases. In general, about 50% of patients with strokes have prior hypertension, whereas perhaps as many as 80% to 90% of those with MID and lacunar states are hypertensive, suggesting that hypertension is a major risk factor for MID. Nevertheless, one must be cautious in treating hypertension in individuals with early MID or lacunar states because too rapid reduction of blood pressure may precipitate additional strokes when the cerebral vasculature is severely impaired.

Some early studies suggested that as many as 50% of elderly patients with dementia had vascular dementia. In the exceptionally well carried out pathologic study of Tomlinson and colleagues,[210] about 18% of patients with senile dementia had primary multiple infarcts, and another 10% had a mixture of vascular disease and AD (MIX). In the Jellinger study, 22.5% had dementia caused by cerebrovascular disease and 15% had MIX. However, in recent clinical studies, as shown in Table 7–5, the percentage with vascular dementia has been reported to be much lower. This probably reflects the marked reduction in large hemispheral strokes that has occurred in the past 20 years, due at least in part to the availability and use of a variety of safe antihypertensive drugs. On the other hand, there appears to have been no decrease, or perhaps even an increase, in small-vessel lesions.[23,122,222] It is possible that

the recent increase in small-vessel lesions is a consequence of the greater longevity of hypertensive individuals.

The occurrence of dementia in association with numerous small infarcts or lacunes was noted by Hachinski and colleagues[79,80] to be one of the most common forms of vascular dementia. They noted that it is characterized by "abrupt episodes which lead to weakness, slowness, dysarthria, dysphagia, small-stepped gait, brisk reflexes and extensor plantar responses." Based on clinical experience, Hachinski developed an ishemic score that has been widely used.[78] Rosen and associates[190] modified the items in this score after a retrospective determination of the history in autopsied patients with AD, MID, and MIX. Both the original and modified scores are in wide use.

The greatest difficulty in diagnosis concerns the mixed cases. Hachinski[79] noted that the the true incidence of vascular dementia would be overestimated clinically because AD and strokes coexist and the symptoms and signs of the latter will be used to explain the patients' mental impairments. This was confirmed in an autopsy series by Rosen and associates[190] who were unable to differentiate between MID and MIX on the basis of the ischemic score. This problem is particularly difficult in elderly populations where the occurrence of stroke rivals that of AD.[109] If there is clearly an insidious onset and if the pattern of neuropsychologic findings is consistent with AD, then even in the presence of multiple overt strokes, MIX can be diagnosed, but the diagnostic accuracy is not high based on autopsy experience, and a biochemical test for AD would be especially valuable in this regard.

The question of whether vascular dementia is overdiagnosed or underdiagnosed has recently been discussed.[25,99,163] On the one hand, patients with severe vascular disease often die much earlier than those with AD; in some cases, small strokes may cause dementia because of strategic location rather than amount of tissue destroyed—for example, bilateral hippocampal strokes. Alternatively, ischemia scores identify only the presence of a stroke and do not distinguish AD patients with a coincidental stroke from patients with vascular disease. In particular, a patient *with early pathologic changes of AD*, who is still able to compensate cognitively, can have his or her dementia become manifest if there is a small stroke. Both arguments are correct; in our experience based on autopsy cases, we have found that vascular dementia has been overdiagnosed.

Binswanger disease is a definitive but somewhat uncommon syndrome occurring most often in hypertensive individuals. In 1894, Binswanger described the gross findings in brains from eight cases to differentiate the condition from neurosyphilis and other dementing illnesses of the elderly; the characteristic features were the enormous enlarged ventricles, lesions in subcortical white matter, and a normal cerebral cortex. Histologically, the white matter shows cystic demyelination but with relative preservation of short association fiber bundles (the U fibers), gliosis, numerous lacunes, and usually one or more larger cerebral infarcts.[29,166] In this disorder, the small arteries show intimal thickening, fibrosis, and often occlusion.[166] In typical cases, clinical features include persistent hypertension, acute strokes, subacute accumulation of neurologic symptoms and signs over weeks to months, plateau periods, lengthy clinical course, dementia, prominent motor signs, pseudobulbar palsy, and hydrocephalus.[29] Interest in the diagnosis of this syndrome was heightened in the 1970s because of the prominent hydrocephalus and the existence of cases with partial syndromes, including large ventricles that appeared to show some improvement after shunting because of the diagnosis of NPH.[44,120]

The diagnosis of Binswanger disease remained a comparatively uncommon one. This state of affairs changed dramatically when higher resolution CT scans and, more particularly, the MRI became available. Rosenberg and colleagues[191] reported a case of Binswanger disease in which the autopsy confirmed both the diagnosis and the extent of the white matter degeneration as shown by CT scan. McQuinn and O'Leary[141] found that diffuse white matter lucencies of <39 Hounsfield units occurred in 11 of 1643 cranial CT scans, and that only 3 of the 11 had the clinical signs of Binswanger disease, a fourth with dementia being neurologically normal; however, 10 of the 11 with white matter changes had unstable blood pressure, hypertension, hypotension, or a combination of these. Severity of CT changes correlated more clearly with blood pressure instability than with clinical encephalopathy. In AD patients, there may be periventricular white matter lucencies on CT scan, pathologic examination of which shows diffuse white matter pallor without infarction or hypertensive vascular changes.[185] With the introduction of the more sensitive T_2 images on MRI scans, it was found that intense bright spots occurred in the white matter of some elderly with vascular dementia; these bright spots were interpreted as diagnostic of subacute arteriosclerotic encephalopathy. Because of the frequent occurrence of these bright T_2 spots, Roman[188] asserted that vascular dementia was a much more common cause of dementia than had been believed. However, it had been found that these white matter changes occurred in asymptomatic individuals.[118] The MRI white matter changes, in fact, occur in many elderly, including normal control subjects (about 10% to 20%), AD patients (20% to 40%), and over 40% in patients with presumed vascular dementia. These changes are more common in patients with vascular risk factors, such as hypertension or diabetes, but also occur in some cognitively normal individuals who are free of vascular risk factors. Hachinski and colleagues[80,93,203] have suggested the use of a neutral term *leuko-araiosis* to describe these MRI changes. Indeed, in attempts to find a pathologic correlate, there appears to be loosening of the myelin, increase in extracellular water, and spotty demyelination associated with these "unidentified bright objects." We recommend that, until this process is better understood, the Hachinski term leuko-araiosis be used. Continued designation by some neuroradiologists of these findings on T_2-weighted MRI images as evidence of arteriosclerotic encephalopathy is unwarranted at our present state of knowledge and has been one factor leading to the overdiagnosis of vascular dementia. The diagnosis of MID should not be made unless there is at least one unequivocal stroke based upon classic clinical findings of the acute onset and later improvement and the presence of a hemiparesis or other appropriate neurologic deficit or a large infact in a "silent" area of the cerebrum present on CT scan or T_1-weighted MRI images or unequivocal radiologic evidence of multiple lacunes together with characteristic clinical findings expected from the location of the lacunes. Such evidence will still not distinguish MID from MIX, and this remains a very high priority area for specific delineation of diagnostic clinical criteria based on autopsy-proved cases.

THE ROLE OF THE PHYSICIAN IN THE MANAGEMENT AND TREATMENT OF THE PATIENT WITH A PROGRESSIVE DEMENTIA

Most often, the diagnostic workup of a patient with dementia will lead to the diagnosis of AD or a related disorder for which no specific treatment is available. If the physician is acting strictly as a consultant, then the family must be given the diagnosis and information as requested and referred back to the primary physician for further management. But if the physician is the principal caregiver to the patient, there is much to be done despite the absence today of specific treatment.

One of the major contributions that can be made by the physician is that of finding secondary conditions that increase cognitive impairment. The most frequent among the metabolic conditions are disturbances in water metabolism; volume depletion, either isotonic or commonly hypertonic, is found primarily in the severely demented; water intoxication is sometimes seen early in dementia, in connection with some dietary fads and is also a common accompaniment of congestive heart failure or administration of medications common in the elderly, most notably diuretics; both can increase cognitive impairment. Hypothyroidism was found in 1.5% of the patients in the Larson series.[125] However, more frequent than such metabolic disorders are the toxic changes that occur secondary to medications that have relatively minor cognitive effects in most normal individuals but can produce major changes in those with dementing disorders. Sedative hypnotic agents related to benzodiazepine can occasionally produce cognitive changes in the normal elderly; their effect is much greater in individuals with an underlying dementia. Similarly, the diazepine-related antianxiety drugs, major and minor tranquilizers, all may have adverse effects in patients with AD or other dementias. Antihypertensives, including the beta blockers that cross the blood-brain barrier, most notably propranolol (the angiotensin-converting enzyme antagonists appear to be relatively safe in this regard); analgesics, especially codeine-containing preparations; calcium channel blockers; and digitalis-related drugs are among those one must be concerned about. Neurologists and geriatricians can help AD patients directly by careful and selective discontinuation of offending medications when medically possible.

At present, there are no FDA-approved drugs to treat the cognitive deficit in AD or other degenerative dementias, or in the case of AD, to stop progression of the disorder. One FDA-approved drug, Hydergine (a nootropic agent), improves the performance of demented patients on a geriatric rating scale but not on specific tests of cognition or memory. Numerous drugs are currently undergoing testing; drugs purported to help memory and other cognitive functions, include cholinomimetic agents, such as physostigmine and tetrahydroaminoacridine (THA), acetylcarnitine, and nootropic agents; and drugs that might improve the survival of central neurons, such as nerve growth factor, gangliosides, and phosphatidyl serine. However, there are drugs available, none ideal, for treating the affective and behavioral side effects that often occur as AD progresses.

Psychotropic Medication for Depression and Agitation

Depression frequently occurs in AD patients, being experienced by at least 40% at some time during the course of the illness. In some patients, there is an excellent response to antidepressant medications. In selecting an antidepressant medication it is important to avoid drugs with anticholinergic effects that can increase the memory deficit and confusion. The traditional standby for use in depressed AD patients has been desimipramine; recent additions have been trazadone and fluoxetine. The two recent drugs are said to act primarily by blocking reuptake of serotonin; however, trazadone has major sedative properties and can be used effectively as a hypnotic, whereas fluoxetine activates some individuals and is given preferentially in the morning.

As AD progresses, personality changes frequently occur, with as many as 67% of affected individuals developing agitation in late stages.[193] Although the major tranquilizers such as thioridazine (Mellaril) and haloperidol often increase cognitive impairment and are poorly tolerated by most de-

mented patients, the physician must sometimes prescribe them for AD patients. These drugs are especially effective in patients with stereotyped paranoid symptomatology or hallucinations; very small doses (e.g., 0.5 to 2 mg haloperidol per day) may be sufficient to get rid of these disturbing symptoms without compromising other functions. Tranquilizers are also needed at times if patients become violent or overly agitated; in these situations again, the smallest possible dose is used, but there is a narrow therapeutic window and sometimes for the protection of the patient and caregiver, doses sufficient to increase cognitive impairment or make the patient lethargic are needed. Whenever possible, alternative tactics should be employed; in some cases, newly designed locked-care facilities permit an agitated patient to wander with minimal or no chemical or direct physical constraint.

General Health and Nutrition

During the initial phase of the illness, AD patients are often in quite good general health and able to continue participating in their customary physical activities. However, as the disorder progresses, and particularly in the very late stages when many are cared for in nursing homes, there is a steady loss of weight. In one study in a geriatric hospital, AD patients weighed 21% less than nondemented patients and 14% less than MID patients and were the only group to continue to lose weight over a 1-year follow-up; the weight loss was not accounted for by an obvious deficit in food intake or by malabsorption[198] nor did serum nutritional markers afford an explanation. It is evident that well-controlled metabolic studies need to be carried out both to provide the clinician with guidelines for dealing with this problem and to determine whether there is indeed a generalized metabolic deficit as some have suggested, a finding that would be important in understanding the pathogenesis of the disease.

Information Resources

Whether acting in the capacity of a one-time consultant or as the principal caregiver, a major role of the physician is to provide the patient and family with information about the diagnosis, prognosis, and community support systems and resources. If the physician is not part of a "team" in which nurses and social workers participate (as described in Chapter 1), the patient and family need to be put into contact with these sources of help. In many communities, informational and other resources specifically targeted for AD and related disorders have been developed. Among the many current sources of help, the Alzheimer Association (formerly the Alzheimer Disease and Related Disorders Association was the first.) The national office of this association* maintains an 800 number and will provide informational material on specific questions of concern to a caregiver or family and will refer the caregiver or family to the local chapter of the association. Local chapters usually provide direct information from experienced caregivers or staff and maintain self-help support groups, the meetings serving as an informal setting for caregivers (and in occasional instances, patients) to exchange information and provide mutual emotional support, often with a professional attending. In addition to the voluntary organization, state governmental agencies, including local Area Agencies on Aging, are often involved in providing information and help to dementia patients. In a number of states, diagnostic and treatment centers have been established with social service and other resources. Nationwide, there are 20 Alzheimer Disease Research Centers supported by grants from the National Institute on Aging; each of these centers has a responsibility to provide education to professionals and caregivers, and most centers provide formal courses open to family members as well as professionals. There are now a number of books directed toward family members; among the books that have received the most widespread acceptance are *The Thirty-six-Hour Day* by Nancy L. Mace and Peter V. Rabins, M.D.,[142] *Understanding Alzheimer's Disease* by Miriam Aronson, Ed.D.,[7] and *Care of Alzheimer Patients: A Manual for Nursing Home Staff* by Lisa Gwyther, ACSW.[75]

When caring for a demented patient, the physician must also be concerned about the caregiver, often a spouse, friend, or adult child. The physical health of caregivers of impaired older adults may be affected; Aronson[7] reported an increase in incidence of hypertension, depression, and heart attack in a cohort of 100 caregivers. There are nearly three times as many stress symptoms, lower life satisfaction, and a markedly reduced ability to pursue social activities or relax in caregivers who live with the patient. More than 50% of such caregivers believed they needed more assistance.[66] Special facilities directed at providing relief to a caregiver, short of institutionalization, are being developed in many communities. These include day-care centers and respite care. When the caregiver situation requires that a nursing home be found, there are now a number of care facilities with special units designed for the AD patient, often with the goals of providing a greater opportunity for the socialization of patients and the freedom to walk and wander within a secured outer perimeter.

Legal Counsel

If the patient is competent at the time of the first examination and a progressive dementing disorder is diagnosed, it is critical to counsel the patient in regard to prognosis and the need to estab-

---

*Alzheimer Association, 70 E. Lake Street, Suite 600, Chicago, IL 60601-5997. The National toll free number is 1-800-621-0379.

lish legal safeguards. One of the most important advances, available in many states, is the *durable power of attorney,* which is available for both financial affairs and health. If a trusted individual is given these powers, then that individual can make decisions in regard to financial and health matters when the patient becomes too impaired to handle his or her own affairs. The durable power of attorney avoids the difficult court proceedings often involved in establishing a conservatorship. In some communities, lawyers specialize in such problems and can provide optimal counsel in this regard.

Is Driving Safe?

In our society, the automobile is an essential element in terms of personal freedom, and removal of driving privileges is difficult for many patients. At the same time, however, patients, their families, and the general public must be protected. Friedland and associates[61] found an eightfold increase in automobile accident rates in AD patients compared with matched controls, an increase that occurred even in mildly to moderately demented individuals. Accidents most frequently occurred at intersections. In part, impairment of geographic knowledge, a frequent deficit in AD patients, may play a role.[12] Some states, including California, now require that demented patients be reported to local health authorities, and the motor vehicle bureau then makes its own determination of whether a driver's license is to be lifted. In states in which the motor vehicle authority is not involved in such determinations, it is the obligation of the physician to counsel the patient and family in this regard.[135]

CONCLUSION

The recent advances in the accuracy of clinical diagnosis of dementia have made its recognition, a major responsi-

bility of the physician, easier to accomplish. Differentiating dementia from delirium and from depression—and realizing that they may often coexist— continues to be crucial, as does the differentiation of dementia from normal mild memory loss. It is important to pinpoint the cause of dementia, in particular because some conditions producing dementia are treatable and even reversible.

The most critical features of the comprehensive workup for the differential diagnosis of dementia include the history, mental status examination, and neurologic examination, as well as appropriate laboratory evaluation. Specific criteria for the diagnosis of definite, probable, and possible AD, established by a joint NINCDS-ADRDA task force, have improved diagnostic accuracy, but AD coexisting with other dementing disorders still remains a diagnostic problem. Among the conditions that can develop in the course of AD are myoclonus, epilepsy, and extrapyramidal findings. Other conditions in which dementia, but not necessarily AD, may develop include PD, PSP, and vascular disease.

When serving as the principal caregiver to the patient with progressive dementia, the physician can often still improve the patient's situation by finding and treating secondary conditions that increase cognitive impairment, prescribing antidepressants and tranquilizers if appropriate, attending to general health and nutrition concerns, and acting as an information resource for the family.

REFERENCES

1. Adams, RA: Disturbances of Cerebrospinal Fluid Circulation, Including Hydrocephalus and Meningeal Reactions. In Adams, RA and Victor, M (eds): Principles of Neurology, ed 4. McGraw-Hill, New York, 1989, pp 507–508.
2. Adams, RD, Fisher, CM, Hakim, S, Ojemann, RG, and Sweet, WH:

Symptomatic occult hydrocephalus with "normal" cerebrospinal fluid pressure. N Engl J Med 273:117–126, 1965.

3. Albert, M, Feldman, RG, and Wills, AL: The "subcortical dementia" of progressive supranuclear palsy. J Neurol Neurosurg Psychiatry 37:121–130, 1974.

4. American Psychiatric Association Task Force on Nomenclature and Statistics: Diagnostic and Statistical Manual of Mental Disorders (DSM-I), ed 1. American Psychiatric Association, Washington, DC, 1952.

5. American Psychiatric Association Task Force on Nomenclature and Statistics: Diagnostic and Statistical Manual of Mental Disorders (DSM-III), ed 3. American Psychiatric Association, Washington, DC, 1980.

6. Armstrong, TP, Hansen, LA, Salmon, D, Maliah, E, Pay, M, and Katzman, R: Documented rapid progression of dementia in a patient with the Lewy body variant of Alzheimer's disease. Abstract: Amer Neurol Assoc, 1989.

7. Aronson, MK (ed): Understanding Alzheimer's Disease. Macmillan, New York, 1988.

8. Barker, MG and Lawton, JS: Nominal aphasia in dementia. Br J Psychiatry 114:1351–1356, 1968.

9. Barnes, RH, Busse, EW, and Friedman, EL: The psychological functioning of aged individuals with normal and abnormal electroencephalograms. II. A study of hospitalized individuals. J Nerv Ment Dis 124:585–593, 1956.

10. Bayles, KA and Boone, DR: The potential of language tasks for identifying senile dementia. J Speech Hear Disord 47:210–217, 1982.

11. Bayles, KA and Tomoeda, CK: Confrontation naming impairment in dementia. Brain Lang 19:98–114, 1983.

12. Beatty, WW and Berstein, N: Geographical knowledge in patients with Alzheimer's disease. J Geriatr Psychiatry Neurol 2:76–82, 1989.

13. Bender, MB: Defects in reversal of serial order of symbols. Neuropsychologia 17:125–138, 1979.

14. Benson, DF: Parkinsonian dementia: Cortical or subcortical? Adv Neurol 40:235–240, 1984.

15. Benson, DF: Commentaries. PET/dementia: An update. Neurobiol Aging 9:87–89, 1988.

16. Berg, L, Danziger, WL, Storandt, M, Coben, LA, Gado, M, Hughes, CP, Knesevich, JW, and Botwinick, J: Predictive features in mild senile dementia of the Alzheimer type. Neurology 34:563–569, 1984.

17. Berlin, L: Presenile sclerosis (Alzheimer's disease) with features resembling Pick's disease. Arch Neurol 61:369–384, 1949.

18. Blessed, G, Tomlinson, BE, and Roth, M: The association between quantitative measures of dementia and of senile change in the cerebral grey matter of elderly subjects. Br J Psychiatry 114:797–811, 1968.

19. Boller, F, Katzman, R, Rascol, A, Signoret, JL, and Christen, Y (eds): Biological Markers of Alzheimer's Disease. Springer-Verlag, Berlin, 1989.

20. Boller, F, Mizutani, T, Roessmann, U, and Gambetti, P: Parkinson disease, dementia, and Alzheimer disease: Clinicopathological correlations. Ann Neurol 7:329–335, 1980.

21. Breen, AR, Larson, EB, Reifler, BV, Vitaliano, PP, and Lawrence, GL: Cognitive performance and functional competence in coexisting dementia and depression. J Am Geriatr Soc 32:132–137, 1984.

22. Brenner, RP, Reynolds, CF, and Ulrich, RF: Diagnostic efficacy of computerized spectral versus visual EEG analysis in elderly normal, demented and depressed subjects. Electroencephalog Clin Neurophysiol 69:110–117, 1988.

23. Broderick, JP, Phillips, SJ, Whisnant, JP, O'Fallon, WM, and Bergstralh, EJ: Incidence rates of stroke in the eighties: The end of the decline in stroke? Stroke 20:577–582, 1989.

24. Brown, RG and Marsden, CD: How common is dementia in Parkinson's disease? Lancet 2:1262–1265, 1984.

25. Brust, JM: Vascular dementia is overdiagnosed. Arch Neurol 45:799–801, 1988.

26. Børgesen, SE: Conductance to outflow of CSF in normal pressure hydrocephalus. Acta Neurochir 71:1–45, 1984.

27. Børgesen, SE and Gjerris, F: The predictive value of conductance to outflow of CSF in normal pressure hydrocephalus. Brain 105:65–86, 1982.

28. Caltagirone, C, Masullo, C, Benedetti, N, and Gainotti, G: Dementia in Parkinson's disease: Possible specific involvement of the frontal lobes. Int J Neurosci 26:15–16, 1985.

29. Caplan, LR and Schoene, WC: Clinical features of subcortical arteriosclerotic encephalopathy (Binswanger disease). Neurology 28:1206–1215, 1978.

30. Celesia, GG and Wanamaker, WM: Psychiatric disturbances in Parkinson's disease. Dis Nerv Syst 33:577–583, 1972.

31. Chui, HC, Teng, EL, Henderson, VW, and Moy, AC: Clinical subtypes of dementia of the Alzheimer type. Neurology 35:1544–1550, 1985.

32. Clarfield, AM: The reversible dementias: Do they reverse? Ann Intern Med 109:476–486, 1988.

33. Coblentz, JM, Mattis, S, Zingesser, LH, Kasoff, SS, Wiseniewski, HM, and Katzman, R: Presenile dementia: Clinical aspects and evaluation of cerebrospinal fluid dynamics. Arch Neurol 29:299–308, 1973.

34. Corsellis, JAN: Mental Illness and the Ageing Brain. Maudsley Monograph, No. 9. Oxford University Press, London, 1962, pp 1–76.

35. Crystal, HA, Horoupian, DS, Katzman, R, and Jotkowitz, S: Biopsy-proved Alzheimer disease presenting as a right patietal lobe syndrome. Ann Neurol 12:186–188, 1982.

36. Cummings, JL and Benson, DF: Dementia: A Clinical Approach. Buttersworth, Boston, 1983, p 40.

37. Cummings, JL and Benson, DF: Subcortical dementia: Review of an emerging concept. Arch Neurol 41:874–879, 1984.

38. Cutler, NR, Haxby, JV, Duara, R, Grady, CL, Moore, AM, Parisi, JE, White, J, Heston, L, and Rapoport, SI: Brain metabolism as measured with PET: Serial assessment in a patient with familial Alzheimer's disease. Neurology (Suppl 1)35:184, 1985.

39. Delaney, P: Dementia: The search for treatable causes. South Med J 75:707–709, 1982.

40. Dementia—Consensus Conference: Differential diagnosis of dementing diseases. JAMA 258:3411–3416, 1987.

41. DePaulo, JR, Jr and Folstein, MF: Psychiatric disturbances in neurological patients: Detection, recognition, and hospital course. Ann Neurol 4:225–228, 1978.

42. Ditter, SM and Mirra, SS: Neuropathologic and clinical features of Parkinson's disease in Alzheimer's disease patients. Neurology 37:754–760, 1987.

43. Dubois, B, Pillion, B, Legault, F, Agid, Y, and Lhermitte, F: Slowing of cognitive processing in progressive supranuclear palsy: A comparison with Parkinson's disease. Arch Neurol 45:1194–1199, 1988.

44. Earnest, MP, Heaton, RK, Wilkinson, WE, and Manke, WF: Cortical atrophy, ventricular enlargement and intellectual impairment in the aged. Neurology 29:1138–1143, 1979.

45. Faden, Al and Townsend, JJ: Myoclonus in Alzheimer disease: A confusing sign. Arch Neurol 33:278–280, 1976.

46. Fillenbaum, GG: Comparison of two brief tests of organic brain impairment, the MSQ and the short portable MSQ. J Am Geriatr Soc 28:381–389, 1980.

47. Fisher, CM: Dementia in Cerebral Vascular Disease. In Toole, JF, Siekert, RG, and Whisnant, JP (eds): Sixth Princeton Conference on Cerebrovascular Disease. Grune & Stratton, New York, 1968, p 232.

48. Fisher, CM: The clinical picture in occult hydrocephalus. Clin Neurosurg 24:270–284, 1977.

49. Folstein, MF, Folstein, SE, and McHugh, PR: "Mini-Mental State": A practical method for grading the cognitive state of patients for the clinician. J Psychiatr Res 12:189–198, 1975.

50. Folstein, MF and McHugh, PR: Dementia Syndrome of Depression. In Katzman, R, Terry, RD, and Bick, KL (eds): Alzheimer's Disease: Senile Dementia and Related Disorders. Aging Series, Vol 7. Raven Press, New York, 1978, pp 87–93.

51. Foster, NL, Chase, TN, Mansi, L, Brooks, R, Fedio, P, Patronas, NJ, and Di Chiro, G: Cortical abnormalities in Alzheimer's disease. Ann Neurol 16:649–654, 1984.

52. Fox, JH, Penn, R, Clasen, R, Martin, E, Wilson, R, and Savoy, S: Pathological diagnosis in clinically typical Alzheimer's disease [letter]. N Engl J Med 313:1419–1420, 1985.

53. Frackowiak, RSJ, Lenzi, GL, Jones, T, and Heather, JD: Quantative measurement of regional cerebral blood flow and oxygen metabolism in man using ^{15}O and positron emission tomography: Theory, procedure and normal values. J Comput Assist Tomogr 4:727–736, 1980.

54. Frackowiak, RSJ, Pozzilli, C, Legg, NJ, Du Boulay, GH, Marshall, J, Lenzi, GL, and Jones, T: Regional cerebral oxygen supply and utilization in dementia: A clinical and physiological study with oxygen-15 and positron tomography. Brain 104:753–778, 1981.

55. Freeman, FR and Rudd, SM: Clinical features that predict potentially reversible progressive intellectual deterioration. J Am Geriatr Soc 33:449–451, 1982.

56. Freyhan, FA, Woodford, RB, and Kety, SS: Cerebral blood flow and metabolism in psychoses of senility. J Nerv Ment Dis 113:449–456, 1951.

57. Friedland, RP: "Normal"-pressure hydrocephalus and the saga of the treatable dementias. JAMA 262:2577–2581, 1989.

58. Friedland, RP, Brun, A, and Budinger, TF: Pathological and positron emission tomographic correlations in Alzheimer's disease. Lancet 1:228, 1985.

59. Friedland, RP, Budinger, TF, Koss, E, and Ober, BA: Alzheimer's disease: Anterior-posterior and lateral hemispheric alterations in cortical glucose utilization. Neurosci Lett 53:235–240, 1985.

60. Friedland, RP, Koss, E, and Jagust, WJ: Lateral hemispheric asymmetries of glucose use in Alzheimer's disease: Relationships to behavior, age of onset and prognosis. J Cereb Blood Flow Metab (Suppl 1)5:S609–S610, 1985.

61. Friedland, RP, Koss, E, and Kumar, A: Motor vehicle crashes in dementia of the Alzheimer's type. Ann Neurol 24:782–786, 1988.

62. Fuld, PA, Katzman, R, Davies, P, and Terry, RD: Intrusions as a sign of Alzheimer dementia: Chemical and pathological verification. Ann Neurol 11:155–159, 1982.

63. Fuld, PA: The Fuld Object Memory Evaluation. Stoelting Instrument Co., Chicago, IL, 1981.

64. Galloway, PG: Antigenic characteristics of neurofibrillary tangles in

progressive supranuclear palsy. Neurosci Lett 91:148–153, 1988.

65. Garcia, CA, Tweedy, JR, and Blass, JP: Underdiagnosis of cognitive impairment in a rehabilitation setting. J Am Geriatr Soc 32:339–342, 1984.

66. George, LK and Gwyther, LP: Caregiver well-being: A multidimensional examination of family caregivers of demented adults. Gerontologist 26:253–259, 1986.

67. Goodin, DS and Aminoff, MJ: Electrophysiological differences between subtypes of dementia. Brain 109:1103–1113, 1986.

68. Goodin, DS and Aminoff, MJ: Electrophysiological differences between demented and nondemented patients with Parkinson's disease. Ann Neurol 21:90–94, 1987.

69. Goodin, DG, Squires, KC, and Starr, A: Long latency event-related components of the auditory evoked potential in dementia. Brain 101:635–648, 1978.

70. Gordon, EB and Sim, M: The E.E.G. in presenile dementia. J Neurol Neurosurg Psychiatry 30:285–291, 1967.

71. Gowers, WR: A Manual of Diseases of the Nervous System. P Blakiston & Son, Philadelphia, 1888.

72. Graff-Radford, NR and Godersky, JC: Normal pressure hydrocephalus: Onset of gait abnormality before dementia predicts a good surgical outcome. Arch neurol 43:940–942, 1986.

73. Graff-Radford, NR, Rezai, K, Godersky, JC, Eslinger, PJ, Damasio, H, and Kirchner, PT: Regional cerebral blood flow in normal pressure hydrocephalus. J Neurol Neurosurg Psychiatry 50:1589–1596, 1987.

74. Groen, JJ and Endtz, LJ: Hereditary Pick's disease: Second re-examination of a large family and discussion of other hereditary cases, with particular reference to electroencephalography and computerized tomography. Brain 105:443–449, 1982.

75. Gwyther, L: Care of Alzheimer Patients: A Manual for Nursing Home Staff. American Health Care Association/Alzheimer's Disease and Related Disorder Association (ADRDA) Inc., New York/Chicago, 1985.

76. Haase, GR: Diseases Presenting as Dementia. In Wells, CE (ed): Dementia, ed 2. FA Davis, Philadelphia, 1977, p 26.

77. Hachinski, VC: Cerebral Blood Flow: Differentiation of Alzheimer's Disease from Multi-Infarct Dementia. In Katzman, R, Terry, R, and Bick, KL (eds): Alzheimer's Disease: Senile Dementia and Related Disorders. Aging Series, Vol 7. Raven Press, New York, 1978, pp 97–104.

78. Hachinski, VC, Iliff, LD, Phil, M, Zilhka, E, Du Boulay, GH, McAllister, VL, Marshall, J, Russell, RWR, and Symond, L: Cerebral blood flow in dementia. Arch Neurol 32:632–637, 1975.

79. Hachinski, VC, Lassen, NA, and Marshall, J: Multi-infarct dementia: Cause of mental deterioration in the elderly. Lancet 2:207–210, 1974.

80. Hachinski, VC, Potter, P, and Merskey, H: Leuko-araiosis. Arch Neurol 44:21–29, 1987.

81. Hakim, AM and Mathieson, G: Dementia in Parkinson disease: A neuropathologic study. Neurology 29:1209–1214, 1979.

82. Hansen, L, Salmon, D, Galasko, D, Masliah, E, Katzman, R, DeTeresa, R, Thal, L, Pay, MM, Hofstetter, R, Klauber, MR, Rice, V, Butters, N, and Alford, M: The Lewy body variant of Alzheimer's disease: A clinical and pathological entity. Neurology 40:1–8, 1989.

83. Hansen, LA, DeTeresa, R, Tobias, H, Alford, M, and Terry, RD: Neocortical morphometry and cholinergic neurochemistry in Pick's disease. Am J Pathol 131:507–518, 1988.

84. Heston, LL, White, JA, and Mastri,

AR: Pick's disease. Arch Gen Psychiatry 44:409–411, 1987.

85. Hietanen, M and Teravainen, H: The effect of age of disease onset on neuropsychological performance in Parkinson's disease. J Neurol Neurosurg Psychiatry 51:244–249, 1988.

86. Hoehn, MM and Yahr, MD: Parkinsonism: Onset, progression and mortality. Neurology 17:427–442, 1967.

87. Horoupian, DS, Pick, P, and Spigland, I: Acquired immuno deficiency syndrome and multiple tract degeneration in a homosexual man. Ann Neurol 15:502–505, 1984.

88. Horoupian, DS, Thal, L, Katzman, R, Terry, RD, Davies, P, Hirano, A, DeTeresa, R, Fuld, PA, Petito, C, Blass, J, and Ellis, JM: Dementia and motor neuron disease: Morphometric, biochemical, and Golgi studies. Ann Neurol 16:305–313, 1984.

89. Hoyer, S: Blood Flow and Oxidative Metabolism of the Brain in Different Phases of Dementia. In Katzman, R, Terry, RD, and Bick, KL (eds): Alzheimer's Disease and Related Disorders, Aging Series, Vol 7. Raven Press, New York, 1978, p 219.

90. Hughes, CP, Berg, L, Danziger, WL, Coben, LA, and Martin, RL: A new clinical scale for the staging of dementia. Br J Psychiatry 40:566–572, 1982.

91. Hussey, F, Schanzer, B, and Katzman, R: A simple constant-infusion manometric test for measurement of CSF absorption. II. Clinical studies. Neurology 20:665–680, 1970.

92. Ingvar, DH, Brun, A, Hagsberg, B, and Gustafson, L: Regional Cerebral Blood Flow in the Dominant Hemisphere in Confirmed Cases of Alzheimer's Disease, Pick's Disease, and Multi-Infarct Dementia: Relationship in Clinical Symptomatology and Neuropathological Findings. In Katzman, R, Terry, RD, and Bick, KL (eds): Alzheimer's Disease: Senile Dementia and Related Disorders. Aging Series, Vol 7. Raven Press, New York, 1978, p 203.

93. Inzitari, D, Diaz, F, Fox, A, Hachinski, VC, Steingart, A, Lau, C, Donald, A, Wade, J, Mulic, H, and Marskey, H: Vascular risk factors and leuko-araiosis. Arch Neurol 44:42–47, 1987.

94. Jagust, WJ, Friedland, RP, Budinger, TF, Koss, E, and Ober, B: Longitudinal studies of regional cerebral metabolism in Alzheimer's disease. Neurology 38:909–912, 1988.

95. Jellinger, K: Neuropathological aspects of dementia resulting from abnormal blood and cerebrospinal fluid dynamics. Acta Neurol Belg 76:83–102, 1976.

96. Jellinger, K: Pathologic correlates of dementia in Parkinson's disease. Arch Neurol 44:690–691, 1987.

97. Joachim, CL, Morris, JH, and Selkoe, DJ: Clinically diagnosed Alzheimer's disease: Autopsy results in 150 cases. Ann Neurol 24:50–56, 1988.

98. Johannesson, G, Hagberg, B, Gustafson, L, and Ingvar, DH: EEG and cognitive impairment in presenile dementia. Acta Neurol Scand 59:225–240, 1979.

99. Joynt, RJ: Vascular dementia: Too much or too little? Arch Neurol 45:801, 1988.

100. Kahn, RL, Goldfarb, AI, Pollack, M, and Peck, A: Brief objective measures for the determination of mental status in the aged. Am J Psychiatry 117:326–328, 1960.

101. Kaszniak, AW, Garron, DC, Fox, JH, Bergen, D, and Huckman, M: Cerebral atrophy, EEG slowing, age, education, and cognitive functioning in suspected dementia. Neurology 29:1273–1279, 1979.

102. Katz, B, Rimmer, S, Iraqui, V, and Katzman, R: Abnormal pattern electroretinogram in Alzheimer's disease: Evidence for retinal ganglion cell degeneration? Ann Neurol 26:221–225, 1989.

103. Katzman, R: Normal Pressure Hydrocephalus. In Wells, CE (ed): Dementia, ed 2. FA Davis, Philadelphia, 1977, pp 69–92.

104. Katzman, R: Clinical Approach to Dementia. In Smith, JL (ed): Neuro-Ophthalmology Focus, 1980. Masson Publ USA, New York, 1980, pp 341–346.

105. Katzman, R: Early detection of senile dementia. Hosp Prac June:61–76, 1981.

106. Katzman, R: Vascular Disease and Dementia. In Yahr, MD (ed): H Houston Merritt Memorial Volume. Raven Press, New York, 1983, pp 153–176.

107. Katzman, R: Clinical Presentation of the Course of Alzheimer's Disease: The Atypical Patient. In von Hahn, HP (ed): Interdisciplinary Topics in Gerontology, Vol 20. S Karger, Basel, 1985, pp 12–18.

108. Katzman, R: Differential Diagnosis of Dementing Illnesses. In Hutton, JT (ed): Neurologic Clinics. WB Saunders, Philadelphia, 1986, pp 329–340.

108a. Katzman, R: Controversies in family practice: Should a major imaging procedure (CT or MRI) be required in the workup of dementia? An affirmative view. J Fam Pract 31:401–405, 1990.

108b. Katzman, R: Unpublished material.

109. Katzman, R, Aronson, M, Fuld, PA, Kawas, C, Brown, T, Morgenstern, H, Frishman, W, Gidez, L, Eder, H, and Ooi, WL: Development of dementia in an 80-year-old volunteer cohort. Ann Neurol 25:317–324, 1989.

110. Katzman, R, Brown, T, Fuld, P, Peck, A, Schechter, R, and Schimmel, H; Validation of a Short Orientation–Memory–Concentration test of cognitive impairment. Am J Psychiatry 140:734–739, 1983.

111. Katzman, R and Hussey, F: A simple constant-infusion manometric test for measurement of CSF absorption. I. Rationale and method. Neurology 20:534–544, 1970.

112. Katzman, R and Kawas, C: The Evolution of the Diagnosis of Dementia: Past, Present, and Future. In Poeck, K and Freund, HJ (eds): Neurology: Clinical Aspects of the Dementias. Springer-Verlag, Berlin/Heidelberg, 1986, pp 43–49.

113. Katzman, R, Lasker, B, and Bernstein, N: Advances in the Diagnosis of Dementia: Accuracy of Diagnosis and Consequences of Misdiagnosis of Disorders Causing Dementia. In Terry, RD (ed): Aging and the Brain, Vol 32. Raven Press, New York, 1988, pp 17–62.

114. Katzman, R, Terry, RD, DeTeresa, R, Brown, T, Davies, P, Fuld, P, Renbing, X, and Peck, A: Clinical, pathological, and neurochemical changes in dementia: A subgroup with preserved mental status and numerous neocortical plaques. Ann Neurol 23:53–59, 1988.

115. Kendell, RE: The stability of psychiatric diagnoses. Br J Psychiatry 124:352–356, 1974.

116. Khachaturian, ZS: Diagnosis of Alzheimer's disease. Arch Neurol 42:1097–1105, 1985.

117. Kiloh, LG: Pseudodementia. Acta Psychiatr Scand 37:336–351, 1961.

118. Kinkel, WR, Jacob, L, Polachini, I, Bates, V, and Heffner, RR: Subcortical arteriosclerotic encephalopathy (Binswanger's disease). Computed tomographic, nuclear magnetic resonance, and clinical correlations. Arch Neurol 42:951–959, 1985.

119. Knights, EG and Folstein, MF: Unsuspected emotional and cognitive disturbances in medical patients. Ann Intern Med 87:723–724, 1977.

120. Koto, A, Rosenberg, G, Zingesser, LH, Horoupian, D, and Katzman, R: Syndrome of normal pressure hydrocephalus possible relation to hypertensive and arteriosclerotic vasculopathy. J Neurol Neurosurg Psychiatry 40:73–79, 1977.

121. Kuhl, DE, Phelps, ME, Markham, CH, Metter, EJ, Riege, WH, and Winter, J: Cerebral metabolism and

atrophy in Huntington's disease determined by 18-FDG and computed tomographic scan. Ann Neurol 12:425–434, 1982.

122. Kuller, LH: Incidence rates of stroke in the eighties: The end of the decline in stroke? (editorial) Stroke 20:841–843, 1989.

123. Larson, EB: Diagnostic tests in the evaluation of dementia: A prospective study of 200 elderly outpatients. Arch Intern Med 146:1917–1922, 1986.

124. Larson, EB, and Clarfield, AM: Controversies in family practice: Should a major imaging procedure (CT or MRI) be required in the workup of dementia? An opposing view. J Fam Pract 31:405–410, 1990.

125. Larson, EB, Kukull, WA, Buchner, D, and Reifler, BV: Adverse drug reactions associated with global cognitive impairment in elderly persons. Ann Intern Med 107:169–173, 1987.

126. Larson, EB, Reifler, BV, Sumi, SM, Canfield, CG, and Chinn, NM.: Diagnostic evaluation of 200 elderly outpatients with suspected dementia. J Gerontol 40:536–543, 1985.

127. Lassen, NA, Munck, O, and Tottey, ER: Mental function and cerebral oxygen consumption in organic dementia. Arch Neurol Psychiatry 77:126–133, 1957.

128. Leverenz, J and Sumi, M: Parkinson's disease in patients with Alzheimer's disease. Arch Neurol 43:662–664, 1986.

129. Lieberman, A, Dziatolowski, M, Kupersmith, M, Serby, M, Goodgold, A, Korein, J, Goldstein, M: Dementia in Parkinson disease. Ann Neurol 6:355–359, 1979.

130. Lijtmaer, H, Fuld, PA, and Katzman, R: Prevalence and malignancy of Alzheimer's disease. Arch Neurol 33:304, 1976.

131. Lindenbaum, J, Healton, EB, Savage, DG, Brust, JCM, Garrett, TJ, Podell, ER, Marcell, PD, Stabler, SP, and Allen, RH: Neuropsychiatric disorders caused by cobalamin deficiency in the absence of anemia or macrocytosis. N Engl J Med 318:1720–1728, 1988.

132. Loranger, AW, Goodell, H, McDowell, FH, Lee, JE, and Sweet, RD: Intellectual impairment in Parkinson's syndrome. Brain 95:405–412, 1972.

133. Love, S, Quijada, S, Saitoh, T, Davies, P, and Terry, RD: Immunohistochemical demonstration of Alz-50 antigen and ubiquitin in Pick bodies and neurofibrillary tangles. Soc Neurosci Abstr 13:1151, 1987.

134. Love, S, Saitoh, T, Quijada, S, Cole, G, and Terry, RD: Alz-50, ubiquitin and tau immunoreactivity of neurofibrillary tangles, Pick bodies and Lewy bodies. J Neuropathol Exp Neurol 47:393–405, 1988.

135. Lucas-Blaustein, MJ, Filipp, L, and Dugan, C: Driving in patients with dementia. J Am Geriatr Soc 36:1087–1091, 1988.

136. Lying-Tunell, U: Psychotic symptoms in normal-pressure hydrocephalus. Acta Psychiatr Scand 59:415–419, 1979.

137. McAdam, W and Robinson, RA: Senile intellectual deterioration and the electroencephalogram: A quantitative correlation. J Ment Sci 102:819–825, 1956.

138. McGeachie, RE, Fleming, JO, Sharer, LR, and Hyman, RA: Diagnosis of Pick's disease by computed tomography. J Comput Assist Tomogr 3:113–115, 1979.

139. McHugh, PR and Folstein, MF: Psychopathology of Dementia: Implications for Neuropathology. In Katzman, R (ed): Congenital and Acquired Cognitive Disorders. Raven Press, New York, 1979, p 17.

140. McKhann, G, Drachman, D, Folstein, M, Katzman, R, Price, D, and Stadlan, EM: Clinical diagnosis of Alzheimer's disease: Report of the NINCDS-ADRDA Work Groups under the auspices of Department of Health and Human Services

Task Force on Alzheimer's Disease. Neurology 34:939–944, 1984.

141. McQuinn, BA and O'Leary, DH: White matter lucencies on computed tomography, subacute arteriosclerotic encephalopathy (Binswanger's disease), and blood pressure. Stroke 18:900–905, 1987.

142. Mace, NL and Rabins, PV: The 36-Hour Day. Johns Hopkins Press, Baltimore, 1981.

143. Mahendra, B: Depression and dementia: The multi-faceted relationship. Psychological Med 15:227–236, 1985.

144. Marsden, C and Harrison, M: Outcome of investigation of patients with presenile dementia. Br Med J 2:249–252, 1972.

145. Martin, WE, Loewenson, RB, and Resch, JA: Parkinson's disease—Clinical analysis of 100 patients. Neurology 23:783–790, 1973.

146. Marttila, RJ and Rinne, UK: Dementia in Parkinson's disease. Acta Neurol Scand 54:431–441, 1976.

147. Mas, JL, Bousser, M-G, Lacombe, C, and Agar, N: Hyperlipidemic dementia. Neurology 35:1385–1387, 1985.

148. Masliah, E, Galasko, D, Wiley, CA, and Hansen, LA: Lobar atrophy with dense core (brainstem type) Lewy bodies in a patient with dementia. Acta Neuropathol 80:453–458, 1990.

149. Mattis, S: Mental Status Examination for Organic Mental Syndrome in the Elderly Patient. In Bellack R and Karasu B (eds): Geriatric Psychiatry. Grune & Stratton, New York, 1976.

150. Mayer-Gross, W and Guttmann, E: The problem of general as against focal symptoms in cerebral lesions: A contribution to general symptomatology. J Ment Sci 82:222–241, 1936.

151. Mayeux, R, Stern, Y, and Spanton, S: Heterogeneity in dementia of the Alzheimer type: Evidence of subgroups. Neurology 35:453–461, 1985.

152. Mesulam, M-M: Slowly progressive aphasia without generalized dementia. Ann Neurol 11:592–598, 1982.

153. Mindham, RHS: Psychiatric symptoms in parkinsonism. J Neurol Neurosurg Psychiatry 33:188–191, 1970.

154. Mitsuyama, Y and Takamiya, S: Presenile dementia with motor neuron disease in Japan—A new entity? Arch Neurol 36:592–593, 1979.

155. Moberg, PJ, Pearlson, GD, Speedie, LJ, Lipsey, JR, Strauss, ME, and Folstein, SE: Olfactory recognition: Differential impairments in early and late Huntington's and Alzheimer's diseases. J Clin Exp Neuropsychol 9:650–664, 1987.

156. Morris, JC, Cole, M, Banker, BQ, and Wright, D: Hereditary dysphasic dementia and the Pick-Alzheimer spectrum. Ann Neurol 16:455–466, 1984.

157. Morris, JC, McKeel, DW, Fulling, K, Torack, RM, and Berg, L: Validation of clinical diagnostic criteria for Alzheimer's disease. Ann Neurol 24:17–22, 1988.

158. Muller, HF and Schwartz, G: Electroencephalograms and autopsy findings in geropsychiatry. J Gerontol 33:504–513, 1978.

159. Murphy, C, Gilmore, MM, Seery, CS, Salmon, DP, Lasker, BR: Olfactory thresholds are associated with degree of dementia in Alzheimer's disease. Neurobiol Aging 11:465–469, 1990.

160. National Institute on Aging Task Force (NIA): Senility reconsidered: Treatment possibilities for mental impairment in the elderly. JAMA 244:259–263, 1980.

161. Neary, D, Snowden, JS, Mann, DMA, Bowen, DM, Sims, NR, Northen, B, Yates, PO, and Davison, AN: Alzheimer's disease: A correlative study. J Neurol Neurosurg Psychiatry 49:229–237, 1986.

162. Nelson, JR and Goodman, SJ: An evaluation of the cerebrospinal fluid infusion test for hydroceph-

alus. Neurology 21:1037–1053, 1971.

163. O'Brien, MD: Vascular dementia is underdiagnosed. Arch Neurol 45:797–798, 1988.

164. O'Connor, KP, Shaw, JC, and Ongley, CO: The EEG and differential diagnosis in psychogeriatrics. Br J Psychiatry 135:156–162, 1979.

165. Obrist, WD: Electroencephalography in Aging and Dementia. In Katzman, R, Terry, RD, and Bick, KL (eds): Alzheimer's Disease: Senile Dementia and Related Disorders. Aging Series, Vol 7. Raven Press, New York, 1978, pp 227–232.

166. Olszewski, J: Subcortical arteriosclerotic encephalopathy: Review of the literature on the so-called Binswanger's disease and presentation of two cases. World Neurol 3:359–374, 1962.

167. Parkinson, J: An Essay on the Shaking Palsy (1817). In Critchley, M (ed): James Parkinson. MacMillan, London, 1955, p 153.

168. Patterson, JV, Michalewski, HJ, and Starr, A: Latency variability of the components of auditory event-related potentials to infrequent stimuli in aging, Alzheimer-type dementia, and depression. Electroencephalogr Clin Neurophysiol (Wien) 71:450–460, 1988.

169. Penttilä, M, Partanen, JV, Soininen, H, and Riekkinen, PJ: Quantitative analysis of occiptal EEG in different stages of Alzheimer's disease. Electroencephalogr Clin Neurophysiol (Wien) 60:1–6, 1985.

170. Perry, EK, Curtis, M, Dick, DJ, Candy, JM, Atack, JR, Bloxham, CA, Blessed, G, Fairbairn, A, Tomlinson, BE, and Perry, RH: Cholinergic correlates of cognitive impairment in Parkinson's disease: Comparisons with Alzheimer's disease. J Neurol Neurosurg Psychiatry 48:413–421, 1985.

171. Pfeffer, RI, Kurosaki, TT, Harrah, CH, Chance, JM, and Filos, S: Measurement of functional activities in older adults in the community. J Gerontol 37:323–329, 1982.

172. Pfeiffer, E: A short portable mental status questionnaire for the assessment of organic brain deficit in elderly patients. J Am Geriatr Soc 23:433–441, 1975.

173. Pollock, M and Hornabrook, RW: The prevalence, natural history and dementia of Parkinson's disease. Brain 89:429–448, 1966.

174. Price, RW, Brew, B, Sidtis, J, Rosenblum, M, Scheck, AC, and Cleary, P: The brain in AIDS: Central nervous system HIV-1 infection and the AIDS dementia complex. Science 239:586–592, 1988.

175. Prohovnik, I, Mayeux, R, Sackeim, HA, Smith, G, Stern, Y, and Alderson, PO: Cerebral perfusion as a diagnostic marker of early Alzheimer's disease. Neurology 38:931–937, 1988.

176. Quinn, NP, Rossor, MN, and Marsden, CD: Dementia and Parkinson's disease—Pathological and neurochemical considerations. Br Med J 42:86–90, 1986.

177. Rabins, PV: The prevalence of reversible dementia in a psychiatric hospital. Hosp Commun Psychiatry 32:490–492, 1981.

178. Rae-Grant, A, Blume, W, Lau, C, Hachinski, VC, Fisman, M, and Merskey, H: The electroencephalogram in Alzheimer-type dementia. A sequential study correlating the electroencephalogram with psychometric and quantitative pathologic data. Arch Neurol 44:50–54, 1987.

179. Rapoport, SI: Positron emission tomography in normal aging and Alzheimer's disease. Gerontology (Suppl 1)32:6–13, 1986.

180. Reding, M, Haycox, J, and Blass, J: Depression in patients referred to a dementia clinic: A three-year prospective study. Arch Neurol 42:894–896, 1985.

181. Reding, M, Haycox, J, Wigforss, K, Brush, D, and Blass, JP: Follow-up of patients referred to a dementia service. J Am Geriatr Soc 32:265–269, 1984.

182. Reifler, BV: Arguments for abandoning the term pseudodementia. J

Am Geriatr Soc 30:665–668, 1982.

183. Reifler, B, Larson, E, and Hanley, R: Coexistence of cognitive impairment and depression in geriatric outpatients. Am J Psychiatry 139:623–626, 1982.

184. Reisberg, B, Ferris, SH, DeLeon, MJ, and Crook, T: The global deterioration scale for assessment of primary degenerative dementia. Am J Psychiatry 139:1136–1139, 1982.

185. Rezek, DL, Morris, JC, Fulling, KH, and Gado, MH: Periventricular white matter lucencies in senile dementia of the Alzheimer type and in normal aging. Neurology 37:1365–1368, 1987.

186. Roberts, MA, McGeorge, AP, and Caird, FI: Electroencephalography and computerized tomography in vascular and non-vascular dementia in old age. J Neurol Neurosurg Psychiatry 41:903–906, 1978.

187. Roca, RP, Klein, LE, Kirby, SM, McArthur, JC, Vogelsang, GB, Folstein, MF, and Smith, CR: Recognition of dementia among medical patients. Arch Intern Med 144:73–75, 1984.

188. Roman, GC: Senile dementia of the Binswanger type: A vascular form of dementia in the elderly. JAMA 258:1728–1788, 1987.

189. Ron, MA, Toone, BK, Garralda, ME, and Lishman, WA: Diagnostic accuracy in presenile dementia. Br J Psychiatry 134:161–168, 1979.

190. Rosen, WG, Terry, RD, Fuld, PA, Katzman, R, and Peck, A: Pathological verification of ischemic score in differentiation of dementias. Ann Neurol 7:486–488, 1980.

191. Rosenberg, GA, Kornfeld, M, Stovring, J, and Bicknell, JM: Subcortical arteriosclerotic encephalopathy (Binswanger): Computerized tomography. Neurology 29:1102–1106, 1979.

192. Roth, M and Hopkins, B: Psychological test performance in patients over sixty. I. Senile psychosis and the affective disorders of old age. J Ment Sci 99:439–449, 1953.

193. Rubin, EH, Morris, JC, and Berg, L: The progression of personality changes in senile dementia of the Alzheimer's type. J Am Geriatr Soc 35:721–725, 1987.

194. St Clair, D, Blackburn, I, Blackwood, D, and Tyrer, C: Measuring the course of Alzheimer's disease: A longitudinal study of neuropsychological function and changes in P3 event-related potential. Br J Psychiatry 152:48–54, 1988.

195. Selkoe, DJ: Amyloid β-protein precursor and the pathogenesis of Alzheimer's disease. Cell 58:611, 1989.

196. Shuttleworth, EC: Atypical presentations of dementia of the Alzheimer type. J Am Geriatr Soc 32:485–490, 1984.

197. Shuttleworth, EC, Huber, SJ, and Paulson, GW: Depression in patients with dementia of Alzheimer type. J Natl Med Assoc 79:733–736, 1987.

198. Singh, S, Mulley, GP, and Losowsky, MS: Why are Alzheimer's patients thin? Age ageing 17:21–28, 1988.

199. Smith, JS and Kiloh, LG: The investigation of dementia: Results in 200 consecutive admissions. Lancet 1:824–827, 1981.

200. Soininen, H, Partanen, J, Riekkinen, P, Laulumaa, V, and Paakkonen, A: Changes in absolute EEG power values in the follow-up of Alzheimer's disease (abstr). Neurology (Suppl 1)39:170, 1989.

201. Sokoloff, L: Cerebral Blood Flow and Metabolism in the Differentiation of Dementias: General Considerations. In Katzman, R, Terry, RD, and Bick, KL (eds): Alzheimer's Disease: Senile Dementia and Related Disorders. Aging Series, Vol 7. Raven Press, New York, 1978, pp 197–212.

202. Steele, JC, Richardson, JC, and Olszewski, J: Progressive supranuclear palsy. Arch Neurol 10:333–359, 1964.

203. Steingart, A, Hachinski, VC, Lau, C, Fox, AJ, Fox, H, Lee, D, Inzitari,

D, and Merskey, H: Cognitive and neurologic findings in demented patients with diffuse white matter lucencies on computed tomographic scan (leuko-araiosis). Arch Neurol 44:36–39, 1987.

204. Sudarsky, L and Simon, S: Gait disorder in late-life hydrocephalus. Arch Neurol 44:263–267, 1987.

205. Sulkava, R, Haltia, M, Paetau, A, Wilkstrom, J, and Palo, J: Accuracy of clinical diagnosis of primary degenerative dementia: Correlation with neuropathological findings. J Neurol Neurosurg Psychiatry 46:9–13, 1983.

206. Sweet, RD, McDowell, FH, Feifenson, JS, Loranger, AW, and Goodell, H: Mental symptoms in Parkinson's disease during chronic treatment with levodopa. Neurology 26:305–310, 1976.

207. Symond, L and Dorsch, NW: Use of long-term intracranial pressure measurement to assess hydrocephalic patients prior to shunt surgery. J Neurosurg 42:258–273, 1975.

208. Taylor, MA, Abrams, R, Faber, R, and Almy, G: Cognitive tasks in the mental status examination. J Nerv Ment Dis 168:167–170, 1980.

209. Tomlinson, BE: Morphological Changes in Dementia in Old Age. In Smith, WL and Kinsbourne, M (eds): Aging and Dementia. Spectrum, New York, 1977, p 24.

210. Tomlinson, BE, Blessed, G, and Roth, M: Observations on the brains of demented old people. J Neurol Sci 11:205–242, 1970.

211. Tomlinson, BE and Henderson, G: Some Quantitative Cerebral Findings in Normal and Demented Old People. In Terry, RD and Gershon, S (eds): Neurobiology of Aging. Aging Series, Vol 3. Raven Press, New York, 1976, pp 183–204.

212. Tomlinson, BE, Irving, D, and Blessed, G: Cell loss in the locus coeruleus in senile dementia of Alzheimer type. J Neurol Sci 49:419–429, 1975.

213. Walshe, FMR: Diseases of the Nervous System. Williams & Wilkins, Baltimore, 1951.

214. Wells, CE (ed): Dementia, ed 2. FA Davis, Philadelphia, 1977.

215. Wells, CE: Diagnostic Evaluation and Treatment in Dementia. In Wells, CE (ed): Dementia, ed 2. FA Davis, Philadelphia, 1977, p 247.

216. Wells, CE: Pseudodementia. Am J Psychiatry 136:895–900, 1979.

217. Whitehead, A: The Clinical Psychologist's Role in Assessment and Management. In Isaacs, AD and Post, F (eds): Studies in Geriatric Psychiatry. John Wiley & Sons, New York, 1978, p 153.

218. Whitehouse, PJ, Hedreen, JC, White, CL, III, and Price, DL: Basal forebrain neurons in the dementia of Parkinson disease. Ann Neurol 13:243–248, 1983.

219. Wikstrom, J, Paetau, A, Palo, J, Sulkava, R, and Haltia, M: Classic amyotrophic lateral sclerosis with dementia. Arch Neurol 39:681–683, 1982.

220. Wilkins, DE, Hallett, M, Berardelli, A, Walshe, T, and Alvarez, N: Physiologic analysis of the myoclonus of Alzheimer's disease. Neurology 34:898–903, 1984.

221. Withers, E and Hinton, J: Three forms of the clinical tests of the sensorium and their reliability. Br J Psychiatry, 119:1–8, 1971.

222. Wolf, PA, D'Agostino, RB, Sytkowski, PA, Kannel, WB, Kase, C S, Stokes, J, III, and Belanger, AJ: Secular trends in risk factors and declining mortality from stroke: The Framingham study. Neurology (Suppl 1)39:284, 1989.

223. Yoshimura, M: Pathological basis for dementia in elderly patients with idiopathic Parkinson's disease. Eur Neurol (Suppl 1)28:29–35, 1988.

Chapter 8

ALZHEIMER DISEASE AND COGNITIVE LOSS

Robert Terry, M.D., and Robert Katzman, M.D.

Alzheimer disease (AD) is now increasingly recognized as one of the major health problems in countries such as the United States that have a growing population of elderly individuals.[321] Lewis Thomas,[329] the scientist and essayist, described AD as "the disease of the century," and a *British Medical Journal* editorial spoke of "the quiet epidemic." AD accounts for at least 65% of cases of senile dementia and is a major public health problem, with between 1.5 and 3 million persons afflicted in the United States today.[96,167,339] AD accounts for 40% to 50% of nursing home admissions[175] and between 120,000 and 200,000 excess deaths per year. The prevalence of AD will triple by the year 2050 if preven-

tion or effective treatment is not discovered.[163] The annual cost of this disease in the United States in 1990 will exceed $80 billion. Thus, the fiscal impact of AD is enormous.

ALZHEIMER DISEASE: AN HISTORICAL NOTE

In 1907, Alois Alzheimer,[6] a psychiatrist and neuropathologist, first used newly available silver stains in studying the brain of a 51-year-old patient with a progressive fatal dementia. He found the neuritic plaques (NP) and first described the neurofibrillary tangles (NFT) of what is now termed *Alzheimer disease.* Because Alzheimer's patient was in her presenium, AD was initially considered to be a presenile dementia with onset before age 65, but Alzheimer subsequently found the same changes in the brain of a patient with senile dementia. For many decades there was intense debate as to the identity of the presenile and senile forms. However, a number of studies have indicated that senile and presenile forms cannot be distinguished on the basis of clinical, pathologic, or chemical findings. The light microscopic aspects and the ultrastructure of the NP and NFT are the same in the presenile form of AD as in senile dementia. This identity of presenile and senile forms of AD is now ac-

207

cepted by almost all neurologists and pathologists.

THE AGE-SPECIFIC PREVALENCE AND INCIDENCE OF DEMENTIA AND ALZHEIMER DISEASE

Accumulating epidemiologic evidence from studies in many countries indicates that both prevalence and incidence rise exponentially with age[68a,129,222,293] as shown in Figure 8–1. The question of whether there is a peak in incidence in the ninth decade is uncertain since the number of subjects living to the tenth decade is very small in the studies cited. In a prospective study of a volunteer cohort initially aged 75 to 85, Katzman and colleagues[171] found that the incidence of new cases of dementia exceeded that of heart attacks and the incidence of new cases of AD was as great as that of stroke (Table 8–1). The best evidence to date suggests that in the tenth decade one third of the population will be cognitively intact, 30% to 40% will have AD, and the remainder will suffer from age-associated memory impairment, vascular dementia, or other disorders,[170] although one study reports that 47% of those over the age of 85 meet the clinical criteria for the diagnosis of AD.[96]

We have reviewed elsewhere the prevalence and malignancy of AD, both the presenile and senile forms of this disorder.[167] Excellent community surveys of organic dementias have been carried out in northern Europe and the United States. The prevalence of *severe dementia*, that is, dementia to such a degree as to significantly impair independent functioning, for persons over age 60 is between 4% and 5% in most studies.[38,95,176,216,246,290] These studies undoubtedly underestimate the amount of dementia today, since they were carried out two or three decades ago, and the mean age of the population over 65 is continually rising. Thus, an early study in Newcastle by Kay and associates[176] yielded a figure of 4.5%, but has been increased to 6.2% in a more recent analysis of the same region.[268] If the age-specific prevalence of dementia in the population continues to hold and no progress is made in prevention or treatment of this disorder, the number of cases will more than double by the year 2025 and more than quintuple by the year 2040 as the "baby boomers" reach maximum susceptibility.[339] The data of Tomlinson and co-workers[331,332] and others[159] indicated that 55% to 65% of all patients with organic dementia have AD (although Tomlinson increased this estimate in a later paper[330]), and the estimate of AD patient numbers in the United States with *severe* dementia is about 900,000 cases in 1990. If there are two patients with mild to moderate dementia for every patient with severe dementia, the total number of AD cases would be about 2.7 million, a number remarkably close to the 3 million obtained if the recent East Boston prevalence figure of 10.3% of those over the age 65 is multiplied by the estimate of persons over age 65 in the United States in 1990.[96] The total with dementia would then be about 4.1 million, a number that might well grow to 20 million by the year 2040 if ways of preventing or treating AD are not found.

One estimate of the malignancy of AD depended on the fact that there is a marked decrease in life expectancy based on the age of onset of these symptoms, as was earlier summarized by

Table 8–1 EVENTS, BRONX AGING STUDY: 434 SUBJECTS FOLLOWED FOR 1584 PERSON-YEARS

	N	Rate/100 Person-Years
Dementia	56	3.5
AD	32	2.0
MID/MIX	15	1.0
Other	9	0.6
Myocardial infarct	50	3.1
Stroke	26	1.6

Note: MID = multi-infarct dementia; MIX = mixed vascular and Alzheimer disease.
Source: Data from Katzman et al.[171]

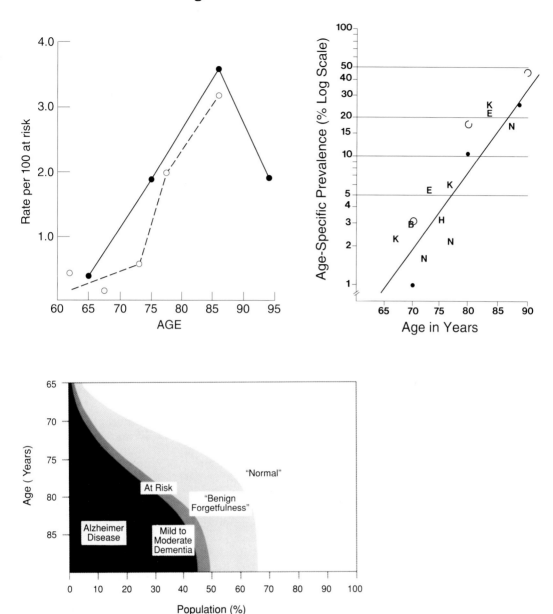

Figure 8–1. *A,* The incidence of development of dementia per 100 individuals at risk per year. ● = Data for women in Lundby study (Hagnell et al,[129]). ○ = Data for men in Baltimore Longitudinal Study (Sluss et al,[297]). (Adapted from Katzman,[170] p 70, with permission.) *B,* Age-specific prevalence of dementia in Shanghai study using the mean of each age group (O) compared to several European studies summarized in figure form by Cross, PS and Gurland, BJ[68a]; Bollerup, B[32a]; Essen-Möller, E[95]; Helgason, H[37a]; Kay, K[176]; and Nielsen, N.[216] The large circles represent the East Boston Study of Evans et al.[96] (Adapted from Zhang et al,[365] p 436) *C,* Changing patterns of cognitive abilities as a function of age. (Adapted from Katzman,[170] p 71)

Wang and Whanger.[344] If one assumes the remaining life span of those with severe dementia would be reduced by half by the presence of AD, then more than 120,000 deaths per year are due to this disorder[167] and if the Evans's estimates of prevalence[96] are correct, then it would be 200,000 per year, placing

AD in a tie with stroke as the third most common cause of death.

THE PATHOLOGY OF ALZHEIMER DISEASE

In considering the pathology of AD, it should be noted that all of the morphologic lesions to be described are found, although to a much lesser degree, in the brain tissue of cognitively normal aged people. It seems probable, therefore, that the disease represents a threshold phenomenon, that is, a situation in which clinical symptoms do not appear until after a certain number of tissue alterations occur. Each person may well have a different threshold based on his or her own reserve. That reserve, in turn, is dependent on the extent of redundancy in the neuronal circuitry, which is related to the number of active synapses subserving each cerebral function. As the number and concentration of structural and chemical abnormalities increase, no functional changes need to be expected until the individual threshold is reached. Thereupon, a further increase in abnormalities results in clinical symptoms, which continue to increase in severity. It is this latter, suprathreshold stage of structural, chemical, and clinical abnormalities that we recognize as disease. It is very probable that most people, even with a few lesions, would not progress significantly, in terms of lesions or symptoms, toward the threshold, even if they were to live much longer.

Loss of Brain Substance, Neurons, and Synapses

The degree of brain atrophy to be found in AD is remarkably variable. In some cases the whole brain weight may be as little as 850 g; but in other cases, similarly demented, the weight has been as high as 1250 g. Certainly 950 to 1100 g is the common range. In a small series of patients aged 70 to 89, but one in which the authors[322] could be confident of the clinical and pathologic normalcy of the control group, the average weight of the AD brain specimens was 1050 g, about 100 g or nearly 9% less than age-matched normal cases. This difference was statistically significant ($P < 0.05$).

This weight loss corresponds principally to shrinkage of cerebral white matter. The cortical ribbon may display significant thinning in a diffuse or a focal fashion, but it is often not apparent at all. Measurements of the cortical thickness in the frontal and superior temporal regions in the same series mentioned above[322] did not demonstrate a statistically significant difference between the mean cortical thickness in the AD cases and that of the controls, although they differed by about 10% (Table 8–2).

Usually, however, the gyri in AD are somewhat narrowed, leaving wider sulci (Fig. 8–2). Similarly, the gyral white matter and centrum ovale are diminished, leaving enlarged lateral ventricles, especially in their frontal and temporal poles (Fig. 8–3). The third ventricle may also participate in this di-

Table 8–2 BRAIN WEIGHT AND CORTICAL THICKNESS

	Normal	AD
Fixed brain weight (g):		
Range	930–1350 (n = 10)	918–1150 (n = 14)
Mean	1152	1055
Thickness (mm):		
Midfrontal cortex	1.71–3.07 (n = 12)	1.57–2.77 (n = 18)
Mean	2.43	2.19
Superior temporal cortex	2.05–3.09	1.44–2.70
Mean	2.49	2.26

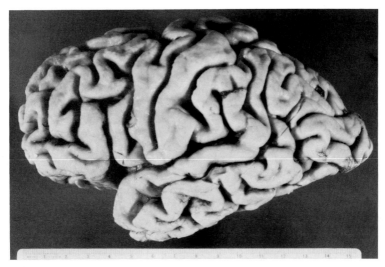

Figure 8–2. The lateral view of the left cerebral hemisphere from a patient with severe AD. The leptomeninges have been stripped away to reveal moderate gyral atrophy and widening of the sulci. The atrophy is quite diffuse but spares to some extent the postcentral gyrus. The fixed weight of this whole brain was 1050 g. (From Katzman and Terry,[173] p 55, with permission.)

latation, and the massa intermedia may be thinned.

Although cerebral atrophy is usually quite diffuse, it is often particularly prominent in the region of the hippocampal gyrus and frontal lobes. The temporal and parietal lobes are frequently involved, but one often sees relative sparing of the paracentral region and the occipital pole. The hippocampus is usually quite atrophic. The basal ganglia and thalami, other than the

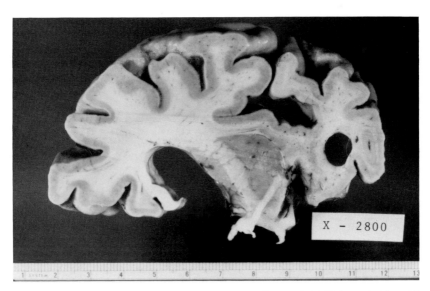

Figure 8–3. A coronal section of the same specimen as in Figure 8–2. Note again the widened sulci, especially on the superior convexity and the insula. The left lateral ventricle, including its temporal horn, is dilated. The cortex is visibly thin in the third frontal gyrus, the temporal insular cortex, and in the rostral hippocampal gyrus. The basal ganglia are intact, but the amygdaloid nucleus just dorsal to the temporal horn is also somewhat shrunken. (From Katzman and Terry,[173] p 56, with permission.)

massa intermedia, are not grossly shrunken. The midbrain and brainstem also appear normal on gross examination. The cerebellum is slightly atrophic as a rule, but probably not more so than in the normal elderly except when the patient has been malnourished. In these latter cases, one quite frequently finds mild atrophy of the folia in the rostral vermis. It is worth re-emphasizing that a gross diagnosis of AD may often be in error because of the great overlap between the atrophy associated with normal aging and that accompanying the disorder.

Although a decrease in tissue water, especially from the extracellular space, may partially account for the loss of brain mass in normal aging, and even more in AD, this is not measurable in the living human under current circumstances. A normal age-related shrinkage of large cortical neurons has been verified in the cerebral cortex, and in some other areas of the central nervous system (CNS) (see Chapter 2), and

is more severe in AD. This latter work has been done by means of computerized image analysis after it was determined with the instrument that almost all recognizable glial somata had a cross-sectional area—in the histologic preparations used for the study—of less than 40 μm^2, whereas more than 95% of neurons had somata greater than 40 μm^2. It was found that the number of glia in the midfrontal region did not change in AD, compared with age-matched normals. In the superior temporal region, the glia were increased by 15% in the diseased group, but this difference was not statistically significant. Small neurons, measuring between 40 and 90 μm^2, were significantly decreased by 11% in the superior temporal gyrus. The most important loss of neurons concerned those that measure more than 90 μm^2. In AD, the frontal area lost 40% of these large neurons and the temporal gyrus lost 46% (Fig. 8–4).[322] The loss of large neurons is greater in the younger patient than in

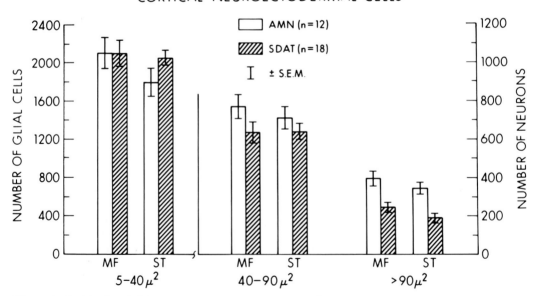

Figure 8–4. The four left bars represent glial cells (<40 μm^2). There are no significant differences between aged-matched normal (AMN) and AD (SADT) in the midfrontal (MF) ad superior temporal (ST) areas. As to neurons, the middle four bars show small neurons that are significantly different ($P < 0.05$) in MF but not in ST. The large neurons in the right four bars display major differences in quantity, significant at the 0.01 level of confidence. (From Katzman and Terry,[173] p 57, with permission.)

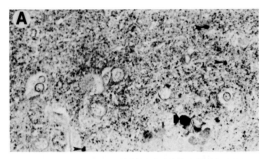

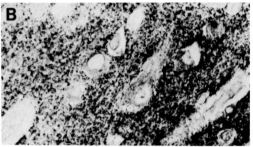

Figure 8–5. Comparison of synaptophysin immunoreactivity between AD (*A*) and normal control (NC) (*B*) in layer 5 of the parietal cortex. In AD the decrease in the neuropil density is due to a diminution in the number of grains, which are presumed to be immunoreactive boutons. Additionally, abnormal dilated terminals are noted in the neuropil (*arrowheads*) and in the plaque (*arrow*). (From Masliah et al,[202] p 236, with permission.)

the older, relative to age-matched controls.[132]

The neuronal loss is thus confined to the pyramidal neurons, particularly in layers III and V. The ratio between small and large neurons rises significantly. A dramatic loss is observed in the synapses as measured immunohistochemically with an antibody to the synaptic vesicle component, synaptophysin (Fig. 8–5).[202] The loss of synapses is present in all layers of the neocortex. Synaptic loss is also present in other structures, including the hippocampus.[130]

As a consequence of the neuronal loss, the neuron-glia ratio has been found to be diminished by 27% in the frontal and 33% in the superior temporal areas.[322] Immunohistologic studies of fibrous astrocytes,[131,132] utilizing an antibody to the glial filament acidic protein (GFAP), revealed no significant dif-

ference in the molecular layer between the controls and the demented cases. However, in the cellular portion of the cerebral cortex, that is, layers II through VI, fibrous astrocytes were increased fourfold in AD. This does not necessarily indicate proliferation of astrocytes, because the change from protoplasmic to fibrous form would give the same results.

Image analysis study[322] showed that neuroectodermal cell bodies occupied 20% less space in AD neocortex than in the normal brain. The increased neuropil volume in the diseased tissue might be occupied by the increased volume of fibrous astrocytes as compared with normal glia, or by increased extracellular space.

Other studies showed that in AD, cortical neuronal configurations also changed as revealed by Golgi preparations.[281] These alterations were similar to those in normal aging (see Chapter 2), but greatly exaggerated. The pyramidal cell bodies of the cortex took on a bumpy outline, or sometimes a bell shape. There was a loss of dendrites, especially from the basilar or horizontal arbor. In the familial form, Scheibel[280] reported a tufting of dendritic outgrowth not found in sporadic cases, but this has not been confirmed. Numbers of dendritic spines are also lost in the process. The number of spines per unit length of dendrite was said to be significantly below that in normal elderly.[206] Synaptic counts were not made, but were presumed low under these circumstances. Two other studies of synapses have also found a marked reduction in these structures.[73,130]

Our own synaptic studies[201] utilized an antibody against synaptophysin, a synapse-specific protein localized in the membrane of the synaptic vesicle, thus demonstrating presynaptic boutons. Densitometric analysis of the immunocytochemical reaction in the AD neocortex provided figures that were about 50% below normal in each layer of the cortex. This work strongly indicates that presynaptic boutons are markedly diminished in the disease.

The decrease is even greater than that of the pyramidal neurons within the same cortical areas. One might, therefore, postulate that the degeneration starts in the axonal terminals and later involves the perikaryon. We found a powerful correlation between scores on in vivo tests of cognition and the density of synapses as measured by microdensitometry of the immunoreaction. The correlation coefficients were higher here than with any other morphologic assay such as plaque or tangle density, brain weight, and the like.

As in the normal elderly, lipofuscin is increased in the neurons of AD, but not beyond that of the normal aged.[195]

NP and NFT

The microscopic lesions on which the diagnosis of AD ultimately rests are NP and NFT. Large concentrations of these lesions in the neocortex have a very high correlation with the presence of dementia.[32] Many cases of AD have great numbers of NP in the neocortex, but only very few or no NFT.[320] Even in these cases, however, the NP are made up of neurites that contain the characteristic abnormal fibers. This form of the disease with many NP and few or no neocortical NFT is found particularly in the very elderly.[320] In this study, there was no significant difference between cases with few or many neocortical NFT in regard to the degree of dementia, degree of neuronal loss, plaque count, or choline acetyltransferase (ChAT) level. Although the rate of change of mental status was somewhat greater, it was not statistically significant. However, Constantinidis[53] reported that AD brains with few neocortical NFT were associated with a shorter clinical course. It cannot be said on this basis, however, that NFT would necessarily have followed had the patient lived longer. Small numbers of NP, it must be remembered, are to be found in the normal elderly neocortex in the great majority of patients reaching their eighth decade (see Chapter 2). In the hippocampus of the normal elderly, there are almost always at least a few NP and NFT. Significant numbers of neocortical NFT are essentially always accompanied by clinical dementia.

In AD, many of both lesions are also to be found in certain deeper gray areas.[153,154] In addition to the hippocampus, there is marked involvement of the entorhinal cortex[150] and often of the amygdala and prepiriform cortex.[251] The olfactory bulb is usually involved.[18,94] The substantia innominata is always affected with neuron loss and NFT[350] presence (although one exception has been noted[227] and may be of great functional significance since this is the major source of the cholinergic input to the neocortex[162]). NFT and NP are also noteworthy in the claustrum, hypothalamus, periaqueductal region, locus ceruleus, and in the pontine tegmentum in the region of the floor of the rostral fourth ventricle, including the raphe cells believed to give rise to the serotonergic system.[146,333] On the other hand, certain other areas are almost invariably spared.

Some very primitive amyloid plaques, visible faintly with thioflavine, more strongly with Bielschowsky or antiamyloid antisera, are found in the striatum, pallidum, and cerebellar molecular layer. The noncholinergic nuclei of the thalamus often contain moderate numbers of NP, which usually have a dense amyloid content. However, the thalamic reticular nucleus, which has a very strong cholinergic input from the nucleus basalis of Meynert (nbM), has only very rare NP.[201] Nevertheless, some Alz-50-positive neurites are present in this reticulate nucleus of the thalamus.[335] It has been suggested that NP develop because of degeneration of neurons in the nbM, but that hypothesis is distinctly weakened by the absence of plaques in the thalamic reticular nucleus because that area is supplied by the same neurons of the nbM that send other efferents to the neocortex. The presence of Alz-50 reactivity, even in the absence of plaques, might be related to the formation of

NFT in the neurons of the nbM, but the presence of the antigen revealed by that immunoreactivity clearly does not lead to NP formation.

Although a diffuse type of plaque may be seen in the cerebellum of AD brains and some normal elderly, using an immunostain to β/A4-amyloid protein epitopes, these deposits do not normally stain with Congo red or thioflavine S, indicating that typical amyloid has not been formed.[361] In some very severely affected cases of AD, there are deposits of dense amyloid in the cerebellar cortex. These are most common in the border region between Purkinje and granule cell layers. Although it was suggested originally that such cerebellar plaques are only in familial cases, this is clearly not accurate. They would seem more related to the severity of disease than to any particular pattern of inheritance. The spinal cord and medulla are essentially free of NP and NFT, and NFT are not to be found in the cerebellum.

Whether they are found in the cortex or deep gray areas or brain stem, NFT occupy the cell body of medium and large neurons. Although they can oc-casionally be seen with routine oversight stains, such as hematoxylin and eosin (H & E) (Fig. 8–6), they are greatly underestimated in frequency or even missed altogether if only these methods are used for histology. The use of either of two major types of relevant special stains is much better. Most commonly used is a silver impregnation such as that of Bielschowsky. Various modifications of these procedures make it possible to use the stains on frozen sections or paraffin- or celloidin-embedded material. In general, the silver stains, which cause a clumping of the abnormal fibers rendering them in black or dark brown, are more complex, more difficult, and more expensive than the less commonly used thioflavine-S stain. While this preparation is slightly inconvenient in that it must be viewed with ultraviolet illumination, the inconvenience is more than compensated by the ease of the technique and the extraordinary resolution and sensitivity to the abnormal structures that it reveals (Fig. 8–7). Another useful technique, the use of Congo red stain, is viewed with polarized illumination.

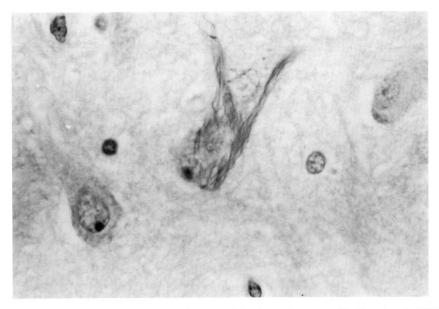

Figure 8–6. A hematoxylin and eosin stain of pyramidal cells, with a neurofibrillary tangle (NFT) in the middle one and two unaffected neurons on either side. This tangle can be seen more clearly than most in H & E stain. (From Katzman and Terry,[173] p 59, with permission.)

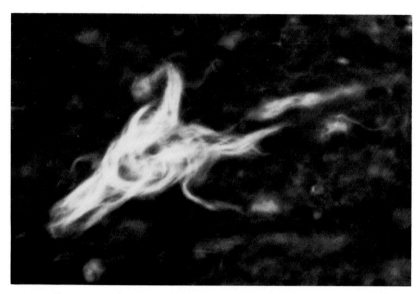

Figure 8–7. A thioflavine S-stained neuron with a well-formed NFT. The paired helical filaments (PHFs) glow bright yellow in ultraviolet illumination. (From Katzman and Terry,[173] p 59, with permission.)

This is also quite sensitive, but sometimes gives false negatives.

With any of these techniques, the NFT appears to the light microscopist as a mass of tangled fibers within the cytoplasm of the affected neurons. Electron microscopy reveals the abnormal fibers making up the NFT each to be composed of a pair of twisted filaments, thus the term *paired helical filaments* (PHF).[178,357] Each element of the pair measures approximately 10 nm in width, and they cross each other at regular 80 nm intervals. Cross sections of the PHF usually have the appearance of an arc with a concentrically placed dot, but a complete circle may be seen. The difference presumably depends on the thickness of the section and the interval of the PHF that it includes. These tangles of PHF traverse the cytoplasm, pushing aside most of its normal constituents. Sometimes a significant number of normal neurofilaments is included among the PHF. These measure 10 nm in width and have short side arms at frequent intervals (Figs. 8–8 and 8–9). Also occasionally seen in the tangle are 15-nm-wide tubules similar

to those found in progressive supranuclear palsy (PSP).

It should be noted that NFT with PHF are not unique to AD but also occur as a prominent feature of dementia pugilistica, Guam-Parkinson-dementia complex, and Down syndrome, and are also found at times in brains of patients with subacute sclerosing leukoencephalopathy, postencephalitic PD, and Kuf's disease.[356]

CHEMICAL
CHARACTERIZATION
OF THE PHF

The chemical characterization of the PHF has been hindered because of the insolubility of PHF in a variety of protein solvents.[289] Brain subcellular fractions enriched in PHF are, however, relatively easy to isolate, and such fractions are highly antigenic. Moreover, antibodies raised to a variety of normal filamentous proteins can readily be tested against both NFT in tissue sections and against purified PHF fractions. It has been shown that antibodies to the higher molecular

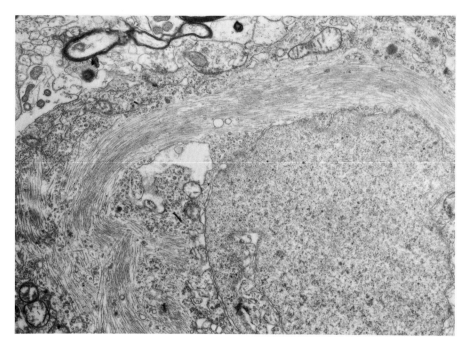

Figure 8–8. An unremarkable neuronal nucleus is at lower right. The cytoplasm is traversed by a large band of abnormal neurofibers, making up the NFT. The other cytoplasmic contents, as well as the surrounding neuropil, are normal. (From Terry and Wisniewski,[324] p 145, with permission.)

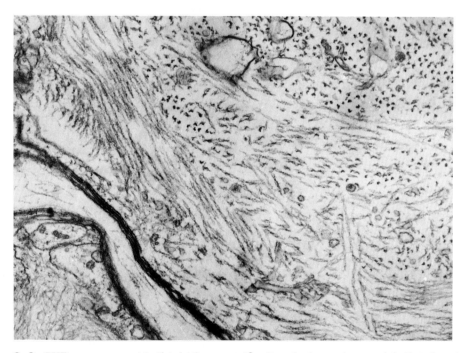

Figure 8–9. PHFs are apparent in this higher magnification electron micrograph both in longitudinal and cross section. In longitudinal section they are seen to cross over at regular 80-nm intervals. Most of the cross sections appear to be crescentic. (From Terry, Gonatas, and Weiss,[319] p 269, with permission.)

weight, phosphorylated, neurofilament proteins and to the microtubule-associated proteins, MAP-2 and tau, immunostain NFT and PHF.[285] In particular, there is now a consensus that tau epitopes are important constituents of PHF.[83] In turn, antibodies raised against PHF fractions stain phosphorylated tau preparations.

Sternberger and colleagues[302] observed that certain antibodies to phosphorylated epitopes of neurofilament proteins stained tangles, whereas antibodies to nonphosphorylated neurofilament proteins stain normal axons. They postulated the existence of an imbalance among specific kinases in the Alzheimer brain. Saitoh and associates have shown that there is a decrease in the activity of protein kinase C (PKC),[52,275] specifically of its β-2 form in Alzheimer neocortex, the other isoenzymes (α, β-1, and γ) being within normal limits.[200] Not only is β-2 PKC immunostaining decreased in neurons in AD brain but also much of the remaining immunostaining is localized extracellularly in NP cores in association with the β/A4-amyloid peptide. Antibodies to casein–kinase II vividly immunostain NFT.[151] One can speculate that these aberrant kinases play a specific role in the pathogenesis of NP and NFT, but this needs to be demonstrated.

The most effective antibodies in detecting NFT and PHF are tau antibodies and Alz-50; the latter is an antibody initially raised against cytoplasmic fractions obtained from AD nbM.[359] Alz-50 reacts with a phosphorylated tau epitope near the carboxy terminal of the tau molecule. Alz-50 and tau antibodies normally stain neuronal somata in early development, the antigen being re-expressed in AD and Down syndrome.[359]

Tau is a relatively heat stable protein isolated initially from purified microtubular fractions. In normal mature tissue, tau or tau fragments are involved in side-arm microtubule attachment. Normally, tau is expressed in neuronal cell bodies in the developing brain but is found primarily as the phosphorylated form in axons in normal adult brain; hence, its presence in NFT[39] in the perikarya is highly abnormal. The tau present in NFT and PHF is known to be highly phosphorylated, but as yet there is no agreement as to whether only one of the four known tau isoforms is present.

Electron microscopic immunocytochemistry conclusively establishes that tau is an important component of the PHF. A current issue is whether the PHF is actually an abnormal polymer of phosphorylated tau or whether there is another protein present that accounts for the helical fibrous structures. A few groups have reported evidence for the presence of the *amyloid β/A4-protein precursor* (APP) in PHF, but this is not a unanimous finding.

Both tau and Alz-50 antigenicity in AD brain are found not only in NFT but also in the degenerating neurites that comprise the NP and in the thickened neurites found in the neocortex independent of the presence of NP and NFT as well as in some neuronal bodies that do not show thioflavine or silver staining, both indicative of NFT. It has been suggested that an increase in tau and Alz-50 immunoreactivity defines the presence of the AD process independently of whether NP or NFT are also expressed, although Probst and colleagues claim that senile plaque neurities do not immunostain with PHF or tau antibodies unless NFT are present in neocortex.[247] However, tau antibodies and Alz-50 also immunostain NFT in PSP and Pick bodies.[189]

Antibodies to ubiquitin, a protein associated with protein degradation, immunostain a variety of structures in degenerating brains, including the Lewy body (LB) in PD, Pick bodies of Pick disease, Mallory bodies of alcoholic liver disease, and Rosenthal fibers in astrocytes as well as NFT in AD.[189,236] The LB is an eosinophilic neuronal inclusion containing neurofilaments[121] often found in the brain stem in PD. In fact, the staining of LB by ubiquitin has made it easy to identify these structures in neocortex where their presence on H & E stains is subtle. This has led to the identification of the LB variant of AD,[134,135,260] a topic described in Chapter 8.

THE NP AND AMYLOID

The plaque of AD is found in the presenium as well as in the senium and is composed of neurites, as opposed to the plaque of multiple sclerosis or of kuru. It was for these reasons that Terry and Wisniewski[325,326] proposed that it be called the *neuritic plaque*, rather than the senile plaque. The number of NP in the neocortex have been well correlated with the presence of dementia by Blessed and associates.[32] This correlation is much less significant if normals are excluded. As indicated above, these NP are found in the neuropil of neocortex, paleocortex, claustrum, nbM, hypothalamus, and in the dorsorostral brainstem.[146] Very rarely, the granular

layer of the cerebellar cortex contains a few typical NP, although NFT are not present in the cerebellum.

The typical mature lesion has a central core of extracellular amyloid fibers, each 9 to 10 nm wide, and with a hollow lumen (Figs. 8–10 and–11). The amyloid core is surrounded by abnormal neurites, which are distended with lamellar lysosomes,[310] mitochondria, and often PHF[319] (Fig. 8–12). Most of the neurites involved in the plaque are, in fact, preterminal axons, and the abnormality may extend into the terminal bouton.[122] Glial fibers extend from adjacent fibrous astrocytic somata into the plaque as a dense mesh.[279] Microglia-like cells are also often present, and occasionally one finds within these latter cells amyloid fibrils that are not surrounded by any membrane, indicating that they have probably been produced by this cell rather than having been phagocytosed by them.[324] The extracellular amyloid need not be compact in all

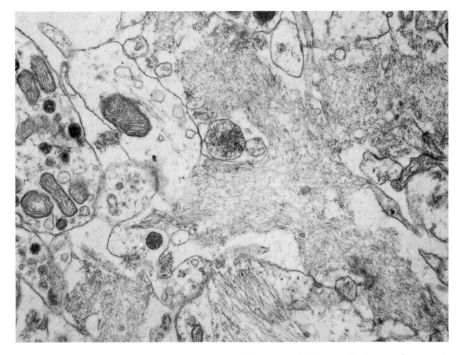

Figure 8–10. The filaments in the center comprise the extracellular amyloid core of a neuritic plaque (NP). Abnormal neurites are apparent at the left, containing degenerating mitochondria and lysosomes. The neurite at bottom contains a small number of PHFs. (From Terry, Gonatas, and Weiss,[319] p 269, with permission.)

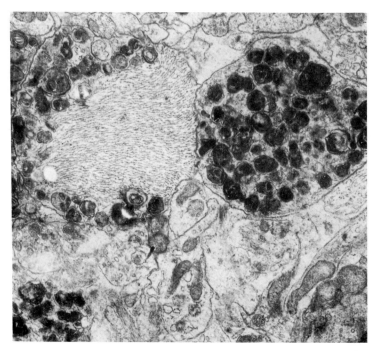

Figure 8–11. Two abnormal neurites comprising part of an NP occupy the center of this electron micrograph. The one on the left contains PHFs and numerous lysosomes. The one on the right is crowded with these organelles. (From Katzman and Terry,[173] p 63, with permission.)

instances but is often dispersed in wisps in the interstices between the cellular elements of the plaque.[87] Most NP are well displayed with Congo red, thioflavine-S, or silver stains (Fig. 8–13).

Rarely, one finds what has been called a hypermature or burned-out plaque.[324] This is made up of a larger compact mass of amyloid surrounded by fibrous astrocytic processes, but without abnormal neurites. The structure of the early plaque is still debated. It has been proposed that the first abnormality is a cluster of neurites that, as they degenerate, attract microglia that then form and deposit the amyloid.[319] On the other hand, it has also been proposed that the amyloid arrives first, either as a local product or penetrating through an adjacent capillary, the wall of which has become permeable for unknown reasons[356] (although not all NP are necessarily associated with a penetrating capillary[213]). Loose deposits of interstitial amyloid are now

considered to be very primitive plaques. Deposits of amyloid precursor peptides in cerebellar molecular layer as well as in forebrain regions are called diffuse plaques and are best recognized immunohistochemically or with Bielschowsky preparations.[360,361] Such deposits have been observed in the cerebral cortex and cerebellum of some nondemented individuals in the absence of plaques or tangles.[74,311]

In amyloid angiopathy, that is, amyloid infiltration of vascular walls, the involved vessels may be small or medium size in the leptomeninges or small arteries within the cortex itself (Fig. 8–14). These abnormalities are to be found in most, but not all, cases of AD.[261] In some instances the amyloid infiltrates the adjacent cerebral parenchyma, where it may be associated with abnormal neurites to comprise a typical NP. Very rarely, amyloid angiopathy may be found without accompanying AD. Even here the amyloid reacts with anti-β-protein antisera. A few cases

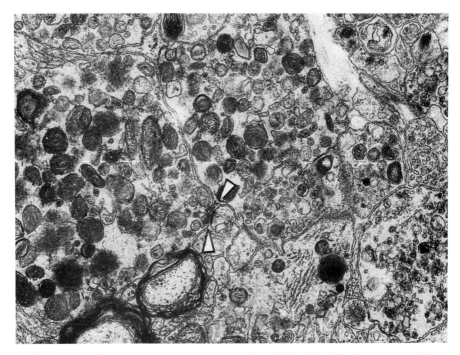

Figure 8–12. Several abnormal neurites are apparent containing lamellar lysosomes and degenerating mitochondria. Another neurite containing PHF is at the bottom. The neurite at the left is a markedly swollen axonal bouton. The normal synaptic membranes, normal gap *(arrows)* and normal dendritic bouton occupy the center. (From Terry and Wisniewski,[325] with permission.)

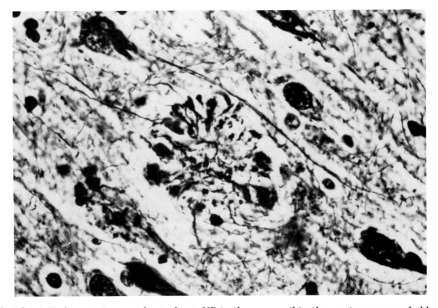

Figure 8–13. A Bodian stain revealing a large NP in the neuropil in the center surrounded by several neurons occupied by NFTs. Both lesions are argentophilic. (From Katzman and Terry,[173] p 64, with permission.)

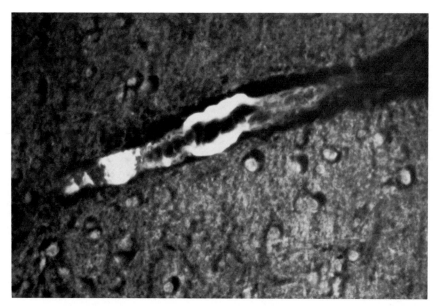

Figure 8–14. Amyloid stained with thioflavine S and photographed with ultraviolet illumination has replaced much of the wall of this cortical vessel in a segmental fashion. The amyloid is white in this representation. (From Katzman and Terry,[173] p 66, with permission.)

have been reported in which cerebral hematoma was apparently caused by bleeding from the affected vessels, especially in combination with surgical intervention or trauma.[334]

Major advances have been made in the past several years in regard to the delineation of the NP and cerebrovascular amyloid present in the AD brain[231]: the amyloid peptide has been sequenced; its precursor protein, the chromosome 21 gene that encodes the precursor protein, and the gene promoter region have been characterized. These advances required the partial characterization of the amyloid peptide, a task complicated by the relative insolubility of these β-pleated fibrils. However, the amyloid found in meningeal blood vessels in selected AD cases proved to be more tractable to solubilization and purification. Thus, the partial characterization of β/A4-amyloid peptide and its amino acid sequence by Glenner and Wong[116] opened the field to the powerful methods of modern molecular biology, because the cerebrovascular amyloid is similar or identical to the NP amyloid. Using the partial amino

acid sequence, various investigators were able to create probes that have led to the identification of the precursor protein mRNA, the corresponding cDNA, and the location of the encoding gene. At the same time, other investigators using antibodies raised against epitopes in various portions of the precursor protein have provided information that has both shed light on the development of plaques and led to new and intriguing questions.

The amyloid fibrils found in the core of the NP and in the walls of some cerebral blood vessels are polymers of a 42- to 43-amino acid peptide, variously termed the β-amyloid peptide, the A-4 peptide, or, currently, the β/A4-peptide.[116,117,203,244,287,288] This peptide is an abnormal degradation product of a precursor protein (the *amyloid β/A4-protein precursor*, or *APP*) present in the membranes of most cells in the body but is in especially high concentration at synaptic junctions. The basic form of the precursor protein is a 695-amino acid residue protein, with an extended extracellular portion, a single transmembrane region, and a short intracel-

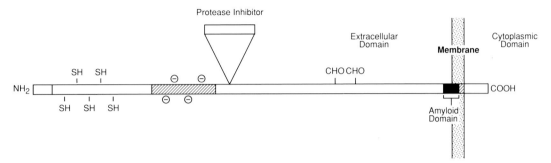

Figure 8–15. Amyloid β-protein precursor (APP), showing the extracellular N-terminal region.

lular carboxy terminal.[91,166,252,272,314] As shown in Figure 8–15 the extracellular N-terminal region contains a cysteine-rich region; next, there is a region of the molecule that contains a number of acidic amino acids; then a lengthy portion with two sites appropriate for N-glycosylation.[91] Although APP is sometimes associated with proteoglycans,[284] the nature of the sugar moieties normally present has not as yet been identified. Significantly, the β-amyloid peptide portion includes part of the transmembrane region and a short extracellular region. This finding is of great importance in terms of the method of production of the β-amyloid peptide. The gene, encoding the precursor molecule, has been found to have 16 exons; the β-amyloid portion is encoded both by portions of exons 14 and 15, the latter encoding the entire transmembrane region.[188] Hence, the β-amyloid peptide cannot be formed by alternative or aberrant splicing but must be a degradation product. Proteolytic enzymes can easily split the β-amyloid peptide from the N-terminal region of the precursor protein; however, the site of proteolysis in the transmembrane region (a site easily susceptible to trypsin and other proteases) is not normally accessible to proteolysis because of the protection afforded by the membrane. The production of β-amyloid must, therefore, involve a perturbation of the membrane with the extracellular accumulation of the precursor molecule due to increased secretion[235] or decreased or abnormal intracellular lysosomal deg-

radation as suggested by G. Cole and T. Saitoh (personal communication).

Two major alternative forms of the precursor molecule have been identified. Both have inserts of a "Kunitz"-type serine protease inhibitor,[179,240,315] the two alternative forms differing in the length of the insert. The 751-amino acid form appears to be more common than the 770-amino acid molecule. Many cells throughout the body produce one or more forms of APP. In peripheral tissues, the Kunitz-containing molecular forms predominate. The primary 695-amino acid APP is produced predominantly by neurons, which also produce comparable quantities of the 751-amino acid form. It is possible that the 695-amino acid APP is particularly affected in AD cortex.[160,161] It is of interest that another serine protease inhibitor, α_1-antichymotrypsin, is also present in association with the brain amyloid deposits in AD.[1]

The gene for APP is located on chromosome 21 in the 21q21 region, immediately adjacent to the portion of the chromosome that is an obligate region for the production of Down syndrome in trisomy 21 (Fig. 8–16).[118,253] There is then an added significance to the site of the gene because all individuals with trisomy 21 develop the pathologic changes of AD, that is, the NP and NFT, by age 50. Recently, Rumble and associates[272] and Giaccone and colleagues[115] have reported that the deposits of extracellular amyloid peptide and APP (as determined by immunohistochemistry) appear in the brains of Down individu-

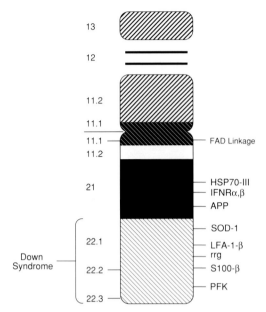

Figure 8–16. The gene for ABPP located on chromosome 21 in the 21q21 region, immediately adjacent to the portion of the chromosome that is an obligate region for the production of Down syndrome in trisomy 21.

als at a much earlier age than do neuritic degeneration and the formation of typical NP. These deposits do not contain amyloid fibrils and, hence, are not stained by Congo red or thioflavine. They are also devoid of degenerating neurities. Similar deposits of amyloid peptide immunoreactivity had previously been found in the brains of cognitively normal elderly patients who did not have AD as well as in AD brains.[311] These deposits may correspond to so-called diffuse plaques observed on Bielschowsky silver stains. Tagliavini and co-workers,[311] Rumble and associates,[272] and Selkoe[286] have suggested the possibility that these deposits precede and could lead to the formation of classical NP and the instigation of the AD process. The early age of onset of AD changes in the Down brains, would, according to this theory, be caused by excess precursor molecule expressed in the Down brain due to the extra APP gene present on the third chromosome 21. In AD, there is not an increased

gene dosage.[214,239,312] However, the APP gene promoter region[277] contains both heat-shock and c-fos elements—as well as numerous GC groups typical of housekeeping genes, that is, genes needed by all cells for maintenance of function. The heat-shock promoter element is known to be responsive not only to rapid increases in temperature but also to hypoxia, trauma, and other stresses. Most groups have not found a consistent change in APP or APP message in AD brain, but one group has reported an increase in the production of the 751-amino acid form as observed by in vitro hybridization.[160,161] If an increase in the production of the precursor protein contributes in any way to the pathogenesis of AD, then one method of preventing or delaying the disorder would be to develop drugs that inhibit the action of the promoters of this protein.

It is in fact likely that the precursor protein is required for the survival or health of many cells.[352] For example, Saitoh and associates[276] have shown that the antisense APP cDNA transfected into fibroblasts impaired the growth of these cells in tissue culture. Conditioned medium from other cells, but particularly cells transfected with the APP cDNA and expressing high levels of APP, was potent in restoring the growth of the antisense-transfected cells. These data also show that APP can be released from cells into the medium; the authors suggest that APP may have an autocrine function, perhaps in growth regulation.

Although APP deposits may precede neuritic involvement in the formation of NP,[90] the presence of APP deposits, however, cannot account solely for the development of NP. These deposits occur in regions of the brain that are usually free of plaques in AD, notably the cerebellum. Moreover, dementia does not appear to develop until there is evidence of neurite involvement with subsequent synaptic loss.[86] The trigger for the latter has not yet been demonstrated.

Other Pathologic Features

GRANULOVACUOLAR BODY

Two other microscopic lesions are almost invariably found only in the hippocampus of patients with AD, or in very small numbers in the normal elderly. The first is the granulovacuolar body of Simchowicz,[294] first described in 1911 (Fig. 8–17A). It consists of a small, dark, basophilic granule lying in a clear vacuole within the cytoplasm of pyramidal cells. Several of these are often present in the cell body. Ball and Lo[19] have established that when large numbers of such affected cells are present, there is a high correlation with dementia. Electron microscopy has shown that the vacuole is bounded by a typical unit membrane, and that the granule is composed of very fine granular material.[325] The presence of tubulin has been demonstrated by immunocytochemistry.[245]

HIRANO BODY

The second such lesion, also essentially limited to the hippocampus, is the Hirano body, which appears as an eosinophilic rod in longitudinal section lying either in or near the cytoplasm of the pyramidal cells (Fig. 8–17A). Its fine structure is that of a close-packed mass of filaments arranged in alternating rows at right angles to each other (Fig. 8–17B). They are intracellular, but more often in neuritic processes than in the perikaryon itself, and were first discovered and described by Hirano[145] in cases of Guam-Parkinson dementia. The lesions are often overlooked by light microscopists because they closely resemble a column of close-packed red blood cells. The filaments react with antiactin.[119,120]

MYELIN

Relatively little research has been done on myelin abnormalities in AD. Both cortex and cerebral white matter often seem pale with myelin stains, and some of this is probably due to loss of myelinated axons caused by degeneration of neuronal perikarya. Neurochemical studies have shown a decrease in white matter cerebroside concentrations, with the demyelination apparent on microscopic examination.[309] Electron microscopy has shown figures typical of secondary wallerianlike degeneration.[319] Rare examples of myelin remodeling with the appearance of primary demyelinization, in which the axon is intact, have also been reported.[319] The large lesions in the deep white matter that are often noted by MRI resemble incomplete infarctions in that the tissue is loosened with rarified myelinated axons and a few macrophages.

CHROMATIN

Crapper and colleagues[63] reported interesting alterations in chromatin chemistry in AD. They found that in the normal elderly 75% of cortical chromatin is euchromatin, and that this falls to 56% in the disease. They also produced neuron-enriched and glia-enriched fractions for further analysis. Here they found that in normal specimens, 82% of neuron-enriched DNA is euchromatin, falling to 39% in AD. This indicates a significant rise in transcriptionally inactive heterochromatin in AD. However, when a labeled nucleotide was added to neuron-enriched euchromatin with RNA polymerase, it was found that incorporation of the nucleotide was equally effective in AD and the normal controls. Furthermore, the chain lengths of RNA so produced were also equal in disease and control.

NUCLEOLUS

Mann and his colleagues[193,194] have shown that neuronal nucleolar volume is decreased by about 40% in biopsied temporal lobe of AD without regard to tangles. In autopsied tissue there was an additional nucleolar shrinkage of

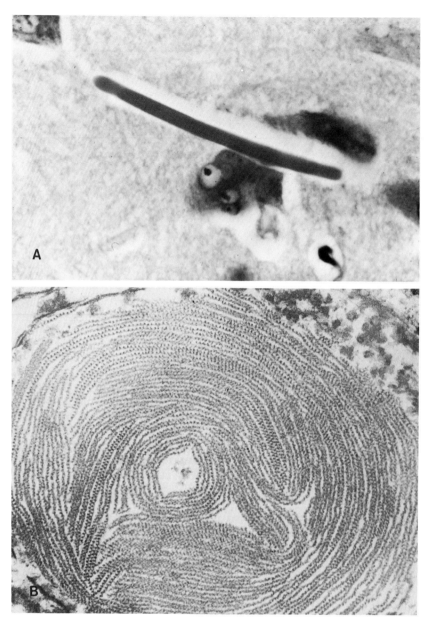

Figure 8–17. *A*, A hematoxylin and eosin preparation of a large rod-shaped Hirano body immediately adjacent to a hippocampal pyramidal cell containing two granulovacuolar bodies. The space surrounding the Hirano body is a shrinkage artifact. *B*, A cross section of a Hirano body. The sheet and perpendicular filament structure are apparent. (From Katzman and Terry,[173] pp 66 and 67, with permission.)

30% in those cells with tangles. They inferred that there is an early reduction in general neuronal protein synthetic capability, and that there is a later additional deterioration associated with the tangle.

CEREBRAL BIOPSY

It is worth noting that cortical biopsy is sometimes required for diagnosis in vivo.[318] In such instances, it is best if the pathologist can attend the surgical procedure so that tissue processing can be started very quickly and atraumatically. At this time, tissue can be prepared for electron microscopy and chemical assay, as well as for light microscopic study. Since plaque and tangle are usually plentiful and very widespread in neocortex, there is a very high probability that the diagnosis can be made definitively when a very small sample of cortical tissue is appropriately studied. Again, thioflavine or silver stains, rather than simple H & E, are most helpful.

Neurotransmitters, Selective Vulnerability, and Cognitive Loss

There is now overwhelming evidence that neurotransmitter alterations found at autopsy in the AD brain are the consequence of the degeneration and loss of specific neuronal systems that are especially vulnerable to the Alzheimer process.[36,169] Although the overall loss of cognitive function is best related to the loss of neocortical (and presumably hippocampal) synapses, loss of particular function has been shown to correlate very well with changes in specific neurotransmitter systems, for example, recent memory and the cholinergic system, and perhaps the serotonergic system and behavior.

THE CHOLINERGIC SYSTEM

The evidence that alterations in neurotransmitter levels are related to the degeneration of specific systems is well illustrated by the findings in the cholinergic system. There is now general consensus that the most important neurotransmitter defect in AD has to do with a deficiency of acetylcholine in the CNS. The earliest evidence came in 1964, when Pope and colleagues[241] reported that acetylcholinesterase levels were lower than normal in the cortex of patients with the disorder. That report

was not followed up for some time, possibly because this hydrolytic enzyme is not specific to neurons. In 1974, Drachman and Leavitt[88,89] published their studies on the effect of the anticholinergic drug scopolamine on normal young volunteers. The investigators found that some of the resulting cognitive deficits in psychometric tests resembled those of AD.

In 1976, Bowen and associates[34] reported very tentatively that some of their AD cases seemed to have low temporal lobe levels of ChAT, the enzyme that is responsible for the synthesis of acetyltransferase from choline and acetyl-coenzyme A. Davies and Maloney[78] reported the first definitive series, stating in late 1976 that there was indeed a very large deficiency of ChAT in the neocortical and hippocampal cortex of both presenile and senile patients with AD. The levels were 70% to 90% below those of normal age-matched controls. This work has been very widely confirmed, most promptly by Perry and associates,[232] and White and co-workers[347] in early 1977. Since that time every laboratory that has assayed CNS tissue for the enzyme has found it to be similarly decreased in the presence of AD. Some find it to be only 50% reduced, but most note that it is more deficient. The severity of the disease has a profound effect on the concentration of ChAT, and this fact may account for the variability among results because, in some series, cases have been selected from the more severe examples, whereas in others, moderate or even mild disorder has been accepted for analysis.

On the basis of animal studies, it had previously been suggested that the major cholinergic input to the neocortex is from neuronal perikarya in the substantia innominata, and more precisely from the nbM.[162] This nucleus, located in part within the substantia innominata in human brain, extends posteriorly to the diagonal band of Broca and the septal area; the rostral portion of this extended nucleus projects to neocortex, the caudal septal portion projects to the hippocampus. Whitehouse and associates[350] have reported a marked deficiency of neurons in the nbM in AD, although there are rare exceptions. Many of the residual neurons here often contain NFT.

In 1978, Perry and associates[234] showed a strong and clear negative correlation between the histologic concentration of cortical NP and the level of cortical ChAT, as well as a correlation between mental test score and the activity of the enzyme. This has been confirmed by others.[172] The loss of cholinergic function in neocortex is present even in biopsy samples from patients with early AD, the samples showing a marked deficiency of both ChAT and acetylcholine synthesis in fresh AD tissue,[295,296] although there is sufficient ChAT remaining in these samples from patients with early AD to synthesize a normal amount of transmitter if all measurable ChAT were available for synthesis. Hence it is likely that much of the enzyme in the tissue was not available for synthesis of the neurotransmitter in these cases with relatively early AD.

A ChAT deficiency is not entirely specific to AD in that Yates and colleagues[364] reported a significant decline in three adult patients with Down syndrome and subsequent AD. Antuono and co-workers[9] mentioned a reduction in Creutzfeldt-Jakob (CJ) disease, but this was not confirmed by Davies and associates.[76] A loss of ChAT in alcoholic dementia has been reported.[218] As indicated below, certain strains of mice inoculated with particular varieties of the scrapie agent developed NP in the cortex.[204] This brain tissue also has depressed levels of ChAT.[204] It is noteworthy that aluminum-treated rabbits with numerous filamentous tangles have normal levels of the enzyme,[143] at least in the acute stage. In PD, ChAT levels are consistently low, especially in the frontal cortex.[271,349] This loss of cortical ChAT is associated with loss of neurons in the basal forebrain in PD.[11] There also may be reduction in ChAT in Pick

disease and PSP,[349] although a change in ChAT in Pick disease has not been found by others.[133]

The degeneration and loss of functional cholinergic terminals in neocortex and hippocampus are not accompanied by any consistent reduction in the postsynaptic muscarinic receptors that make up the major part of the cholinergic receptor system in the cortex. Most investigators have found concentrations of this receptor, as identified by QNB-binding, to be normal in AD.[80,232] Reisine and colleagues[249] found them to be diminished by about 50% in the hippocampus, at the same time reporting normal levels in the frontal cortex. The hippocampus may not be a good indicator, since its tissue is so sensitive to coincident disorders such as anoxia or brain swelling. Also aberrant sprouting of hippocampal cholinergic terminals sometimes occurs in AD.[110,112,114] Recent subclassification of the muscarinic receptor into M1 and M2 subtypes indicated there may be some loss of the M2 receptor in AD.[199] Nevertheless, that loss, if it occurs, is small in comparison to the loss of the primary cholinergic neuron. Thus, insofar as there is a cholinergic deficit, it appears that pharmacologic tools to correct this particular biochemical loss would be useful.

Nicotinic receptors are thought to be, at least in part, presynaptic. They are significantly reduced in AD neocortex whether measured by binding of tritiated α-bungarotoxin, nicotine, or acetylcholine.[75,177,348,349] As would be predicted, cortical nicotinic receptors are also reduced in PD and PSP.[349]

These data thus suggest that major functional deficiencies in cognitive abilities in AD, especially abilities in which recent memory plays an important part, might in large part be ascribed to the loss of cholinergic activity in the neocortex and hippocampus. Attempts to increase the synthesis of acetylcholine by increasing the dietary intake of the acetylcholine precursor choline, or the choline-containing lipid lecithin, in a manner analogous to the use of L-dopa in PD have not met with significant success.[51,56,99,210,328] The other precursor of the transmitter, acetyl-coenzyme A, must also be considered here, but this is not directly accessible for therapy, although it might be increased by drugs that activate intermediary metabolism. It is assumed that the functional and biochemical deficiency of ChAT that occurs in AD is at fault in the failure of substrate therapy.

A second therapeutic approach has to do with inhibiting the normal hydrolysis of acetylcholine. Despite their peripheral side effects, such esterase blockers as physostigmine have met with partial success in selected patients in improving memory by prolonging the activity of endogenous transmitter.[81,327] Longer acting drugs of this kind such as slow release physostigmine and tetrahydroaminoacridine[308] are undergoing extensive clinical evaluation. A third possible mode of treatment involves utilization of an analogue of acetylcholine to substitute for the natural transmitter, since the muscarinic receptors are present at normal concentration even in advanced AD, but cholinergic agonists such as arecholine have not been successful. Another approach would be to increase the sensitivity of the central muscarinic receptors in order to get more effect from the same small amount of acetylcholine or to increase the release of acetylcholine.

In regard to the latter concept, galanin is a neuropeptide of special interest. Galanin inhibits acetylcholine release and in experimental situations impairs memory in aged animals. It has been colocalized to some of the cholinergic neurons in the nbM and has also been identified in neurites forming NP,[182] but neither neocortical nor nbM galanin concentrations are reduced in AD[20]; in fact, in some instances galanin concentrations have been found to be increased in AD nbM. In the nbM galanin is present in small noncholinergic fusiform cells as well as in some of the large cholinergic cells. These fusiform cells have long dendrites and act as local circuit neurons presumably inhibiting the functional activity of remaining intact cholinergic neurons.[45,46] Theoretically, blocking the action of galanin could increase activity in remaining cholinergic cells, but whether this finding can lead to useful therapy remains to be determined.

Perhaps the boldest suggestion in regard to the treatment of the dying cholinergic system is to attempt to "rescue" it by the administration of nerve growth factor (NGF). Although NGF was initially discovered as a neurotrophic factor for peripheral autonomic and sensory neurons, the basal nucleus cholinergic system also requires the presence of this factor to survive. In animals who have undergone fimbria-fornix transections, a procedure that cuts the septal-hippocampal cholinergic projection and leads to the disappearance of the septal cholinergic neurons, administration of NGF promotes not only survival but also neurite outgrowth from these cells.[107,137,354] In a subset of aged rats whose ability to learn the Morris water maze is impaired, and who show a loss of ChAT in hippocampus similar to patients with AD, the intraventricular administration of NGF not only increases ChAT in the cortex and hippocampus but also improves maze learning ability.[108] Whether similar improvements would occur in AD patients is not known, but there may be clinical trials in the not too distant future if experimental studies continue to be promising. It is now possible to insert the NGF gene into various cells including autologous fibroblasts, a method that would provide a continuous source of NGF, if the latter were helpful.[109]

Acetylcholinesterase has been found to be reduced in AD by several investigative groups.[241] Perry and associates[237] noted that some NP and some NFT in the normal aged hippocampus stain histochemically for this hydrolase. The reactivity of these lesions was reduced in AD, as was the activity of the adjacent tissue. The staining of hippocampal tangles suggested to these authors that tangle formation in these pyramidal cells might be related in some fashion to disturbed cholinoreceptive function.

AMINERGIC TRANSMITTERS

Three of the four major monamine projection systems to the neocortex and hippocampus are involved by the Alzheimer process to varying degrees. Highly significant changes occur regularly in the serotonin system, whose cell bodies are in the dorsal raphe; frequent but not consistent alterations are observed in the noradrenergic system arising from the neurons in the locus ceruleus and in the adrenergic system, whose cells of origin are in the medulla. There is considerable disagreement as to the extent of involvement of the dopaminergic system that arises from the substantia nigra, and the medially placed dopaminergic cells that give rise to the mesolimbic projection. In considering the frequency of involvement of the serotonergic, noradrenergic, and cholinergic projection systems, Benton and colleagues[27] have referred to AD as a disorder of the isodendritic core of the brain.

The serotonergic projection system from the dorsal raphe to the cortex and hippocampus is frequently involved in AD. Yamamora and Hirano[362] documented the presence of NFT in the dorsal raphe neurons. Serotonin (5-hydroxytryptamine [5-HT]) is reduced from 40% to 60% in AD frontal and temporal cortex as compared with age-matched controls.[33,72,225,265] The principal metabolite of 5-HT, 5-hydroxyindoleacetic acid, is also reduced. In biopsy tissue from AD patients, both 5-HT uptake and content were reduced.[33] It may be concluded that there is substantial damage to serotonergic neurons in AD. Palmer and associates[225] and Sparks and colleagues[300] suggested that the loss of 5-HT in the frontal lobe and hypothalamus, respectively, might relate to behavioral changes that occur in AD.

Using appropriate ligands, investigators have shown that there is a consistent reduction in both S_1 and S_2 serotonin receptors in AD cortex and hippocampus.[33,72,233,267] Cross and colleagues[65,67] found no change in ligand binding to α_1-adrenergic, α_2-adrenergic, β-adrenergic, benzodiazepine, or γ-aminobutyric acid (GABA) receptors in the neocortex or hippocampus in AD, but they did find a selective loss of serotonergic S_1 and especially S_2 receptors in the AD hippocampus and temporal lobe cortex. The decrease in serotonin receptors was a relatively early change, but there was no correlation with the clinical assessment of the degree of dementia or with the severity of pathologic changes.

Noradrenaline (NA) is most easily assayed by quantification of the enzyme dopamine β-hydroxylase (DBH), which changes dopamine to NA. Davies and Maloney[78] reported the enzyme to be present in normal concentrations in AD. Adolfsson and associates[2] found NA to be low in putamen and frontal cortex, but normal in hippocampus, cingulate gyrus, caudate nucleus, hypothalamus, thalamus, mesencephalon, and pons. Cross and colleagues[66] reported significantly reduced levels of DBH in temporal, frontal, and hippocampus cortex. It has been found that most patients with AD and without PD have diminished numbers of neurons in the locus ceruleus.[192,333] Since these pigmented neurons are believed to be the source of neocortical NA, their loss may account for the alterations found in some specimens.

Noradrenaline is histofluorescent under appropriate conditions.[97] Berger and colleagues[28] so examined sections of biopsied frontal cortex in AD and reported that noradrenergic fibers were largely absent, while abnormal varicosities were found near NP.

Burke and colleagues[42] found that phenylethanolamine N-methyltransferase (PNMT) activity, the rate-limiting enzyme involved in the synthesis of epinephrine (adrenaline) and a specific marker for epinephrine neurons, was reduced 37% to 48% in AD brains in areas affected by the Alzheimer process but not in the cerebellum. The degree of decrease in PNMT activity in the hippocampus correlated significantly with the degree of dementia in the small series of AD brains studied.

There has been much disagreement in regard to assay results of brain dopamine. As reviewed by Gottfries,[123] the basal ganglia of patients with senile dementia are said to contain about 55% of normal levels of dopamine, and the dopamine metabolite, homovanillic acid (HVA), is reduced to 70% of that found in age-matched normals. Gottfries[124] also reported lowered HVA in the cerebrospinal fluid (CSF) of patients with presenile AD. On the other hand, Parkes and co-workers[226] did not confirm this decrease in the CSF. However, Adolfsson[2] did not find significant differences in dopamine levels in the caudate or putamen, but reported statistical decreases in the thalamus and pons. While these alterations were statistically significant, at least two points might be kept in mind in their consideration. First, Hornykiewicz's early findings[147] in regard to the nigrostriatal system in PD indicated that abnormal function could be expected only when transmitter levels were reduced well below 50% of normal. Second, the specimens analyzed by the Scandinavian groups have not been subjected to postmortem microscopic study.[2] It is not impossible, therefore, that some specimens with PD have mistakenly been assayed as unmixed AD, and that other specimens with subclinical but significant alterations of the latter disease might have been included in the normal series.

In regard to monoamine oxidase in AD, it has been reported that the isoenzyme acting on β-phenylethylamine as a substrate was elevated in hippocampus, neocortex, and caudate. The other two isoenzymes, acting on tryptamine and on serotonin, respectively, were normal.[3]

γ-AMINOBUTYRIC ACID

The widespread inhibitory transmitter γ-aminobutyric acid (GABA) has been assayed in AD by analyzing its synthesizing enzyme, glutamic acid decarboxylase (GAD). It was first reported to be reduced in AD,[35] but the same authors soon recognized that the enzyme was altered by various premortem factors such as bronchopneumonia, and they subsequently stated[34] that GAD is normal in AD when the specimens were carefully screened to rule out the circumstances causing irrelevant depression. In a study of surgical biopsy samples there was no deficit in GABA concentration[190]; however, a modest loss of GABA in the neocortex, particularly in the temporal cortex, is likely to be real after the agonal changes have been taken into account.[10,190] There is little change in $GABA_A$ or $GABA_B$ receptors in the neocortex or hippocampus in AD.[65,111] However, Chu and colleagues[48] reported a highly localized reduction of $GABA_A$ and $GABA_B$ receptors in stratum moleculare of the dentate gyrus and in CA1 pyramidal cell regions that might reflect neuronal pathologies in CA1 and dentate gyrus and in the projections from the entorhinal cortex, the latter associated with memory impairment in AD.

GLUTAMIC ACID

Glutamic acid as a neurotransmitter is difficult to study since it is also a normal metabolite in intermediary metabolism. It is of undoubted importance in AD since many of the large pyramidal cells in both the association cortex and limbic cortex that are affected pathologically in AD may be glutaminergic. For example, the entorhinal projection to the dentate gyrus by way of the perforant pathway is severely affected in AD. Hyman and colleagues[149] microdissected a portion from the terminal zone in the molecular layer of the dentate gyrus and found an almost 80% reduction in glutamate. In addition to measurements of glutamate content, investigators have utilized direct and indirect measures of glutamate uptake as a method of determining the integrity of the glutamate neuron and its presynaptic processes.[60,67,68,136,224] These studies indicate a substantial reduction in glutamatergic neural processes in specific regions, particularly in temporal cortex. In contrast, studies of postsynaptic receptors, measured either by L-glutamate binding or specific NMDA ligands, have given conflicting data.[111,126] It may be concluded, however, that postsynaptic NMDA receptors are not altered significantly.[59,60,111] Thus, the concept that the release of glutamic acid as an excitatory neurotransmitter with the capacity to kill cells might play a role in the pathogenesis of AD[126] appears to be unlikely.[60] But there is little doubt that disruption of glutamatergic pathways may lead to learning and memory deficits since these neurons are an important component of the corticocortical association neurons as well as the entorhinal system.

NEUROPEPTIDES

It was not until 1980 that data concerning neuropeptides in relation to AD began to appear in the literature. The greatest deficit among peptides in AD neocortex and hippocampus is that of somatostatin (SS); a close second is the neuropeptide, corticotropin-releasing factor (CRF) (Table 8–3). Vasoactive intestinal polypeptide (VIP) concentrations have been found to be normal.[264] This peptide is present in small cortical neurons, and these cells are not greatly decreased in AD.[322] On the other hand, SS, which is also present in smaller cortical neurons, is reduced. The reduction in SS in autopsy brain was first reported by Davies and associates[77,79] and has been confirmed in many laboratories.[23,24,263] The finding of Beal and as-

Table 8–3 CHEMICAL PATHOLOGY OF AD

Neurotransmitter		Change		Pathologic Correlates	
				Nucleus of Origin (Cell Loss and NFT)	**Terminal Field (NP)**
Cholinergic	↓	40%–90%	(15 labs)	Basal nucleus	Cerebral cortex
Somatostatin	↓	49%–90%	(6 labs)	Cerebral cortex	Cerebral cortex
CRF	↓	40+%	(2 labs)	Temporal pole	Cerebral cortex
Glutamate	↓	40+%	(4 labs)	Pyramidal cells	Cerebral cortex
				Entorhinal cortex	Hippocampus
Serotonin	↓	40+%	(4 labs)	Dorsal raphe	Cerebral cortex, hippocampus
Noradrenalin		Variable		Locus cruleus	Cerebral cortex, hippocampus
Substance P		Variable		?	Cerebral cortex

SUBSTANTIALLY UNCHANGED OR CONFLICTING DATA

Galanin
GABA
Dopamine
Vasopressin
Oxytocin
Enkephalin
Neurotensin
Cholecystokinin
Vasoactive intestinal peptide
Neuropeptide Y
Thyrotropin-releasing hormone
Luteinizing hormone-releasing hormone

Key: NFT = neurofibrillary tangles; NP = neuritic plaques; CRF = corticotropin releasing factor; NA = noradrenaline; GABA = γ-aminobutyric acid; ? = location unknown.

sociates[25] of a similar reduction of two prosomatostatin-derived peptides, SS-28 and SS-14, in AD cerebral cortex supports the contention that the loss of the peptide is caused by degeneration of SS cortical neurons and terminals. A loss of SS receptors has been reported.[24] Roberts and colleagues demonstrated that some NFT occurred in SS neurons in AD cerebral cortex.[255] Joynt and McNeill[164] used immunohistochemical methods to visualize SS cells in AD frontal cortex and found them to be shrunken and irregularly shaped. However, Francis and colleagues[103] did not find consistent changes in SS-like immunoreactivity in frontal or temporal lobe surgical biopsies at a time when cholinergic markers were definitely reduced, indicating that changes in neocortical SS do not occur at the earliest stages in many AD patients. Their data suggest that when changes in brain SS did occur, the changes were correlated with deficits in verbal tasks including a measure of language comprehension. A correlation between CSF somatostatin levels and cognitive performance, especially verbal and visual spatial, was observed in a small series of AD patients and controls.[312]

CRF-like immunoreactivity is also significantly reduced in AD neocortex, a finding first reported by Bissette and colleagues.[31] This reduction is substantial, over 40%, and has been confirmed by others.[85,243,351] Again CRF is localized to smaller neurons, not the large neocortical pyramidal neurons. Receptors to both SS and CRF are also reduced in AD cortex.[26,85] In contrast to the decreases in SS and CRF, which appear to be quite reproducible, a moderate 20% to 40% reduction in substance P (SP) immunoreactivity in AD neocortex and hippocampus has been found by two groups,[21,69] a finding not confirmed by others.[98,363] There is also controversy in regard to neuropeptide Y, which has been reported to be increased, decreased, and unchanged.[22] A variety of other neuropeptides has been found to be normal or not consistently reduced by various investigators; these include arginine vasopressin, enkephalins, neurotensin, cholecystokinin, thyrotropin-releasing hormone, and luteinizing hormone-releasing hormone.* It has been reported that some enkephalin- or VIP- immunoreactive hippocampal pyramidal cells contain NFT.[185,312]

NPs and Neurotransmitters

Modern immunohistochemical methods combined with thioflavine or other markers of the NP have provided striking visual evidence for the presence of specific transmitter systems in individual neurites that form the NP. GABA neurites have been labeled with antibody to glutamic acid decarboxylase,[343] cholinergic neurites with the antibody to ChAT,[14,180] noradrenergic neurites with antibody to dopamine-β-hydroxylase, and the neuropeptides somatostatin, substance P, and neuropeptide Y with antibodies to appropriate epitopes.[15,16] It has become evident that in a single NP multiple transmitter systems may contribute individual neurites,[13,342] including neurites from transmitter systems with unaltered concentrations in the AD brain such as VIP.[303,304] These findings put aside an earlier hypothesis that NP are formed from the degeneration and contraction of cholinergic neurites. Rather, it is now probable that the plaque core forms a nidus that leads to the degeneration of surrounding neurites.

Dementia in AD Is Correlated with Pathologic Changes

Whether the degree of clinical dementia is correlated with these pathologic changes has, in the past, been held in serious question by many investigators. For many years the belief that there was no such correlation led to the supposition that the pathologic changes of AD had little to do with clinical symptomatology. When Alzheimer

---

*References 98, 106, 263, 264, 266, 363.

found that the NP and NFT demonstrated on silver stain in presenile dementia also occurred in senile dementia, he assumed a unity of the two diseases, and this was widely accepted by pathologists during the first third of the century. However, in a study based on pathologic material at the Foxborough State Hospital, Rothschild[270] clearly differentiated between vascular changes in the brain and AD changes in what he termed senile psychosis. He reported that in his material he could find cases in which there were extensive changes in the brain with reportedly good function prior to death, and other cases with severe psychoses in which there were relatively few changes in the brain. Similar discrepancies had been reported by others.[113] Rothschild[270] concluded,

> In the light of the conception advocated here the pathologic changes no longer appear as the sole determining factor or even necessarily as the most important factor in the occurrence of senile psychosis. The person's capacity to compensate for a certain amount of tissue damage becomes of immediate importance. Depending on this capacity, one person with senile changes in the brain may show no clinical abnormalities, another may develop a psychosis which shows little evidence of compensatory mechanism, and between the two extremes, all gradations will be observed.

This view, repeatedly promulgated by Rothschild, gained widespread credence. As late as 1964, a statement that there is "no significant relation between brain alterations, thinking and behavior" was attributed to workers in the Duke Longitudinal Study.[191]

The pendulum had now swung. Clinical studies suggested an identity of AD and the major form of senile dementia.[215] Pathologic studies by Corsellis,[58] Malamud,[191] and prospective clinicopathologic studies by Tomlinson and associates[331] and Blessed and colleagues[32] then led to a reversal of Rothschild's interpretation. There are three elements involved in this reversal. The first is the recognition, beginning in the

1950s, that most cases of dementia can be differentiated clinically from cases of functional senile psychosis; moreover, the functional psychoses with late onset have a much greater longevity than patients with senile dementias of an organic nature.[267] It is quite probable, for example, that in the studies of Rothschild, which depended on state hospital records, such distinctions were not accurately made. A second factor was a closer interpretation of the pathologic data. Some atrophy of the brain, some neuronal loss, as well as the presence of hippocampal tangles and a few generalized senile plaques, are part of the normal aging process. The more specific changes associated with AD are the increased number and diffusion of plaques, as well as tangles, in the cortex. A third factor was that the work of Rothschild and others was not prospective and did not measure intellectual function prior to autopsy examination of brains.[248,270] In a prospective clinicopathologic study, carried out by Blessed and colleagues,[32,331] mental status tests and functional evaluations were carried out in a chronic hospital population in which the presence of other diseases would likely lead to demise and the possibility of subsequent neuropathologic examination. On the basis of the autopsy materials obtained from this series, it was possible to demonstrate that there is, indeed, a correlation between cognitive decline and the presence of large numbers of plaques or the presence of NFT in the cortex. Finally, the demonstration that the ultrastructure of the changes in the brain of senile demented patients was identical to that of younger patients clinched the argument.[319] In the late 1970s, a consensus developed in this regard,[167,174] and by 1980 the identity was recognized in the diagnostic scheme developed by the American Psychiatric Association.[8]

Nevertheless, one must assume, a priori, that there would be subclinical cases of AD; that is, cases in which there were plaques and tangles in the brain without extensive cognitive decline. Some AD patients with diffuse pathology present with focal symptoms, the remainder of the neocortex still functioning above a detectable threshold.[70,71] As noted previously, diffuse plaques are occasionally present in the brains of nondemented individuals under the age of 65.[337] In a study of 137 autopsies obtained from a nursing home in which regular clinical evaluations were carried out, 10 subjects were identified with numerous neocortical plaques but retained cognition as measured by a mental status test.[175] On the average these subjects were 86.7 years old. The brains of the subset with neocortical plaques and retained cognition weighed more than did brains from demented AD patients but also more than did brains from cognitively intact subjects without AD or other neuropathologic changes. There was also a greater number of large neurons, especially in parietal cortex as determined by computer-assisted morphometry. One possibility is that these patients had early AD changes but were protected cognitively by the presence of a greater reserve of large neurons. Synapse counts were not done in this series, but one can postulate that this number would also have been normal since the number of synapses in neocortex appears to show the best correlation with cognitive measures. These findings do not, however, alter our belief that the essential element in AD is the underlying neuronal pathology. If we are to prevent or cure this disorder, we must deal with the events that produce the NFT and NP, and cause loss of cells and synapses and the other morphologic and chemical abnormalities. Treatment of the disease would deal with the effects of these lesions.

ETIOLOGY AND RISK FACTORS

The etiology of AD remains unknown. In two situations, Down syndrome and a subset of familial cases with apparent autosomal dominant onset, genetic factors are clearly predominant. But even among identical twins, the concordance is only 50% to 60% as will be described later. Hence, there must be important environmental or other risk factors that are not yet understood. In this section we will discuss evidence concerning genetic, chromosomal, and a variety of other proposed etiologic or risk factors.

Genetic Factors

The existence of a genetic factor in AD appears to be well established. Many families have been reported with apparently autosomal dominant transmission in several generations. An increase in risk for AD among first-degree relatives of AD probands who were under the age of 75 at onset of illness is well established both in studies utilizing clinically diagnosed probands[7,37,144,257] and in the studies based on autopsy-confirmed probands.[139–142,186,345] A study involving subjects who were aged 75 to 84 at entry did not find an increase in the history of dementia among first-degree relatives of those who developed AD.[17,171] Clinically, there are many sporadic cases with no family history of the disease despite reasonable longevity in parents. In two well-conducted case control studies, 60% of AD patients had no evidence of family aggregation.[7,144,257]

In an analysis of the kindred of patients with senile dementia, Larsson and associates[186] suggested the existence of a predisposing autosomal dominant gene with a gene frequency at 12%. This gene was postulated to have an age-related penetrance, reaching 40% at age 90. Similar results have been reported by others.[37,209,345] Thus, Martin and associates projected that 41% of the relatives of 22 rigorously diagnosed AD subjects would have contracted AD if they lived to age 83, against 23% of the relatives of nondemented controls.[198] The apparently sophisticated mathematics used in these various studies has been challenged by others.[298] The projections that have been made of the family history data to the ninth and tenth decade are questionable because the prevalence of AD at age 90 in the general population is between 30% and 50%.[96,170]

Another informative source is twin studies. In a study of 2926 twin pairs over the age of 60, Kallman[165] found a 42.8% concordance of AD or senile dementia in monozygotic twins, as compared to an 8.9% concordance in parents. Jarvik[155–158] reported a concordance of 61% for organic brain syndrome in elderly monozygotic twin pairs. Thus, these findings strongly implicate a genetic factor, but the same data strongly implicate an environmental or systemic factor. A concordance rate of 40% to 60% in monozygotic twins is not high compared with many other diseases, and it indicates an important role for a nongenetic factor. The finding of autopsy-proved AD in two identical twins with onset almost 15 years apart suggests that even in genetic cases, nongenetic factors play a crucial role.[54] The nature of these nongenetic factors, however, discussed below as "Other Risk Factors," is at present poorly understood.

Major advances in the understanding of AD are occuring with the application of the techniques of gene mapping and molecular genetics to familial cases. The present evidence indicates at least three different gene sites. One specific mutation at site APP717 has been found on the APP gene in a very small subset with early-onset AD.[117a] A second locus for early-onset families appears to be on the long arm of chromosome 21, distinct from and closer to the centromere than the APP gene.[273,316,340] However, both loci have been excluded as a site of an AD gene in another group of families,[30] the so-called Volga German families, as well as in studies of families with late-onset AD.[262,282] In the late-onset cases, a locus on the long arm of chromosome 19 has been published.[262]

Chromosomal Factors

The possibility that chromosomal abnormalities may predispose toward AD has drawn considerable attention.[155–157] Individuals with Down syndrome who live more than 30 to 40 years almost invariably develop morphologic and biochemical changes of AD—NP, cerebrovascular β-amyloid peptide, NFT, loss of ChAT—in cerebral cortex and hippocampus.[43,93,115,223,364] This is usually, but not always, accompanied by clinical changes, suggesting further cognitive impairment in these already impaired persons.[358] Heston[139,140] found an increase in Down syndrome and lymphomas and leukemias in relatives of patients with AD, especially in familial cases, but other investigators have been unable to confirm this.[41] Nevertheless, abnormal karyotypes do not appear to be reproducibly present in AD,[41,217,219,306] and early reports of increased dosage for the β-amyloid gene[84] have been denied.[214,274,313]

Aluminum

Over 20 years ago it was found that the injection of small quantities of aluminum salts into the rabbit intrathecal space or into the cerebral parenchyma induced the formation of NFT, especially in certain susceptible areas of the CNS.[181,323] Not all species react in the same fashion. While superficially resembling the human lesions of AD, these tangles are significantly different in that they are made up of masses of morphologically and chemically normal neurofilaments. Human neurons in culture respond to aluminum by forming filamentous tangles rather than those made up of PHF.[61,62]

Stimulated by those early reports, Crapper[62] examined AD specimens from the Toronto region for their aluminum content and found it to be significantly elevated, but McDermott and co-workers,[205] using New York specimens, disagreed. Most recently, Markesberry[197] has found that brain aluminum levels increase with age, but are not abnormally elevated in AD specimens from Kentucky assayed by neutron activation. The latter workers suggested that the concentration of aluminum in the brain is related to age and to its level in local drinking water, rather than to disease. On the other hand, Perl and colleagues[228-230] have found that the aluminum is located in the cytoplasm of neurons with tangles rather than in adjacent normal neurons. These last findings suggest a true relationship between tangle and aluminum. If total tissue aluminum is not increased while the concentration is high in NFT, however, then it must be low outside the NFT. This implies that the metal is adsorbed by the NFT as a secondary event. Candy and colleagues[44] reported very high concentrations of aluminum in the core of plaques using a sophisticated magnetic resonance spectral technique, but this has not been confirmed by others using equally sensitive methods (Perl, personal communication).

Crapper and associates suggest that the metal binds to neuronal chromatin and changes its ability in regard to the initiation of protein synthesis. Conceivably, this might result in less transcription activity or it might allow derepression of genetic material, which then starts the processing of a more or less abnormal protein.

There is no consistent epidemiologic evidence to suggest that the ingestion of aluminum antacids or the direct application of aluminum to the skin (as in aluminum antiperspirants) is a risk factor for AD. Dialysis encephalopathy, which occurred in many dialysis patients in the late 1970s and early 1980s, was likely due to aluminum toxicity resulting from the large amount of aluminum antacids used then by many dialysis centers to reduce phosphate; this condition, however, was reversible when recognized and treated, unlike AD.[4,5,12,207,259,283,301] Although a small number of patients undergoing dialysis were later found at autopsy to show NFT, there are no data to indicate that this was greater than that expected in the general population. Flaten[100] has noted a geographic association of aluminum level in drinking water and death certificate reports of AD in Norway. However, the aluminum content of drinking water is determined in many areas by the decision of local health authorities in regard to the use of aluminum water purification and is more likely to be used in more urbanized areas. Because the diagnosis and reporting of AD will vary considerably depending on the sophistication and specialization of the medical profession, it is possible that such epidemiologic studies might be biased.

Virus

Evidence concerning the relationship of virus to AD is weak. The most direct evidence was the report that concerned the transmission of two of six familial cases to subhuman primates by means of cerebral inoculation.[336] Nearly 40 sporadic cases had been tried without success. The two familial cases caused a spongy encephalopathy in the recipient primates, rather than plaques and tangles. Ultimately this report was retracted, since it could not be repeated even with the same tissue samples.[125] Our own inference was that a laboratory error had taken place.

It has been shown that certain strains of the scrapie agent inoculated into particular strains of mice cause the appearance of NP in addition to spongy encephalopathy in the recipient murine brain.[355] These plaques are made of an amyloid core (prion peptides rather than APP peptides) and abnormal neurites containing degenerating mitochondria and lamellar lysosomes. The lesion lacks the characteristic PHF of human AD but is otherwise remarkably similar. The plaques tend to cluster around a stab would, indicating that an altered blood-brain barrier might be significant.[356]

Manuelides and associates[196] reported that buffy-coat cells from AD relatives inoculated intracerebrally into hamsters caused spongy encephalopathy. They suggested that a CJ-like agent "may be involved in at least some form of AD." This finding has not been corroborated.

Autoimmunity

Another hypothesis is that AD might be an autoimmune disease. There is little direct evidence to support this hypothesis. There is amyloid present in the core of the NP, but it is not derived from serum immunoglobulin. There have been various reports of a decrease in specific immunoglobulins in AD,[92,317] but these findings were not replicated in a careful case control study.[208] We found an increase in immunosuppression in AD patients, but this may well be secondary to hypothalamic involvement, rather than a primary event.[208] Immunosuppression is usually decreased in autoimmune disease.

If AD were an autoimmune disorder, one might expect to find a relationship to specific HLA haplotypes. Indeed, increases in HLA B7, BW15, and CW3 frequency have been reported,[50,250,341] but other groups have been unable to confirm these changes.[138,305,346,353]

Even though it is unlikely that autoimmunity is the primary etiologic factor in AD, it is reasonable to expect that during the course of a neurodegenerative disease such as AD, antibodies to components of degenerating neurons would develop. Chapman and associates[47] have reported the existence of antibodies in the sera of AD patients that bind specifically to the purely cholinergic neurons of the electric fish. One might anticipate that other specific antibodies will be found in AD sera. Such antibodies might find some use as a diagnostic marker.

Risk Factors: Epidemiologic Studies

Epidemiologic studies have proved invaluable in identifying risk factors for many chronic diseases; perhaps the best examples are cardiovascular disease and atherosclerosis. It has been disappointing that despite a number of well-conducted case control studies, longitudinal studies, and community surveys, easily modifiable risk factors have not been found. Thus, Rocca and associates[257,258] have noted that in a number of case control studies,[7,29,104,144] "possible risk factors such as previous diseases, surgical interventions, anesthesia, presence of specific disease among relatives, extreme temperatures, x-ray studies, behavior patterns, stressful life events" were found not to be significantly associated with AD with the exception of thyroid disease, which was found to be a risk factor in only one study.[144] Also, a history of exposure to organic solvents or lead is not a risk factor.[291,292] One risk factor that has been found in more than one well-conducted case control study is head injury. Thus, Heyman, Mortimer, and others[104,144,212] found that serious head injuries up to 35 years before the onset of AD occurred in 15% to 20% of AD patients, whereas such injuries had occurred in only 5% of carefully matched controls. It should be noted that boxers with the "punch drunk syndrome" develop not only NFT (but in a distribution typical of dementia pugilistica rather than AD) but also diffuse plaques.[254] Some case control studies have also reported that parental age, birth order, and thyroid disease are risk factors in younger patients, but this has not been confirmed by others.[7,49,57,82,144,338,345]

In case control studies, clinically diagnosed AD patients are compared with controls, often matched for age, gender, ethnicity, education, and sometimes general health (e.g., not in hospitals). Among the problems with this technique when applied to AD is the difficulty in deciding how controls should be matched to cases and whether the data should be obtained from case and control subjects or from informants. The greatest difficulty, however, is that demographic items used in matching cases and controls may, in fact, be risk factors. Three such demographic items are age, gender, and education.

Age is the dominant risk factor for dementia and AD as was discussed earlier and shown in Figure 8–1. Age as a risk factor is found both on community surveys and longitudinal studies.* In all but one study using current diagnostic criteria, AD occurs more commonly in women (with relative risks as high as 3:1), taking age into account; this appears to be especially significant over the age of 75.[17,40,96,209,238,307,365]

Several previous attempts to look at the socioeconomic status and the personality structure prior to the development of AD have been unavailing. The work of Roth[269] in the 1950s and Post[242] failed to find any relationship among dementia, other psychiatric disorders, or prior personality. AD occurs in persons of every socioeconomic status and education level. A striking example is that of the Nobel laureate George Beadle, one of the pioneers of the molecular genetic revolution and a president of the University of Chicago who died at age 85 of AD.

A striking effect of education on the prevalence of dementia has recently been shown in a community survey of 5055 elderly carried out in the Jing-An district of Shanghai.[365] More than 26% of the sample had had no education whatsoever, and the prevalence of dementia among the noneducated was significantly greater than among those with even an elementary school education, particularly in women over the age of 75 (Table 8–4). Conversely, among individuals who had had at least a sixth-grade education, cognitive impairment in the elderly was found to be almost identical in the Shanghai cohort and in a Finnish cohort.[278]

Many of the available community surveys of dementia have been carried out in northern Europe, the United States, and Japan. Surprising differences, in the order of 2:1, have been found in regard to the age-specific prevalence of dementia in various studies,[257] even when carried out by a collaborating group of investigators. For example, Copeland and associates found the prevalence of dementia in New York to be twice that of London.[55] The highest prevalence figures are from the east Boston study.[96] It is likely that much of this difference is due to ascertainment criteria, since many studies identify a "questionable" group. Some surveys exclude subjects in nursing homes, a procedure that drastically reduces the prevalence rate. As discussed, differing educational levels affect prevalence. It is also possible that there is differential mortality among AD patients in different societies. It will be important to carry out cross-cultural studies, taking these factors into account to determine if in addition there are nutritional, environmental, or other factors that can be unmasked.

The available data thus suggest the possibility that different risk factors are important in younger and older individuals and in women as compared to men. For example, in the Bronx Aging Study, myocardial infarct (MI) is a highly significant risk factor in elderly women.[17]

These various risk factors are summarized in Table 8–5. One could postulate that a common theme tying together age, low education, head injury, and MI is a loss of synaptic reserve, giving rise to symptoms years earlier in the presence of the same number of plaques and tangles. Alternatively, however, certain of these conditions might in some unknown way set off the AD process. For example, head injury also produces dementia pugilistica in which typical NFT without NP are observed but in a different distribution

---

*References 96, 127, 129, 211, 216, 238, 257, 297, 365.

**Table 8–4 AGE-SPECIFIC PREVALENCE OF
DEMENTIA (BY GENDER AND EDUCATION)**

Age and Education	Men		Women	
	Sample Screened	Age-Specific Prevalence	Sample Screened	Age-Specific Prevalence
55–64 yr				
> 6 yr*	419	0.48	292	0.68
≤ 6 yr†	189	0.53	360	0.56
No ed‡	26	0.00	211	0.00
Total	634	0.47	863	0.46
65–74 yr				
> 6 yr	504	0.00	263	0.38
≤ 6 yr	397	1.00	438	0.68
No ed	91	0.00	491	2.65
Total	992	0.40	1192	1.42
75–84 yr				
> 6 yr	208	3.37	101	3.96
≤ 6 yr	219	3.16	211	12.64
No ed	98	9.18	378	18.07
Total	525	4.36	690	14.33
85+ yr				
> 6 yr	25	12.00	16	18.75
≤ 6 yr	16	18.75	27	22.22
No ed	17	23.53	54	32.27
Total	58	17.24	97	27.80
Total	2208		2842	

*Middle school or greater education.
†Elementary school (< 6 years) education.
‡No education.

than in AD, more often affecting basal ganglia and giving rise to parkinsonian like symptoms.

ALZHEIMER DISEASE AND CEREBRAL ARTERIOSCLEROSIS

Just a few years ago many physicians labeled any elderly person with mental deterioration as a case of cerebral arteriosclerosis. Indeed, when one looks at the arteries of individuals of advanced age, one frequently finds arteriosclerosis, but this clearly is not correlated with the presence or absence of dementia.[58] Persons with advanced AD often have minimal atheromatous change in their intracranial vessels.

The clinical pathologic correlations of Tomlinson and associates[330–333] pro-

vided the critical evidence that dementia during life was correlated with overt pathologic changes in brain parenchyma—the number of plaques per unit area in cerebral cortex in AD, the volume of cerebral hemisphere in-

Table 8–5 RISK FACTORS IN AD

ALL AGES: EXPONENTIAL FUNCTION OF AGE

Onset before Age 75	Onset after Age 75
Family history	Gender: female
APP 717 gene, chromosome 21	
2nd FAD gene on chromosome 21	Education
Gene on other chromosome (19)	MI (clinical + silent)
Head injury; boxers	
(Thyroiditis; parental age)	

FAD = familial Alzheimer disease.

farcted in vascular dementia—rather than the degree of arteriosclerosis in cerebral arteries, or any presumed cerebral ischemia.

These concepts have been further strengthened by studies of cerebral metabolism and blood flow in dementia. Dementia is regularly accompanied by a decrease in both cerebral blood flow and cerebral oxygen metabolism as measured in vivo by the nitrous oxide and xenon techniques.[105,148,152,187,220, 221,299] However, this decrease is secondary to the decrease in neuronal activity and is not a consequence of ischemia, since the arteriovenous oxygen difference is the same in persons with dementia and normal controls. These somewhat indirect measures have been dramatically confirmed[101,102] by positron emission tomography (PET) with ^{15}O, which shows that there is no change in oxygen extraction by cerebral cortex in AD.

On the other hand, multiple strokes are correlated with dementia, forming a distinct group of patients with senile dementia.[128] There are two forms of vascular disease that produce dementia most commonly.[168] The first is multiple strokes, or MID, and the second is the lacunar state. The latter is a condition in which there are multiple small lacunae, or cavities, usually in the basal ganglia and other periventricular areas, which are associated with hypertension in a very high percentage of cases. In general, about 50% of patients with strokes have prior hypertension, while perhaps as much as 80% to 90% of those with MID and lacunar states are hypertensive. Nevertheless, one must be cautious in treating hypertension in individuals with early MID or lacunar states, since too rapid reduction of blood pressure may precipitate even more strokes when the cerebral vasculature is severely impaired. From the data of Tomlinson and colleagues,[331] about 18% of patients with senile dementia have primary multiple infarcts, and another 10% have mixed vascular disease and AD.

ALZHEIMER DISEASE AND NORMAL AGING

When one considers the creative talents of Eubie Blake, Konrad Adenauer, Pablo Casals, Rebecca West, or Pablo Picasso when they were in their late 80s or mid-90s, it is evident that one need not belong to the genetic isolates in mountainous regions of South America or the Indian subcontinent to maintain intellectual vigor in late old age. Longitudinal studies have shown that many individuals maintain full cognitive function as they age (see Chapter 2). Some of the intellectual decline believed to have been demonstrated by earlier cross-sectional studies of intellect in aged individuals appears to represent a secular or generational change due, in part, to the extraordinary educational differences between persons in different decades of life in the United States at present. Nevertheless, it is an accepted part of our tradition, and apparent to anyone with older relatives or friends, that some degree of slowing of intellectual processes and some degree of mild forgetfulness, such as the inability to find the correct word, remember the name of an acquaintance, or recollect details of a recent event, is not, by itself, prognostic of a progressive deterioration. Kral[183,184] labeled such forgetfulness "benign senescent forgetfulness," indicating that it was a normal concomitant of aging. The term *age-associated memory impairment* has now replaced Kral's term.[64] The memory deficit in normal aging is discussed in detail in Chapter 2.

CURRENT PROGRESS AND DIRECTIONS

Major advances have been made in recent years in understanding the pathogenesis or underlying mechanism of the disorder. We can now speak in quantitative terms of neuron and synaptic loss and alterations, of lesion frequency and substructure, and of physiologically significant biochemical alterations.

The cause of the disorder, which is of course the most important problem in terms of prevention or cure, is still a very clouded issue. Significant progress may be noted in terms of understanding the molecular nature of the abnormal proteins that accumulate in plaques and tangles. Slow virus has been related only through the scrapie model, but this sort of agent is under serious consideration. Latent conventional virus infection is another possibility on which more work will undoubtedly be forthcoming. The aluminum story is becoming increasingly clear and does not seem to be a primary cause of the disorder.

The interest in AD has risen as a result of the recognition that "senility," the progressive mental deterioration occurring in some elderly, is not just "aging," but is most often the result of a pathologic process identical to that of AD occurring in the presenium. There is now a consensus that the clinical syndrome of senile dementia can be associated with several organic disorders, but the most important form is identical to the pathology of AD. A consensus has developed that AD is an age-related disease, but not an inevitable consequence of aging and that it is distinct from the normal aging of the brain. Still, there are some investigators who argue that anyone living past 120 years would develop AD changes in the brain, an argument that cannot be settled since the longest longevity yet recorded is 120 years.[205a] However, available epidemiologic data are contrary to the latter argument. A major factor in developing a consensus was the demonstration in 1968 by Blessed and colleagues[32] that the intellectual decline in AD is correlated with the extent of the pathologic changes in the brain.

During the past 14 years, extraordinary advances have been made in understanding the neurotransmitter and molecular changes that occur in the AD brain. The technology of modern biology is now being successfully applied to AD, since developments have reached a point that makes the disease accessible to these approaches. One familial gene present in a limited number of families has been localized to chromosome 21, and other familial genes are still being sought. The gene for the precursor protein for the amyloid peptide that accumulates in the core of the NP as well as the walls of some blood has been sequenced. Major advances have been made in understanding the proteins that form PHFs. It has become apparent, however, that in addition to genetic factors there are as yet unknown metabolic or environmental factors that predispose to AD. Epidemiologic approaches have begun to provide clues in this regard.

A variety of diseases are responsible for the remaining 35% of cases of senile dementia. The second most important of these is senile dementia associated with vascular disease, an entity that includes MID and lacunar states, but it is agreed that AD is not caused by cerebral arteriosclerosis. A newly emerging cause of dementia in younger individuals is AIDS encephalopathy.

By treating AD as a disease rather than as an inevitable consequence of aging, we have brought to bear the investigative techniques of modern biomedical research. These investigations are beginning to provide the first understanding of the molecular pathology of the disease. Much remains to be done to determine the etiologies and risk factors, to understand fully the pathogenetic mechanisms, and to develop ultimately prevention as well as rational therapy to stop the progression of this malignant disorder.

REFERENCES

1. Abraham, CR, Selkoe, DJ, and Potter, H: Immunochemical identification of the serine protease inhibitor alpha antichymotripsin in the brain amyloid deposits of Alzheimer's disease. Cell 52:487–501, 1988.

2. Adolfsson, R, Gottfries, CG, Oreland, L, Roos, BE, and Winblad, B: Reduced Levels of Catecholamines in the Brain and Increased Activity of Monoamine Oxidase in Platelets in Alzheimer's Disease: Therapeutic Implications. In Katzman, R, Terry, RD, and Bick, KL (eds): Alzheimer's Disease: Senile Dementia and Related Disorders. Aging Series, Vol 7. Raven Press, New York, 1978, p 441.

3. Adolfsson, R, Gottfries, CG, Oreland, L, Wiberg, A, and Winblad, B: Increased activity of brain and platelet monoamine oxidase in dementia of Alzheimer type. Life Sci 27:1029–1034, 1980.

4. Alfrey, AC, Hegg, A, and Craswell, P: Metabolism and toxicity of aluminum in renal failure. Am J Clin Nutr 33:1509–1516, 1980.

5. Alfrey, AC, LeGendre, GR, and Kaehny, WD: The dialysis encephalopathy syndrome: Possible aluminum intoxication. N Engl J Med 294:184–188, 1976.

6. Alzheimer, A: Uber eine eigenartige Erkrankung der Hirnrinde Algemeine Zeitschrift Psychiatrie 64:164, 1907.

7. Amaducci, L, Fratiglioni, L, Rocca, WA, Fieschi, C, Livrea, P, Pedone, D, Bracco, L, Lippi, A, Gandolfo, C, Bino, G, Precipe, M, Bonatti, ML, Girotti, F, Carella, F, Tavolato, B, Ferla, S, Lenzi, GL, Carolei, A, Gambi, A, Grigoletto, F, and Schoenberg, BS: Risk factors for clinically diagnosed Alzheimer's disease: A case-control study of an Italian population. Neurology 36:922–931, 1986.

8. American Psychiatric Association: Diagnostic and Statistical Manual of Mental Disorders, ed 3. American Psychiatric Association, Washington, DC, 1980, p 494.

9. Antuono, P, Sorbi, S, Bracco, L, Fusco, T, and Amaducci, L: A discrete sampling technique in senile dementia of the Alzheimer type and alcoholic dementia: Study of the cholinergic system. In Amaducci, L, Davison, AN, and Antuono, P (eds): Aging of the Brain and Dementia. Aging Series, Vol 13. Raven Press, New York, 1980, p 151.

10. Arai, H, Kobayshi, K, Ichimiya, Y, Kosak, K, and Iizyka, RA: Preliminary study of free amino acids in the postmortem temporal cortex from Alzheimer-type dementia patients. Neurobiol Aging 5:319–321, 1984.

11. Arendt, T, Bigl, V, Arendt, A, and Tennstedt, A: Loss of neurons in the nucleus basalis of Meynert in Alzheimer's disease, paralysis agitans and Korsakoff's disease. Acta Neuropathol 61:101–108, 1983.

12. Arieff, AI and Mahoney, CA: Pathogenesis of dialysis encephalopathy. Neurobehav Toxicol Teratol 5:641–644, 1983.

13. Armstrong, DM, Benzing, WC, Evan, J, Terry, RD, Shields, D, and Hansen, LA: Substance P and somatostatin coexist within neuritic plaques: Implications for the pathogenesis of Alzheimer's disease. Neuroscience 3:663–671, 1989.

14. Armstrong, DM, Bruce, G, Hersh, LB, and Terry, RD: Choline acetyltransferase immunoreactivity in neuritic plaques of Alzheimer brain. Neurosci Lett 71:229–234, 1986.

15. Armstrong, DM, LeRoy, J, Shields, D, and Terry, RD: Somatostatin-like immunoreactivity within neuritic plaques. Brain Res 338:71–79, 1985.

16. Armstrong, DM and Terry, RD: Substance P immunoreactivity within neuritic plaques. Neurosci Lett 58:139–144, 1985.

17. Aronson, MK, Ooi, WL, Morgenstern, H, Hafner, A, Masur, D, Crystal, H, Frishman, WH, Fisher, D, and Katzman, R: Women, myocardial infarction and dementia

in the very old. Neurology 40:1102–1106, 1990.

18. Averbach, P: Two new lesions in Alzheimer's disease. Lancet 2:1203, 1983.

19. Ball, MJ and Lo, P: Granulovacuolar degeneration in the aging brain and in dementia. J Neuropathol Exp Neurol 36:474–487, 1977.

20. Beal, MF, Clevens, RA, Chattha, GK, MacGarvey, UM, Mazurek, MF, and Gabriel, SM: Galanin-like immunoreactivity is unchanged in Alzheimer's disease and Parkinson's disease dementia cerbral cortex. J Neurochem 51:1935–1941, 1988.

21. Beal, MF and Mazurek, MF: Substance P-like immunoreactivity is reduced in Alzheimer's disease cerebral cortex. Neurology 37:1205–1209, 1987.

22. Beal, MF, Mazurek, MF, Chattha, GK, Svendsen, CN, Bird, ED, and Martin, JB: Neuropeptide Y immunoreactivity is reduced in cerebral cortex in Alzheimer's disease. Ann Neurol 20:282–288, 1986.

23. Beal, MF, Mazurek, MF, and Martin, JB: Somatostatin immunoreactivity is reduced in Parkinson's disease dementia with Alzheimer's changes. Brain Res 397:386–388, 1986.

24. Beal, MF, Mazurek, MF, and McKee, MA: The regional distribution of somatostatin and neuropeptide Y in control and Alzheimer's disease striatum. Neurosci Lett 79:201–206, 1987.

25. Beal, MF, Mazurek, MF, Svendsen, CN, Bird, ED, and Martin, JB: Widespread reduction of somatostatin-like immunoreactivity in the cerebral cortex in Alzheimer's disease. Ann Neurol 20:489–496, 1986.

26. Beal, MF, Mazurek, MR, Tran, VT, Chattha, G, Bird, ED, and Martin JB: Reduced numbers of somatostatin receptors in the cerebral cortex in Alzheimer's dis-

ease. Science 229:289–291, 1985.

27. Benton, JS, Bowen, DM, Allen, SJ, Haan, EA, Neary, D, Davison, AN, Murphy, RP, and Snowden, JS: Alzheimer's disease as a disorder of isodendritic core. Lancet 1:456, 1982.

28. Berger, B, Escourolle, R, and Moyne, MA: Axones catecho-laminergiques du cortex cerebral humain: Observation, en histofluorescence, de biopsies cerebrales dont 2 case de maladie d'Alzheimer. Rev Neurol (Paris) 132:183–194, 1976.

29. Bharucha, NE, Schoenberg, BS, Kokmen, E: Dementia of Alzheimer's type: A case-control study of association with medical conditions and surgical procedures. Neurology (Suppl 2)33:85, 1983.

30. Bird, TD, Sumi, SM, Nemens, EJ, Nochlin, D, Schellenberg, G, Lampe, TM, Sadovnick, A, Chui, H, Miner, GW, and Tinklenberg, J: Phenotypic heterogeneity in familial Alzheimer's disease: A study of 24 kindreds. Ann Neurol 25:12–25, 1989.

31. Bissette, G, Reynolds, GP, Kitts, CD, Widerlov, E, and Nemeroff, CPB: Corticotropin-releasing factor-like immunoreactivity in senile dementia of the Alzheimer type. JAMA 254:3067–3069, 1985.

32. Blessed, G, Tomlinson, BE, and Roth, M: The association between quantitative measurements of dementia and of senile changes in the cerebral gray matter of elderly subjects. Br J Psychiatry 114:797–811, 1968.

32a. Bollerup, TR: Prevalence of mental illness among 70-year-olds domiciled in nine Copenhagen suburbs: The Glostrup Survey. Acta Psychiatr Scand 51:327–339, 1975.

33. Bowen, DM, Allen, SJ, Benton, JS, Goodhardt, MJ, Haan, EA, Palmer, AM, Sims, NR, Smith, CCT, Spillane, A, Esiri, MM,

Neary, D, Snowdon, JS, Wilcock, GK, and Davison, AN: Biochemical assessment of serotonergic and cholinergic dysfunction and cerebral atrophy in Alzheimer's disease. J Neurochem 41:266–272, 1983.

34. Bowen, DM, Smith, CB, White, P, and Davison, AN: Neurotransmitter-related enzymes and indices of hypoxia in senile dementia and other abiotrophies. Brain 99:459–496, 1976.

35. Bowen, DM, Smith, CB, White, P, and Davison, AN: Senile Dementia and Related Abiotrophies: Biochemical Studies on Histologically Evaluated Human Postmortem Specimens. In Terry, RD and Gershon, S (eds): Neurobiology of Aging. Aging Series, Vol 3. Raven Press, New York, 1976, p 361.

36. Bowen, DM, Spillane, JA, Curzon, G, Meier-Ruge, W, White, P, Goodhardt, MJ, Iwangoff, P, and Davison, AN: Accelerated ageing or selective neuronal loss as an important cause of dementia? Lancet 1:11-14, 1979.

37. Breitner, JCS, Murphy, EA, Silverman, JM, Mohs, RC, and Davis, KL: Age-dependent expression of familial risk in Alzheimer's disease. Am J Epidemiol 128:536–548, 1988.

38. Bremer, J: A social psychiatric investigation of a small community in northern Norway. Acta Psychiatr Neurol Scand (Suppl)62:1–166, 1951.

39. Brion, JP, Passareiro, H, Nunez, J, and Flament-Durand, J: Mise en evidence immunologique de la proteine tau au niveau des lesions de degenerescence neurofibrillaire de la maladie d'Alzheimer. Arch Biol (Bruxelles) 95:229–235, 1985.

40. Broe, GA, Ajhtar, AJ, Andrews, GR, Caird, FI, Gilmore, AJJ, and McLennan, WJ: Neurological disorders in the elderly at home. J Neurol Neurosurg Psychiatry 39:362–366, 1976.

41. Brun, A, Gustafson, L, and Mittelman, F: Normal chromosome banding pattern in Alzheimer's disease. Gerontology (Basel) 24:369, 1978.

42. Burke, WJ, Chung, HD, Nakra, BRS, Grossberg, GT, and Joh, TH: Phenylethanolamine N-methyltransferase activity is decreased in Alzheimer's disease brains. Ann Neurol 22:278–280, 1987.

43. Burger, PC and Vogel, FS: The development of the pathologic changes of Alzheimer's disease and senile dementia in patients with Down's syndrome. Am J Pathol 73:457–476, 1973.

44. Candy, JM, Klinowski, J, Perry, RH, Perry, EK, Fairbairn, A, Oakley, AE, Carpenter, TA, Attack, JR, Blessed, G, and Edwardson, JA: Aluminosilicates and senile plaque formation in Alzheimer's disease. Lancet 1:354–357, 1986.

45. Chan-Palay, V: Neurons with galanin innervate cholinergic cells in the human basal forebrain and galanin and acetylcholine coexist. Brain Res Bull 21:465–472, 1988.

46. Chan-Palay, V: Galanin hyperinnervates surviving neurons of the human basal nucleus of Meynert in dementias of Alzheimer's and Parkinson's disease: A hypothesis for the role of galanin in accentuating cholinergic dysfunction in dementia. J Comp Neurol 273:543–557, 1988.

47. Chapman, J, Bachar, O, Korczlyn, AD, Werman, E, and Michaelson, DM: Antibodies to cholinergic neurons in Alzheimer's disease. J Neurochem 51:479–485, 1988.

48. Chu, DCM, Penney, JF, Jr, and Young, AB: Quantitative autoradiography of hippocampal GABA$_B$ and GABA$_A$ receptor changes in Alzheimer's disease.

Neurosci Lett 82:246–252, 1987.

49. Cohen, D, Eisdorfer, C, and Leverenz, J: Maternal age as a risk factor in Alzheimer's dementia. J Am Geriatr Soc 30:656–659, 1982.

50. Cohen, D, Eisdorfer, C, and Walford, R: HLA antigens and patterns of cognitive loss in dementia of the Alzheimer's type. Neurobiol Aging 2:27–32, 1981.

51. Cohen, EL and Wurtman, RJ: Brain acetylcholine: Control by dietary choline. Science 191:561–562, 1976.

52. Cole, G, Dobkins, KR, Hansen, LA, Terry, RD, and Saitoh, T: Decreased levels of protein kinase C in Alzheimer brain. Brain Res 452:165–174, 1988.

53. Constantinidis, J: Is Alzheimer's Disease a Major Form of Senile Dementia? Clinical, Anatomical, and Genetic Data. In Katzman, R, Terry, RD, and Bick, KL (eds): Alzheimer's Disease: Senile Dementia and Related Disorders Aging Series, Vol 7. Raven Press, New York, 1978, p 15.

54. Cook, RH, Schenck, SA, and Clark, DB: Twins with Alzheimer's disease. Arch Neurol 38:300–301, 1981.

55. Copeland, JRM, Gurland, BJ, Dewey, ME, Kelleher, MJ, Smith, AMR, and Davidson, IA: Is there more dementia, depression and neurosis in New York? A comparative study of the elderly in New York and London using the computer diagnosis AGECAT. Br J Psychiatry 151:466–473, 1987.

56. Corkin, S: An acetylcholine, aging, and Alzheimer's disease: Implications for treatment. Trends Neurosci 4:287–290, 1981.

57. Corkin, S, Growdon, JH, and Rasmussen, L: Parental age as a risk factor in Alzheimer's disease. Ann Neurol 13:674–676, 1983.

58. Corsellis, JAN: Mental illness and the Ageing Brain. Maudsley Monograph, No 9. Oxford University Press, London, 1962.

59. Cowburn, RF, Hardy, JA, Briggs, RS, and Roberts, PJ: Characterization, density and distribution of kainate receptors in normal and Alzheimer's diseased human brain. J Neurochem 52:140–147, 1989.

60. Cowburn, RF, Hardy, JA, Roberts, PJ, and Briggs, RS: Presynaptic and postsynaptic glutamatergic function in Alzheimer's disease. Neurosci Lett 86:109–113, 1988.

61. Crapper, DR, Karlik, S, and Deboni, U: Aluminum and Other Metals in Senile (Alzheimer's) Dementia. In Katzman, R, Terry, RD, and Bick, KL (eds): Alzheimer's Disease: Senile Dementia and Related Disorders. Aging Series, Vol 7. Raven Press, New York, 1978, p 471.

62. Crapper, DR, Krishnan, SS, and Dalton, AJ: Brain aluminum distribution in Alzheimer's disease and experimental neurofibrillary degeneration. Science 180:511–513, 1973.

63. Crapper, DR, Quittkat, S, and Deboni, U: Altered chromatin conformation in Alzheimer's disease. Brain 102:483–495, 1979.

64. Crook, T, Bartus, RT, Ferris, SH, Whitehouse, P, Cohen, GD, and Gershon, S: Age-associated memory impairment: Proposed diagnostic criteria and measures of clinical change: Report of a National Institute of Mental Health work group. Dev Neuropsychol 2:261–276, 1986.

65. Cross, AJ, Crow, TJ, Johnson, JA, Perry, EK, Perry, RH, Blessed, G, and Tomlinson, BE: Studies on neurotransmitter receptor systems in neocortex and hippocampus in senile dementia of the Alzheimer-type. J Neurol Sci 64:109–117, 1984.

66. Cross, AJ, Crow, TJ, Perry, EK, Perry, RH, Blessed, G, and Tom-

linson, BE: Reduced dopamine beta-hydroxylase activity in Alzheimer's disease. Br Med J 282:93–94, 1981.

67. Cross, AJ, Crow, TJ, and Peter, TJ: Cortical Neurochemistry in Alzheimer-Type Dementia. In Swaab, DR (ed): Progress in Brain Research, Vol 70. Elsevier, New York, 1986, p 153.

68. Cross, AJ, Slater, P, Candy, JM, Perry, EK, and Perry, RH: Glutamate deficits in Alzheimer's disease. J Neurol Neurosurg Psychiatry 50:357–358, 1986.

68a. Cross, PS and Gurland, BJ: The Epidemiology of Dementing Disorders: Report to the United States Congress, Office of Technology Assessment, 1986.

69. Crystal, HA and Davis, P: Cortical substance P-like immunoreactivity in cases of Alzheimer's disease and senile dementia of the Alzheimer type. J Neurochem 38:1781–1784, 1982.

70. Crystal, HA, Dickson, D, Fuld, P, Masur, D, Scott, MA, Mehler, M, Masdu, J, Kawas, C, Aronson, M, and Wolfson, L: Clinicopathologic studies in dementia: nondemented subjects with pathologically confirmed Alzheimer's disease. Neurology 38:1682–1687, 1988.

71. Crystal, HA, Houroupian, DS, Katzman, R, and Jotkowits, S: Biopsy-proved Alzheimer disease presenting as a right parietal lobe syndrome. Ann Neurol 12:186–188, 1982.

72. D'Amato, RJ, Zweig, RM, Whitehouse, PJ, Wenk, GL, Singer, HS, Mayeux, R, Price, DL, and Snyder, SH: Aminergic systems in Alzheimer's disease and Parkinson's disease. Ann Neurol 22:229–236, 1987.

73. Davies, CA, Mann, DMA, Sumpter, PQ, and Yates, PO: A quantitative morphometric analysis of the neuronal and synaptic content of the frontal and temporal cortex in patients with Alzhei-

mer's disease. J Neurol Sci 78:151–164, 1987.

74. Davies, LKH, Wolska, B, Hilbich, C, Multhaup, G, Martins, R, Simms, GL, Beyreuther, K, and Masters, CL: A4 amyloid protein deposition and the diagnosis of Alzheimer's disease. Neurology 38:1688–1693, 1988.

75. Davies, P and Feisullin, S: Postmortem stability of alpha bungarotoxin binding sites in mouse and human brain. Brain Res 216:449–454, 1981.

76. Davies, P, Katz, D, and Crystal, H: Choline Acetyltransferase, Somatostatin, and Substance P in Selected Cases of Alzheimer's Disease. In Corkin, S, Davis, KL, Growdon, JH, and Usdin, E (eds): A Report of Progress in Research. Aging Series, Vol 19. Raven Press, New York, 1982, p 9.

77. Davies, P, Katzman, R, and Terry, RD: Reduced somatostatin-like immunoreactivity in cerebral cortex from cases of Alzheimer disease and Alzheimer senile dementia. Nature 288:279–280, 1980.

78. Davies, P and Maloney, AJR: Selective loss of central cholinergic neurons in Alzheimer's disease. Lancet 2:1403, 1976.

79. Davies, P and Terry, RD: Cortical somatostatin-like immunoreactivity in cases of Alzheimer's disease and senile dementia of the Alzheimer type. Neurobiol Aging 2:9–14, 1981.

80. Davies, P and Verth, AH: Regional distribution of muscarinic acetylcholine receptor in normal and Alzheimer's type dementia brains. Brain Res 138:385–392, 1977.

81. Davis, KL, Mohs, RC, Davis, BM, Levy, M, Rosenberg, GS, Horvath, TB, DeNigris, Y, Ross, A, Decker, P, and Rothpearl, A: Cholinomimetic Agents and Human Memory: Clinical Studies in Alzheimer's Disease and

Scopolamine Dementia. In Crook, T and Gershon, S (eds): Strategies for the Development of an Effective Treatment for Senile Dementia. Mark Posley Associates, New Canaan, CT, 1981, p 53.

82. De Braekeleer, M, Froda, S, Gautrin, D, Tetreault, H, and Gauvreau, D: Parental age and birth order in Alzheimer disease: A case-control study in the Saguenay-Lac-St-Jean Area (Quebec, Canada). Can J Neurol Sci 15:139–141, 1988.

83. Defossez, A, Belauviain, JC, Delacourte, A, and Mazzuca, M: Alzheimer's disease: A new evidence for common epitopes between microtubule associated protein Tau and paired helical filaments: Demonstration at the electron microscope level by a double immunogold labelling. Virchows Arch [Pathol Anat] 413:141–145, 1988.

84. Delabar, JM, Goldgaber, D, Lamour, Y, Nicole, A, Huret, J-L, DeGrouchy, J, Brown, P, Gajdusek, C, and Sinet, P-M: β-Amyloid gene duplication in Alzheimer's disease and karyotypically normal Down syndrome. Science 235:1390–1392, 1987.

85. DeSouza, EB, Whitehouse, PJ, Kuhar, MJ, Price, DL, and Vale, WW: Reciprocal changes in corticotropin releasing factor (CRF)-like immunoreactivity and CRF receptors in cerebral cortex of Alzheimer's disease. Nature 319:593–595, 1986.

86. Dickson, DW, Farlo, J, Davies, P, Crystal, H, Fuld, PA, and Yen, SC: Alzheimer's disease: A double labeling immunohistochemical study of senile plaques. Am J Pathol 132:86–101, 1988.

87. Divry, P: Cerebral ageing. J Belge Neurol Psychiatry 47:65, 1947.

88. Drachman, D: Scopolamine-Induced Dementia. In Katzman, R, Terry, RD, and Bick, KL (eds): Alzheimer's Disease: Senile Dementia and Related Disorders. Aging Series, Vol 7. Raven Press, New York, 1978, p 143.

89. Drachman, DA and Leavitt, J: Human memory and the cholinergic system. Arch Neurol 30:113–121, 1974.

90. Duyckaerts, C, Delaere, P, Poulain, V, Brion, JP, and Hauw, JJ: Does amyloid precede paired helical filaments in the senile plaque? A study of 15 cases with graded intellectual status in aging and Alzheimer disease. Neurosci Lett 91:354–359, 1988.

91. Dyrks, T, Weidemann, A, Multhaup, G, Salbaum, JM, Lemaire, HG, Kang, J, Muller-Hill, B, Masters, CL, and Beyreuther, K: Identification, transmembrane orientation and biogenesis of the amyloid A4 precursor of Alzheimer's disease. EMBO J 7:949–957, 1988.

92. Eisdorfer, C, Cohen, D, and Buckley, CE: Serum immunoglobulins and cognition in the impaired elderly. In Katzman, R, Terry, RD, and Bick, KL (eds): Alzheimer's Disease: Senile Dementia and Related Disorders. Aging Series, Vol 7. Raven Press, New York 1978, p 401.

93. Ellis, WG, McCulloch, JR, and Corley, CL: Presenile dementia in Down's syndrome: Ultrastructural identity with Alzheimer's disease. Neurology 24:101–106, 1974.

94. Esiri, MM and Wilcock, GK: The olfactory bulbs in Alzheimer's disease. J Neurol Neurosurg Psychiatry 47:56–60, 1984.

95. Essen-Möller, E: Individual traits and morbidity in a Swedish rural population. Acta Psychiatr Neurol Scand (Suppl 100)31:1–160, 1956.

96. Evans, DA, Funkenstein, HH, Albert, MS, Scherr, PA, Cook, NR, Chown, MJ, Hebert, LE, Hennedens, CH, and Taylor, JO: Prevalence of Alzheimer's disease in a community population of older

persons. Higher than previously reported. JAMA 262:2551–2556, 1989.

97. Falck, B, Hillarp, NA, Thieme, G, and Torp, A: Fluorescence of catecholamines and related compounds condensed with formaldehyde. J Histochem Cytochem 10:348–354, 1962.

98. Ferrier, IN, Cross, AF, Johnson, JA, Roberts, GW, Crow, TJ, Corsellis, JAN, Lee, YC, O'Shaughnessy, D, Adrian, TE, McGregor, GP, Baracese-Hamilton, AJ, and Bloom, SR: Neuropeptides in Alzheimer type dementia. J Neurol Sci 62:159–170, 1983.

99. Fisman, M, Merskey, H, Helmes, E, McCready, J, Colhoun, EH, and Rylett, BJ: Double blind study of lecithin in patients with Alzheimer's disease. Can J Psychiatry 26:426–428, 1981.

100. Flaten, TP: Geographical associations between aluminum in drinking water and registered death rates with dementia (including Alzheimer's disease) in Norway. Proceedings of the Second International Symposium on Geochemistry and Health, 1987.

101. Frackowiak, RSJ, Lenzi, GL, and Jones, T: Quantitative measurement of regional cerebral blood flow and oxygen metabolism in man using ^{15}O and positron emission tomography: Theory, procedure and normal values. J Comput Assist Tomogr 4:727–736, 1980.

102. Frackowiak, RSJ, Pozzilli, C, Legg, CJ, Boulay, GH, Marshall, J, Lenzi, GL, and Jones, T: Regional cerebral oxygen supply and utilization in dementia: A clinical and physiological study with oxygen ^{15}O and positron tomography. Brain 104:753–778, 1981.

103. Francis, PT, Bowen, DM, Lowe, SL, Neary, D, Mann, DMA, and Snowden, JS: Somatostatin content and release measured in cerebral biopsies from demented patients. J Neurol Sci 78:1–16, 1987.

104. French, LR, Schuman, LM, Mortimer, JA, Hutton, JT, Boatman, RA, and Christians, B: A case-control study of dementia of the Alzheimer type. Am J Epidemiol 121:414–421, 1985.

105. Freyhan, FA, Woodford, RB, and Kety, SS: Cerebral blood flow and metabolism in psychoses of senility. J Nerv Mental Dis 113:449–456, 1951.

106. Fujiyoshi, K, Suga, H, Okamoto, K, Nakamura, S, and Kameyama, M: Reduction of arginine-vasopressin in the cerebral cortex in Alzheimer type senile dementia. J Neurol Neurosurg Psychiatry 50:929–932, 1987.

107. Gage, FH, Armstrong, DM, Williams, LR, and Varon, S: Morphological response of axotomized septal neurons to nerve growth factor. J Comp Neurol 269:147–155, 1988.

108. Gage, FH, Björklund, A, Stenevi, U, Dunnet, SB, and Kelly, PAT: Intrahippocampal septal grafts ameliorate learning impairments in aged rats. Science 225:533–536, 1984.

109. Gage, FH, Rosenberg, MB, Tuszynski, MH, Yoshida, K, Armstrong, DM, Hayes, R, and Friedmann, T: Gene Therapy in the CNS: Intracerebral Grafting of Genetically Modified Cells. In Phelps, CH, Coleman, P, and Higgins, G (eds): Progress in Brain Research, Vol 86. Elsevier, New York, 1990, pp 205–217.

110. Geddes, JW, Anderson, KJ, and Cotman, LCW: Senile plaques as aberrant sprout-stimulating structures. Exp Neurol 94:767–776, 1986.

111. Geddes, JW, Chang-Chui, H, Cooper, SM, Lotte, IT, and Cotman, CW: Density and distribution of NMDA receptors in the human hippocampus in Alzheimer's

disease. Brain Res 399:156–161, 1986.

112. Geddes, JW, Monaghan, DT, Cotman, CW, Lott, IT, Kim, RC, and Chui, LHC: Plasticity of hippocampal circuitry in Alzheimer's disease. Science 230:1179–1181, 1985.

113. Gellerstedt, N: Zur Kenntnis der Hirnverandungen bei der normalen Altersinvolution. Upsala Laekarefoerenings Foerhandlingar 38:193, 1932/1933.

114. Gertz, HJ, Cervos-Navarro, J, and Ewald, V: The septo-hippocampal pathway in patients suffering from senile dementia of Alzheimer's type. Evidence for neuronal plasticity. Neurosci Lett 76:228–232, 1987.

115. Giaccone, G, Tagliavini, F, Linoli, G, Bouras, D, Frigeri, OL, Frangione, B, and Bugiani, O: Down patients: Extracellular preamyloid deposits precede neuritic degeneration and senile plaques. Neurosci Lett 97:232–238, 1989.

116. Glenner, GG and Wong, CW: Alzheimer's disease: Initial report of the purification and characterization of a novel cerebrovascular amyloid protein. Biochem Biophys Res Commun 120:885–890, 1984.

117. Glenner, GG and Wong, CW: Alzheimer's disease and Down's syndrome: Sharing of a unique cerebrovascular amyloid fibril protein. Biochem Biophys Res Commun 122:1131–1135, 1984.

117a. Groate, A, Chartier-Harlin, M-C, Mullan, M, Brown, J, Crawford, F, Fidani, L, Giuffra, L, Haynes, A, Irving, N, James, L, Mant, R, Newton, P, Rooke, K, Roques, P, Talbot, C, Pericak-Vance, M, Roses, A, Williamson, R, Rossor, M, Owan, M, and Hardy, J: Segregation of a missense mutation in the amyloid precursor protein gene with familial Alzheimer's

disease. Nature 349:704–706, 1991.

118. Goldgaber, D, Lerman, MI, McBride, OW, Saffiotti, U, and Gajdusek, DC: Characterization and chromosomal localization of a cDNA encoding brain amyloid of Alzheimer's disease. Science 235:877–880, 1987.

119. Goldman, JE: The association of actin with Hirano bodies. J Neuropathol Exp Neurol 42:146–152, 1983.

120. Goldman, JE and Yen, SH: Cytoskeletal protein abnormalities in neurodegenerative disease. Ann Neurol 19:209–223, 1986.

121. Goldman, JE, Yen, SH, Chiu, FC, and Peress, NS: Lewy bodies of Parkinson's disease contain neurofilament antigens. Science 221:1082–1084, 1983.

122. Gonatas, NK, Anderson, W, and Evangelista, I: The contribution of altered synapses in the senile plaque. An electron-microscopic study in Alzheimer's dementia. J Neuropathol Exp Neurol 26:25–39, 1967.

123. Gottfries, CG: Amine Metabolism in Normal Ageing and in Dementia Disorders. In Roberts, PJ (ed): Biochemistry of Dementia. John Wiley & Sons, Chichester, 1980, p 213.

124. Gottfries, CG, Gottfries, I, and Roos, BE: Homovanillic acid and 5-hydroxyindoleacetic acid in the cerebrospinal fluid of patients with senile dementia, presenile dementia and parkinsonism. J Neurochem 16:1341–1345, 1969.

125. Goudsmit, J, Morrow, CH, Asher, DM, Yanagihara, RT, Masters, CL, Gibbs, CJ, and Gajdusek, DC: Evidence for and against the transmissibility of Alzheimer disease. Neurology 30:945–950, 1980.

126. Greenamyre, JT, Penny, JB, Young, AB, D'Amato, CJ, Hicks, SP, and Shoulson, I: Alteration in L-glu-

tamate binding in Alzheimer's and Huntington's diseases. Science 227:1496–1499, 1985.

127. Gruenberg, EM: A Mental Health Survey of Older Persons. In Hoch, PC and Zubin, J (eds): Comparative Epidemiology of the Mental Disorders. Grune & Stratton, New York, 1961, p 13.

128. Hachinski, V: Cerebral Blood Flow: Differentiation of Alzheimer's Disease from Multi-infarct Dementia. In Katzman, R, Terry, RD, and Bick KL (eds): Alzheimer's Disease: Senile Dementia and Related Disorders. Aging Series, Vol 7. Raven Press, New York, 1978, p 97.

129. Hagnell, O, Lanke, J, Rorsman, B, and Ojesjo, L: Does the incidence of age psychosis decrease? Neuropsychobiology 7:201–211, 1981.

130. Hamos, JE, DeGennaro, LJ, and Drachman, DA: Synaptic loss in Alzheimer's disease and other dementias. Neurology 39:355–361, 1989.

131. Hansen, LA, Armstrong, DM, and Terry, RD: An immunohistochemical quantification of fibrous astrocytes in the aging human cerebral cortex. Neurobiol Aging 8:1–6, 1987.

132. Hansen, LA, DeTeresa, R, Davies, P, and Terry, RD: Neocortical morphometry, lesion counts, and choline acetyltransferase levels in the age spectrum of Alzheimer's disease. Neurology 38:48–54, 1989.

133. Hansen, LA, DeTeresa, R, Tobias, H, Alford, M, and Terry, RD: Neocortical morphometry and cholinergic neurochemistry in Pick's disease. Am J Pathol 131:507–518, 1989.

134. Hansen, LA, Masliah, E, Terry, RD, and Mirra, SS: A neuropathological subset of Alzheimer's disease with concomitant Lewy body disease and spongiform

change. Acta Neuropathol 78:194–201, 1989.

135. Hansen, L, Salmon, D, Galasko, D, Masliah, E, Katzman, R, DeTeresa, R, Thal, L, Pay, MM, Hofstetter, R, Klauber, MR, Rice, V, Butters, N, and Alford, M: The Lewy body variant of Alzheimer's disease: A clinical and pathological entity. Neurology 40:1–7, 1989.

136. Hardy, JA, Cowburn, RF, Barton, A, Reynolds, G, Lofdahl, E, O'Carroll, AM, Wester, P, and Winblad, B: Glutamate deficits in Alzheimer's disease. J Neurol Neurosurg Psychiatry 50:356–357, 1987.

137. Hefti, F and Weiner, WJ: Nerve growth factor (NGF) promotes survival of forebrain cholinergic neurons in an animal model of Alzheimer's disease. Neurology (Suppl 1)36:226, 1986.

137a. Helgason, T: Epidemiology of Mental Disorders in Iceland: A Geriatric Follow-up (Preliminary Report). In De La Fuenta, R and Weissman, E (eds): Proceedings of the Fifth Congress of Psychiatry, Mexico, 1971. Excerpta Medica, Amsterdam, 1973, p 350.

138. Henschke, PJ, Bell, DA, and Cape, RDT: Alzheimer's disease and HLA. Tissue Antigens 12:132–135, 1978.

139. Heston, LL: Alzheimer's disease, trisomy 21, and myelo-proliferative disorders: Associations suggesting a genetic diathesis. Science 196:322–323, 1977.

140. Heston, LL: Alzheimer's Disease and Senile Dementia: Genetic Relationships to Down's Syndrome and Hematologic Cancer. In Katzman, R (ed): Congenital and Acquired Cognitive Disorders. Association for Research in Nervous and Mental Disease, Vol 57. Raven Press, New York, 1979, p 167.

141. Heston, LL, Mastri, AR, Anderson, VE, and White, J: Dementia of

the Alzheimer type: Clinical genetics, natural history and associated conditions. Arch Gen Psychiatry 38:1085–1090, 1981.

142. Heston, LL and White, J: Pedigrees of 30 families with Alzheimer's disease: Associations with defective organization of microfilaments and microtubules. Behav Genet 8:315–331, 1978.

143. Hetnarski, B, Wisniewski, HM, Iqbal, K, Dziedzic, JD, and Lajtha, A: Central cholinergic activity in aluminum-induced neurofibrillary degeneration. Ann Neurol 7:489–490, 1980.

144. Heyman, A, Wilkinson, WE, Stafford, JA, Helms, MJ, Sigmon, AG, and Weinberg, T: Alzheimer's disease: A study of epidemiologic aspects. Ann Neurol 15:335–341, 1986.

145. Hirano, A, Dembitzer, HM, Kurland, LT, and Zimmerman, HM: The fine structure of some intraganglionic alterations: Neurofibrillary tangles, granulo-vacuolar bodies and "rod-like" structures as seen in Guam amyotrophic lateral sclerosis and parkinsonism-dementia complex. J Neuropathol Exp Neurol 27:167–182, 1968.

146. Hirano, A and Zimmerman, HM: Alzheimer's neurofibrillary changes: A topographic study. Arch Neurol 7:227–242, 1962.

147. Hornykiewicz, O: Dopamine in basal ganglia. Br Med Bull 29:172–178, 1973.

148. Hoyer, S: Blood Flow and Oxidative Metabolism of the Brain in Different Phases of Dementia. In Katzman, R, Terry, RD, and Bick, KL (eds): Alzheimer's Disease and Related Disorders. Aging Series, Vol 7. Raven Press, New York, 1978, p 219.

149. Hyman, BT, Van Hoesen, GW, and Damasio, AR: Alzheimer's disease: Glutamate depletion in the hippocampal perforant path-

way zone. Ann Neurol 22:37–40, 1987.

150. Hyman, BT, Van Hoesen, GW, Damasio, AR, and Barnes, CL: Alzheimer's disease: Cell-specific pathology isolates the hippocampal formation. Science 225:1168–1170, 1984.

151. Iimoto, D, Masliah, E, DeTeresa, R, Terry, RD, and Saitoh, T: Aberrant casein kinase II in Alzheimer's disease. Brain Res 507: 273–280, 1989.

152. Ingvar, DH, Brun, A, Hagsberg, B, and Gustafson, L: Regional Cerebral Blood Flow in the Dominant Hemisphere in Confirmed Cases of Alzheimer's Disease, Pick's Disease, and Multi-infarct Dementia: Relationship in Clinical Symptomatology and Neuropathological Findings. In Katzman, R, Terry, RD, and Bick, KL (eds): Alzheimer's Disease: Senile Dementia and Related Disorders. Aging Series, Vol 7. Raven Press, New York, 1978, p 203.

153. Ishii, T: Distribution of Alzheimer neurofibrillary tangles in the brain stem and hypothalamus of senile dementia. Acta Neuropathol (Berl) 6:181–187, 1966.

154. Ishino, H and Otsuki, S: Frequency of Alzheimer's neurofibrillary tangles in the basal ganglia and brain stem in Alzheimer's disease. Folia Psychiatr Neurol Japonica 929:279–287, 1975.

155. Jarvik, LF: Genetic Factors and Chromosomal Aberrations in Alzheimer's Disease, Senile Dementia, and Related Disorders. In Katzman, R, Terry, RD, and Bick, KL (eds): Alzheimer's Disease: Senile Dementia and Related Disorders. Aging Series, Vol 7. Raven Press, New York, 1978, p 273.

156. Jarvik, LF, Altshuler, KZ, Kato, T, and Blumner, B: Organic brain syndrome and chromosome loss in aged twins. Dis Nerv Syst 32:159–170, 1971.

157. Jarvik, LF and Kato, T: Chromosomes and mental changes in octogenarians—Preliminary findings. Br J Psychiatry 115:1193–1194, 1969.

158. Jarvik, LF, Ruth, V, and Matsuyama, SS: Organic brain syndrome and aging: A six year follow-up of surviving twins. Arch Gen Psychiatry 37:280–286, 1980.

159. Jellinger, J: Neuropathological aspects of dementias. Acta Neurol Belg 76:83–102, 1976.

160. Johnson, SA, Pasinetti, GM, May, PC, Ponte, PA, Cordell, B, and Finch, CE: Selective reduction of mRNA for the beta-amyloid precursor protein that lacks a Kunitz-type protease inhibitor motif in cortex from Alzheimer brains. Exp Neurol 102:264–268, 1988.

161. Johnson, SA and Finch, CE: Alzheimer's disease does not alter the proportion of hippocampal neurons with APP-695 or APP-751 mRNA. Soc Neurosci Abstr 15:1379, 1989.

162. Johnston, MV, McKinney, M, and Coyle, JT: Evidence for a cholinergic projection to neocortex from neurons in basal forebrain. Proc Natl Acad Sci USA 76:5392–5396, 1979.

163. Jorm, AF, Korten, AE, and Jacomb, PA: Projected increases in the number of dementia cases for 29 developed countries: Application of a new method for making projections. Acta Psychiatr Scand 78:493–500, 1976.

164. Joynt, RJ and McNeill, TH: Neuropeptides in aging and dementia. Peptides (Suppl 1)5:269–274, 1984.

165. Kallmann, FJ: Genetic Aspects of Mental Disorders in Later Life. In Kaplan, OJ (ed): Mental Disorders in Later Life, ed 2. Stanford University Press, Stanford, 1956, p 26.

166. Kang, J, Lemaire, H-G, Unterbeck, A, Salbaum, MJ, Masters, CL, Grzeschik, K-H, Multhaup, G, Beyreuther, K, and Müller-Hill, B: The precursor of Alzheimer's disease amyloid A4 protein resembles a cell-surface receptor. Nature 325:733–736, 1987.

167. Katzman, R: The prevalence and malignancy of Alzheimer disease. Arch Neurol 33:217–218, 1976.

168. Katzman, R: Vascular Disease and Dementia. In H Houston Merritt Memorial Volume. Raven Press, New York, 1983, p 153.

169. Katzman, R: Alzheimer's disease. N Engl J Med 314:964–973, 1986.

170. Katzman, R: Alzheimer's Disease as an Age-Dependent Disorder, Research and the Ageing Population. Ciba Foundation Symposium 134. Wiley, Chichester, 1988, p 69.

171. Katzman, R, Aronson, M, Fuld, PA, Kawas, C, Brown, T, Morgenstern, H, Frishman, W, Gidez, L, Eder, H, and Ooi, WL: Development of dementia in an 80-year-old volunteer cohort. Ann Neurol 25:317–324, 1989.

172. Katzman, R, Brown, T, Fuld, P, Thal, L, Davies, P, and Terry, RD: Significance of Neurotransmitter Abnormalities in Alzheimer's Disease. In Martin, JB and Barchas, J (eds): Neuropeptides in Neurologic and Psychiatric Disease. Association for Research in Nervous and Mental Disease, Vol 64. Raven Press, New York, 1986, p 279.

173. Katzman, R and Terry, RD (eds): The Neurology of Aging. FA Davis, Philadelphia, 1983.

174. Katzman, R, Terry, RD, and Bick, KL (eds): Alzheimer's Disease: Senile Dementia and Related Disorders. Aging Series, Vol 7. Raven Press, New York, 1978, p 1.

175. Katzman, R, Terry, RD, DeTeresa, R, Brown, LT, Davies, P, Fuld, P, Renbing, X, and Peck, A: Clinical pathological and neurochemical changes in dementia: A subgroup with preserved mental status and numerous neocorti-

cal plaques. Ann Neurol 23:53–59, 1988.

176. Kay, DWK, Beamish, P, and Roth, M: Old age mental disorders in Newcastle-upon-Tyne: I. A study of prevalence. Br J Psychiatry 110:146–158, 1964.

177. Kellar, KJ, Whitehouse, PJ, Martin-Barrows, AM, Marcus, K, and Price, DL: Muscarinic and nicotinic cholinergic binding sites in Alzheimer's disease cerebral cortex. Brain Res 436:62–68, 1987.

178. Kidd, M: Paired helical filaments in electron microscopy in Alzheimer's disease. Nature 197:192–193, 1963.

179. Kitaguchi, N, Takahashi, Y, Tokushima, Y, Shiojiri, S, and Hiratak, I: Novel precursor of Alzheimer's disease amyloid protein shows protease inhibitory activity. Nature 331:530–532, 1988.

180. Kitt, CA, Price, DL, Struble, RG, Cork, LC, Wainer, BH, Becher, MW, and Mobley, WC: Evidence for cholinergic neurites in senile plaques. Science 226:1443–1445, 1984.

181. Klatzo, I, Wisniewski, H, and Streicher, E: Experimental production of neurofibrillary degeneration. I. Light microscopic observations. J Neuropathol Exp Neurol 24:187–199, 1965.

182. Kowall, NW and Beal, MF: Galanin-like immunoreactivity is present in human substantia innominata and in senile plaques in Alzheimer's disease. Neurosci Lett 98:118–123, 1989.

183. Kral, VA: Senescent forgetfulness: Benign and malignant. Can Med Assoc J 86:257–260, 1962.

184. Kral, VA: Benign Senescent Forgetfulness. In Katzman, R, Terry, RD, and Bick, KL (eds): Alzheimer's Disease: Senile Dementia and Related Disorders. Aging Series, Vol 7. Raven Press, New York, 1978, p 47.

185. Kulmala, HK: Some enkephalin or VIP immunoreactive hippocam-pal pyramidal cells contain neurofibrillary tangles in the brains of aged humans and persons with Alzheimer's disease. Neurochem Pathol 3:41–51, 1985.

186. Larsson, T, Sjogren, T, and Jacobson, G: Senile dementia. Acta Psychiatr Scand (Suppl 167) 39:3–259, 1963.

187. Lassen, NA, Munck, O, and Tottey, ER: Mental function and cerebral oxygen consumption in organic dementia. AMA Arch Neurol Psychiatry 77:126–133, 1957.

188. Lemaire, HG, Salbaum, JM, Multhaup, G, Kang, J, Bayney, RM, Unterbeck, A, Beyreuther, K, and Müller-Hill, B: The PreA4(695) precursor protein of Alzheimer's disease A4 amyloid is encoded by 16 exons. Nucleic Acids Res 17:517–522, 1989.

189. Love, S, Saitoh, T, Quijada, S, Cole, GM, and Terry, RD: Alz-50, ubiquitin and tau immunoreactivity of neurofibrillary tangles, Pick bodies and Lewy bodies. J Neuropathol Exp Neurol 47:393–403, 1988.

190. Lowe, SL, Francis, PT, Procter, AW, Palmer, AM, Davison, AN, and Bowen, DM: Gamma-aminobutyric acid concentration in brain tissue at two stages of Alzheimer's disease. Brain 111:785–799, 1988.

191. Malamud, N: A comparative study of the neuropathologic findings in senile psychoses and in "normal" senility. J Am Geriatr Soc 13:112–117, 1965.

192. Mann, DMA, Lincoln, J, Yates, PO, Stamp, JE, and Toper, S: Changes in the monoamine containing neurons of the human CNS in senile dementia. Br J Psychiatry 136:533–541, 1980.

193. Mann, DMA, Neary, D, Yates, PO, Lincoln, J, Snowden, JS, and Stanworth, P: Neurofibrillary pathology and protein synthetic capability in nerve cells in Al-

zheimer's disease. Neuropathol Appl Neurobiol 7:37–47, 1981.

194. Mann, DMA, Neary, D, Yates, PO, Lincoln, J. Snowden, JS, and Stanworth, P: Alterations in protein synthetic capability of nerve cells in Alzheimer's disease. J Neurol Neurosurg Psychiatry 44:97–102, 1981.

195. Mann, DMA and Sinclair, KGA: The quantitative assessment of lipofuscin pigment, cytoplasmic RNA and nucleolar volume in senile dementia. Neuropathol Appl Neurobiol 4:129–135, 1978.

196. Manuelidis, EE, de Figueiredo, JM, Kim, JH, and Fritch, WW: Transmission studies from blood of Alzheimer disease patients and healthy relatives. Proc Natl Acad Sci USA 85:4898–4901, 1988.

197. Markesbery, WR, Ehmann, WD, Houssain, TIM, Alanddin, M, and Goodin, DT: Brain trace element levels in Alzheimer's disease by instrumental neutron activation analysis. J Neuropathol Exp Neurol 40:359, 1981.

198. Martin, RL, Gerteis, G, and Gabrielli, WF: A family-genetic study of dementia of Alzheimer type. Arch Gen Psychiatry 45:894–900, 1988.

199. Mash, DC, Flynn, DD and Potter, LT: Loss of M2 muscarine receptors in the cerebral cortex in Alzheimer's disease and experimental cholinergic denervation. Science 228:1115–1117, 1985.

200. Masliah, E, Iimoto, DS, Hansen, LA, Terry, RD, Halliday, WC, and Saitoh, T: Casein kinase II-like immunoreactivity is associated with neurofibrillary tangles. Submitted.

201. Masliah, E, Terry, RD, and Buzsaki, G: Thalamic nuclei in Alzheimer disease: Evidence against the cholinergic hypothesis of plaque formation. Brain Res 493:240–246, 1989.

202. Masliah, E, Terry, RD, DeTeresa, R, and Hansen, LA: Immunohisto-chemical quantification of the synapse related protein synaptophysin in Alzheimer disease. Neurosci Lett 103:234–238, 1989.

203. Masters, CL, Simms, G, Weinman, NA, Multhaup, G, McDonald, BL, and Beyreuther, K: Amyloid plaque core protein in Alzheimer disease and Down syndrome. Pro Natl Acad Sci USA 82:4245–4249, 1985.

204. McDermott, JR, Fraser, H, and Dickinson, AG: Reduced choline acetyltransferase activity in scrapie mouse brain. Lancet 2:318–319, 1978.

205. McDermott, JR, Smith, AI, Iqbal, K, and Wisniewski, HM: Aluminum in Alzheimer's disease. Lancet 2:710–711, 1977.

205a. McFarlan, D (ed): Guinness Book of World Records; Bantam Books, New York, 1991, p 22.

206. Mehraein, P, Yamada, M, and Tarnowska-Dziduszko, E: Quantitative Study on Dendrites and Dendritic Spines in Alzheimer's Disease and Senile Dementia. In Kreutzberg, GW (ed): Physiology and Pathology of Dendrites: Advances in Neurobiology, Vol 12. Raven Press, New York, 1975, p 453.

207. Miline, FJ, Sharf, B, Bell, P, and Meyers, AM: The effect of low aluminum water and desferrioxamine on the outcome of dialysis encephalopathy. Clin Nephrol 20:202–207, 1983.

208. Miller, AE, Neighbour, A, Katzman, R, Aronson, M, and Lipkowitz, R: Immunologic studies in senile dementia of the Alzheimer type: Evidence for enhanced suppressor cell activity. Ann Neurol 10:506–510, 1981.

209. Mohs, RC, Breitner, JCS, Silverman, JM, and Davis, KL: Alzheimer's disease morbid risk among first-degree relatives approximates 50% by 90 years of age. Arch Gen Psychiatry 44:405–408, 1987.

210. Mohs, RC, Davis, KL, Tinklenberg, JR, and Hollister, LE: Choline chloride effects on memory in the elderly. Neurobiol Aging 1:21–25, 1980.

211. Molsa, PK, Marttila, RJ, and Rinne, UK: Epidemiology of dementia in a Finnish population. Acta Neurol Scand 65:541–552, 1982.

212. Mortimer, JA, French, LR, Hutton, JT, and Schuman, LM: Head injury as a risk factor for Alzheimer's disease. Neurology 35:264–267, 1985.

213. Mountjoy, CQ, Tomlinson, BE, and Gibson, PH: Amyloid and senile plaques and cerebral blood vessels—A semi-quantitative investigation of a possible relationship. J Neurol Sci 57:89–103, 1988.

214. Murdoch, GH, Manuelidis, L, Kim, JH, and Manuelidis, EE: Beta-amyloid gene dosage in Alzheimer's disease. Nucleic Acids Res 16:357, 1988.

215. Newton, RD: The identity of Alzheimer's disease and senile dementia and their relationship in senility. J Mental Sci 94:225–248, 1948.

216. Nielsen, J: Geronto-psychiatric period—Prevalence investigation in a geographically delimited population. Acta Psychiatr Scand 38:307–339, 1963.

217. Nielsen, J: Chromosomes in senile, presenile and arteriosclerotic dementia. J Gerontol 25:312–315, 1970.

218. Nordberg, A, Adolfsson, R, Aquilonius, SM, Marklund, S, Oreland, L, and Winblad, B: Brain Enzymes and Acetylcholine Receptors in Dementia of Alzheimer Type and Chronic Alcohol Abuse. In Amaducci, L, Davison, AN, and Antuono, P (eds): Aging of the Brain and Dementia. Aging Series, Vol 13. Raven Press, New York, 1980, p 169.

219. Nordenson, I, Adolfsson, R, Beckman, G, Bucht, G, and Winblad, B: Chromoabnormality in de-mentia of the Alzheimer type. Lancet 1:481–482, 1980.

220. Obrist, WD: Noninvasive Studies of Cerebral Blood Flow in Aging. In Katzman, R, Terry, RD, and Bick, KL (eds): Alzheimer's Disease: Senile Dementia and Related Disorders. Aging Series, Vol 7. Raven Press, New York, 1978, p 213.

221. Obrist, WD: Cerebral Circulatory Changes in Normal Aging and Dementia. In Hoffmeister, F and Muller, C (eds): Brain Function in Old Age. Springer-Verlag, New York, 1979, p 278.

222. O'Connor, DW, Pollitt, PA, Hyde, JB, Fellows, JL, Miller, ND, Brook, CPB, Reiss, BB, and Roth, M: The prevalence of dementia as measured by the Cambridge Mental Disorders of the Elderly Examination. Acta Psychiatr Scand 79:190–198, 1989.

223. Owens, D, Dawson, JC, and Lowsin, S: Alzheimer's disease in Down's syndrome. Am J Ment Defic 75:606–612, 1971.

224. Palmer, AM, Procter, AW, Stratman, GC, and Bowen, DM: Excitatory amino acid releasing and cholinergic neurons in Alzheimer's disease. Neurosci Lett 66:199–204, 1986.

225. Palmer, AM, Statmann, GC, Procter, AW, and Bowen, DM: Possible neurotransmitter basis of behavioral changes in Alzheimer's disease. Ann Neurol 23:616–620, 1988.

226. Parkes, JD, Marsden, CD, Rees, JE, Curzon, G, Kantamaneni, BD, Knill-Jones, R, Akbar, A, Das, S, and Kataria, M: Parkinson's disease, cerebral arteriosclerosis and senile demential. Q J Med 43:49–61, 1973.

227. Pearson, RCA, Sofroniew, MV, Cuello, AC, Powell, TPS, Eckenstein, F, Esiri, MM, and Wilcock, GK: Persistence of cholinergic neurons in the basal nucleus in a brain with senile dementia of the Alzheimer's type demon-

strated by immunohistochemical staining for choline acetyltransferase. Brain Res 289: 375–379, 1983.

228. Perl, DP: Relationship of aluminum to Alzheimer's disease. Environ Health Perspect 63:149–153, 1985.

229. Perl, DP and Brody, AR: Alzheimer's disease: X-ray spectrometric evidence of aluminum accumulation in neurofibrillary tangle-bearing neurons. Science 208:207–209, 1980.

230. Perl, DP and Pendlebury, WW: Aluminum neurotoxicity—Potential role in the pathogenesis of neurofibrillary tangle formation. Can J Neurol Sci 13:441–445, 1986.

231. Perry, EK and Perry, RH: New insights into the nature of senile (Alzheimer-type) plaques. Trends Neurosci 8:301–303, 1985.

232. Perry, EK, Perry, RH, Blessed, G, and Tomlinson, BE: Necropsy evidence of central cholinergic deficits in senile dementia. Lancet 1:189, 1977.

233. Perry, EK, Perry, RH, Candy, JM, Fairbairn, AF, Blessed, G, Dick, DJ, and Tomlinson, BE: Cortical serotonin-S_2 receptor binding abnormalities in patients with Alzheimer's disease: Comparisons with Parkinson's disease. Neurosci Lett 51:353–357, 1984.

234. Perry, EK, Tomlinson, BE, Blessed, G, Bergmann, K, Gibson, PH, and Perry, RH: Correlation of cholinergic abnormalities with senile plaques and mental test scores in senile dementia. Br Med J 2:1457–1459, 1978.

235. Perry, G: Amyloid precursor protein in senile plaques of Alzheimer disease. Lancet 2:746, 1988.

236. Perry, G, Friedman, R, Shaw, G, and Chau, V: Ubiquitin is detected in neurofibrillary tangles and senile plaque neurites of Alzheimer disease brains. Proc Natl Acad Sci USA 84:3033–3036, 1987.

237. Perry, RH, Blessed, G, Perry, EK, and Tomlinson, BE: Histochemical observations and cholinesterase activities in the brains of elderly normal and demented (Alzheimer type) patients. Age Ageing 9:9–16, 1980.

238. Pfeffer, RI, Afifi, AA, and Chance, JM: Prevalence of Alzheimer's disease in a retirement community. Am J Epidemiol 125:420–436, 1987.

239. Podlisny, MB, Lee, G, and Selkow, DJ: Gene dosage of the amyloid β precursor protein in Alzheimer's disease. Science 238:669–671, 1987.

240. Ponte, P, Gonzalez-DeWhitt, P, Schilling, J, Miller, J, Hsu, D, Greenberg, B, Davis, K, Wallace, W, Lieberburg, I, Fuller, F, and Cordell, B: A new A4 amyloid mRNA contains a domain homologous to serine proteinase inhibitors. Nature 331:525–527, 1988.

241. Pope, A, Hess, HH, and Lewin, E: Microchemical pathology of the cerebral cortex in presenile dementias. Trans Am Neurol Assoc 89:15–16, 1964.

242. Post, F: The development of progress of senile dementia in relationship to the functional psychiatric disorders of later life. In Muller, C and Ciompi, L (eds): Senile Dementia. Williams & Wilkins, Baltimore, 1968, p 85.

243. Powers, RE, Walker, LC, DeSouza, EB, Vale, WW, Struble, RG, Whitehouse, PJ, Price, DL: Immunohistochemical study of neurons contain corticotropin-releasing factor in Alzheimer's disease. Synapse 1:405–410, 1987.

244. Prelli, F, Castano, E, Glenner, GG, and Fangione, B: Differences between vascular and plaque core amyloid in Alzheimer's disease. J Neurochem 51:648–651, 1988.

245. Price, DL, Altschuler, RJ, Struble, RG, Casanova, MF, Cork, LC, and Murphy, DB: Sequestration of tubulin in neurons in Alzheimer's disease. Brain Res 385:305–310, 1986.

246. Primrose, EJR: Psychological Illness: A Community Study. JB Lippincott, Philadelphia, 1962, p 1.

247. Probst, A, Anderton, BH, Brion, JP, and Ulrich, J: Senile plaque neurites fail to demonstrate anti-paired helical filament and anti-microtubule-associatedprotein-tau immunoreactive proteins in the absence of neurofibrillary tangles in the neocortex. Acta Neuropathol 77:430–436, 1989.

248. Raskin, N and Ehrenberg, R: Senescence, senility and Alzheimer's disease. Am J Psychiatry 113:133–137, 1956.

249. Reisine, TD, Yamamura, HI, Bird, ED, Spokes, E, and Enna, SJ: Pre- and postsynaptic neurochemical alterations in Alzheimer's disease. Brain Res 159:477–481, 1978.

250. Renvoize, EB, Hambling, HM, Pepper, MD, and Rajah, SM: Possible association of Alzheimer's disease with HLA-BW 15 and cytomegalovirus infection. Lancet 1:1238, 1979.

251. Reyes, PF, Golden, GT, Fagel, PL, Farielio, RG, Katz, L, and Carner, E: The prepiriform cortex in dementia of the Alzheimer type. Arch Neurol 44:1644–1645, 1987.

252. Robakis, NK, Ramakrishna, N, Wolfe, G, and Wisniewski, HM: Molecular cloning and characterization of a cDNA encoding the cerebrovascular and the neuritic plaque amyloid peptides. Proc Natl Acad Sci USA 84:4190–4194, 1987.

253. Robakis, N, Wisniewski, HM, Jenkins, EC, Devine-Gage, EA, Houck, E, Yao, X-L, Ramakrishna, N, Wolfe, G, Silverman, WP, and Brown, WT: Chromosome 21q21 sublocalization of gene encoding beta-amyloid peptide in cerebral vessels and neuritic (senile) plaques of people with Alzheimer disease and Down syndrome. Lancet 2:384–385, 1987.

254. Roberts, GW, Allsop, D, and Bruton, C: The occult aftermath of boxing. Neuropathol Appl Neurobiol 15:273–274, 1989.

255. Roberts, GW, Crow, TJ, and Polak, JM: Location of neuronal tangles in somatostatin neurons in Alzheimer's disease. Nature 314:92–94, 1985.

256. Roberts, GW, Lofthouse, R, Alizop, D, Landon, M, Kidd, M, Pruisner, SB, and Crow, TJ: CNS amyloid proteins in neurodegenerative disease. Neurology 38:1534–1540, 1988.

257. Rocca, WA, Amaducci, LA, and Schoenberg, BS: Epidemiology of clinically diagnosed Alzheimer's disease. Ann Neurol 19:415–424, 1986.

258. Rocca, WA, Bonaiuto, S, Lippi, A, Luciani, P, Turtu, F, Cavarzeran, F, and Amaducci, L: Prevalence of clinically diagnosed Alzheimer's disease and other dementing disorders: A door-to-door survey in Appignano, Macerata Province, Italy. Neurology 40:626–631, 1990.

259. Rosati, G, De Bastiani, P, Gilli, P, and Paolino, E: Oral aluminum and neuropsychological functioning—A study of dialysis patients receiving aluminum hydroxide gels. J Neurol 223:251–257, 1980.

260. Rosenblum, WI and Ghatak, NR: Lewy bodies in the presence of Alzheimer's disease. Arch Neurol 36:170–171, 1979.

261. Rosenblum, WI and Haider, A: Negative correlations between parenchymal amyloid and vascular amyloid in hippocampus. Am J Pathol 130:532–536, 1988.

262. Roses, AD, Pericak-Vance, MA, Clark, CM, Gilbert, JR, Yamaoka, LH, Haynes, CS, Speer,

MC, Gaskell, PC, Hung, WY, Trofatter, JA, Earl, NL, Lee, JE, Alberts, MJ, Dawson, DV, Bartlett, RJ, Siddique, T, Vance, JM, Conneally, PM, Heyman, AL: Linkage studies of late-onset familial Alzheimer's disease. Adv Neurol 51:185–196, 1990.

263. Rossor, MN, Emson, PC, Mountjoy, CQ, Roth, M, and Iversen, LL: Reduced amounts of immunoreactive somatostatin in the temporal cortex in senile dementia of Alzheimer type. Neurosci Lett 20:373–377, 1980.

264. Rossor, M, Fahrenkrug, J, Emson, P, Iversen, LL, and Roth, M: Reduced cortical choline acetyltransferase activity in senile dementia of Alzheimer type is not accompanied by changes in vasoactive intestinal polypeptide. Brain Res 201:249–253, 1980.

265. Rossor, M, Iversen LL: Non-cholinergic neurotransmitter abnormalities in Alzheimer's disease. Br Med Bull 42:70–74, 1986.

266. Rossor, MN, Iversen, L, Mountjoy, CQ, Roth, M, Hawthorn, J, Ang, VY, and Jenkins, JS: Arginine vasopressin and choline acetyltransferase in brains of patients with Alzheimer type senile dementia. Lancet 2:1367–1368, 1980.

267. Rossor, MN, Iversen, LL, Reynolds, GP, Mountjoy, CQ, and Roth, M: Reduced binding of 3H ketanserin to cortical 5-HT2 receptors in senile dementia of the Alzheimer type. Neurosci Lett 44:47–51, 1984.

268. Roth, M: The Diagnosis of Senile and Related Forms of Dementia. In Katzman, R, Terry, RD and Bick, KL (eds): Alzheimer's Disease: Senile Dementia and Related Disorders. Aging Series, Vol 7. Raven Press, New York, 1978, p 71.

269. Roth, M and Kay, DWK: Affective disorders arising in the senium. II. Physical disability as an etiological factor. J Ment Sci 102:141–150, 1956.

270. Rothschild, D: Pathologic changes in senile psychoses and their psychobiologic significance. Am J Psychiatry 93:757–788, 1937.

271. Ruberg, M, Ploska, A, and Javoy-Agid, F: Muscarinic binding and choline acetyltransferase activity in parkinsonian subjects with reference to dementia. Brain Res 232:129–139, 1982.

272. Rumble, B, Retallack, R, Hibich, C, Simms, G, and Multhaup, GB: Amyloid A4 protein and its precursor in Down's syndrome and Alzheimer's disease. N Engl J Med 320:1446–1452, 1989.

273. St George-Hyslop, PH, Tanzi, RE, Polinsky, RJ, Haines, JL, Nee L, Watkins, PC, Myers, RH, Feldman, RG, Pollen, D, Drachman, D, Growdon, J, Bruni, A, Foncin, J-F, Salmon, D, Frommelt, P, Amaducci, L, Sorbi, S, Placentini, S, Stewart, GD, Hobbs, WJ, Conneally, PM, and Gusella, JF: The genetic defect causing familial Alzheimer's disease maps on chromosome 21. Science 235:885–890, 1987.

274. St. George-Hyslop, PH, Tanzi, RE, Polinsky, RJ, Neve, RL, Pollen, D, Drachman, D, Growden, J, Cupples, LA, Nee, L, Myers, RH, O'Sullivan, D, Watkins, PC, Amos, JA, Deutsch, CK, Bodfish, JW, Kinsbourne, M, Feldman, RG, Bruni, A, Amaducci, L, Foncin, J-F, and Gusella, JF: Absence of duplication of chromosome 21 genes in familial and sporadic Alzheimer's disease. Science 238:664–666, 1987.

275. Saitoh, T, Cole, G, and Huynh, TV: Aberrant Protein Kinase C Cascaded in Alzheimer's Disease. In Lauder, JM, (ed): Molecular Aspects of Development and Aging of the Nervous System. Plenum Press, New York, 1990, pp 301–310.

276. Saitoh, T, Sundsmo, M, Roch, J-M, Kimura, N, Cole, G, Schubert, D, Oltersdorf, T, and Schenk, DB: Secreted form of amyloid β-protein precursor is involved in the

growth regulation of fibroblasts. Cell 58:615–622, 1989.

277. Salbaum, JM, Weidemann, A, Lemaire, HL, Masters, CL, and Beyreuther, K: The promoter of Alzheimer's disease amyloid A4 precursor gene. EMBO J 7:2807–2813, 1988.

278. Salmon, DP, Riekkinen, PJ, Katzman, R, Zhang, M, Jin, H, and Yu, E: Cross-cultural studies of dementia: A comparison of mini-mental state examination performance in Finland and China. Arch Neurol 46:769–772, 1989.

279. Schechter, R, Yen, SH, and Terry, RD: Fibrous astrocytes in senile dementia of the Alzheimer type. J Neuropathol Exp Neurol 40:95–101, 1981.

280. Scheibel, AB: Dendritic Changes in Senile and Presenile Dementias. In Katzman, R (ed): Congenital and Acquired Cognitive Disorders. ARNMD, Vol 57. Raven Press, New York, 1979, p 107.

281. Scheibel, ME and Scheibel, AB: Structural Changes in the Aging Brain. In Brody, H, Harman, D, and Ordy, JM (eds): Clinical, Morphological and Neurochemical Aspects in the Aging Central Nervous System. Aging Series, Vol 1. Raven Press, New York, 1975, p 11.

282. Schellenberg, GD, Bird, TD, Wijsman, EM, Moore, DK, Boehnke, M, Bryant, EM, Lampe, TH, Nochlin, D, Sumi, SM, Deeb, SS, Beyreuther, K, and Martin, GM: Absence of linkage of chromosome 21q21 markers to familial Alzheimer's disease. Science 241:1507–1510, 1988.

283. Scholtz, CL, Swash, M, Gray, A, Kogeorgos, J, and Marsh, F: Neurofibrillary neuronal degeneration in dialysis dementia: A feature of aluminum toxicity. Clin Neuropathol 6:93–96, 1987.

284. Schubert, D, Schroeder, R, LaCorbiere, M, Saitoh, T, and Cole, G: Amyloid β-protein precursor

is possibly a heparan sulfate proteoglycan core protein. Science 241:223–241, 1988.

285. Selkoe, DJ: Altered structural proteins in plaques and tangles: What they tell us about the biology of Alzheimer's disease. Neurobiol Aging 7:425–432, 1986.

286. Selkoe, DJ: Aging, amyloid and Alzheimer's disease. N Engl J Med 320:1484–1486, 1989.

287. Selkoe, DJ and Abraham C: Plaque amyloid in Alzheimer's disease (AD): Purification by flow cytometry and protein characterization. Neurology 35(Suppl 1):217, 1985.

288. Selkoe, DJ, Abraham, CR, Podlisny, MB, and Duffy, LK: Isolation of low-molecular-weight protein from amyloid plaque fibers in Alzheimer's disease. J Neurochem 46:1820–1834, 1986.

289. Selkoe, DJ, Ihara, Y, and Salazar, FJ: Alzheimer's disease: Insolubility of partially-purified paired helical filaments in sodium dodecyl sulfate and urea. Science 215:1243–1245, 1982.

290. Sheldon, JH: The Social Medicine of Old Age. Oxford University Press, London, 1948.

291. Shalat, SL, Seltzer, B, and Baker, EL, Jr: Occupational risk factors and Alzheimer's disease: A case-control study. J Occup Med 30:934–936, 1988.

292. Shalat, SL, Seltzer, B, Pidcock, C, and Baker, EL, Jr: Risk factors for Alzheimer's disease. Neurology 37:1630–1633, 1987.

293. Shibayama, G, Kasahara, Y, and Kobayash, H: Prevalence of dementia in a Japanese elderly population. Acta Psychiatr Scand 74:144–151, 1988.

294. Simchowicz, T: Histopathologische Studien uber die senile Demenz. In Nissl, F and Alzheimer, A (eds): Histologie und Histopathologische Arbeiten uber die Grosshirnrinde, Vol 4. Fisher, Jena, Germany, 1911, p 267.

295. Sims, NR, Bowen, DM, and Davison, AN: [^{14}C]Acetylcholine synthesis and [^{14}C]carbon dioxide production from [U-^{14}C]glucose by tissue prisms from human neocortex. Biochem J 196:867–876, 1981.

296. Sims, NR, Bowen, DM, Smith, CCT, Flack, DHA, Davison, AN, and Snowden, JS: Glucose metabolism and acetylcholine synthesis in relation to neuronal activity in Alzheimer's disease. Lancet 1:333–335, 1980.

297. Sluss, TK, Gruenberg, EM, and Kramer, M: The Use of Longitudinal Studies in the Investigation of Risk Factors for Senile Dementia-Alzheimer Type. In Mortimer, JA and Schuman, LM (eds): The Epidemiology of Dementia. Oxford University Press, London, 1981, p 132.

298. Sobel, E, Davanipour, Z, and Alter, MG: Genetic analysis of late-onset diseases using first-degree relatives. Neuroepidemiology 7:81–88, 1988.

299. Sokoloff, L: Cerebral Circulatory and Metabolic Changes Associated with Aging. In Millikan, CH (ed): Cerebrovascular Disease. ARNMD, Vol 41. Williams & Wilkins, Baltimore, 1961, p 237.

300. Sparks, DL, DeKosky, ST, and Markesbery, WR: Alzheimer's disease: Aminergic-cholinergic alterations in hypothalamus. Arch Neurol 45:994–999, 1988.

301. Sprague, SM, Corwin, HL, Wilson, RS, Mayor, GH, and Tanner, CM: Encephalopathy in chronic renal failure responsive of deferoxamine therapy—Another manifestation of aluminum neurotoxicty. Arch Intern Med 146:2063–2064, 1986.

302. Sternberger, NH, Sternberger, LA, and Ulrich, J: Aberrant neurofilament phosphorylation in Alzheimer disease. Proc Natl Acad Sci USA 82:4274–4276, 1985.

303. Struble, RG, Cork, LC, Whitehouse, PJ, and Price, DL: Cholinergic

innervation in neuritic plaques. Science 216:413–415, 1982.

304. Struble, RG, Powers, RE, Casanova, MF, Kitt, CA, Brown, EC, and Price, DL: Neuropeptidergic systems in plaques of Alzheimer's disease. J Neuropathol Exp Neurol 46:567–584, 1987.

305. Sulkava, R, Koshimies, S, Wikstrom, J, and Palo, J: HLA antigens in Alzheimer's disease. Tissue Antigens 16:191–194, 1980.

306. Sulkava, R, Rossi, K, and Knutuila, S: No elevated sister chromatid exchange in Alzheimer's disease. Acta Neurol Scand 59:156–159, 1978.

307. Sulkava, R, Wikstrom, J, Aromaa, A, Raitasalo, R, and Lehtinen, V: Prevalence of severe dementia in Finland. Neurology 35:1025–1029, 1985.

308. Summers, WK, Majovski, LV, Marsh, GM, Tachiki, K, and Kling, A: Oral tetrahydroaminoacridine in long-term treatment of dementia, Alzheimer type. N Engl J Med 315:241–1245, 1986.

309. Suzuki, K, Katzman, R, and Korey, SR: Chemical studies on Alzheimer's disease. J Neuropathol Exp Neurol 24:211–224, 1965.

310. Suzuki, K and Terry, RD: Fine structural localization of acid phosphatase in senile plaques in Alzheimer's presenile dementia. Acta Neuropathol (Berl) 8:276–284, 1967.

311. Tagliavini, F, Giaccone, G, Frangione, B, and Bugiani, O: Preamyloid deposits in the cerebral cortex of patients with Alzheimer's disease and nondemented individuals. Neurosci Lett 93:191–196, 1988.

312. Tamminga, CA, Foster, NL, Fedio, P, Bird, ED, and Chase, TN: Alzheimer's disease: Low cerebral somatostatin levels correlate with impaired cognitive function and cortical metabolism. Neurology 37:161–165, 1987.

313. Tanzi, RE, Bird, ED, Latt, SA, and Neve, RL: The amyloid β-protein

gene is not duplicated in brains from patients with Alzheimer's disease. Science 238:666–669, 1987.

314. Tanzi, RE, Gusella, JF, Watkins, PC, Bruns, GA, St. George-Hyslop, P, Van Keuren, ML, Patterson, D, Pagan, S, Kurnit, DM, and Neve, RL: Amyloid β-proetin gene: cDNA, mRNA distribution, and genetic linkage near the Alzheimer locus. Science 235:880–884, 1987.

315. Tanzi, RE, McClatchey, AI, Lamperti, ED, Villa-Komaroff, L, Gusella, JF, and Neve, RL: Protease inhibitor domain encoded by an amyloid protein precursor mRNA associated with Alzheimer's disease. Nature 331:528–530, 1988.

316. Tanzi, RE, St George-Hyslop, PH, Haines, JL, Polinsky, RJ, Nee, L, Foncin, J-F, Neve, RL, McClatchey, AI, Conneally, PM, and Gusella, JF: The genetic defect in familial Alzheimer's disease is not tightly linked to the amyloid β-protein gene. Nature 329:156–157, 1987.

317. Tavalato, B and Argentiero, V: Immunological indices in presenile Alzheimer's disease. J Neurol Sci 46:325–331, 1980.

318. Terry, RD: The Value of Cerebral Biopsy. In Fields, WS (ed): Neurological Diagnostic Techniques: Thirteenth Annual Houston Neurological Scientific Symposium. Charles C Thomas, Springfield, IL, 1966, p 69.

319. Terry, RD, Gonatas, NK, and Weiss, M: Ultrastructural studies in Alzheimer's presenile demenita. Am J Pathol 44:269–297, 1964.

320. Terry, RD, Hansen, LA, DeTeresa, R, Davies, P, Tobias, H, and Katzman, R: Senile dementia of the Alzheimer type without neocortical neurofibrillary tangles. J Neuropathol Exp Neurol 46: 262–268, 1987.

321. Terry, RD and Katzman, R (eds): Senile Dementia of the Alzheimer Type: Defining a Disease. In The Neurology of Aging. FA Davis, Philadelphia, 1983, p 51.

322. Terry, RD, Peck, A, and DeTeresa, R: Some morphometric aspects of the brain in senile dementia of the Alzheimer type. Ann Neurol 10:184–192, 1981.

323. Terry, RD and Pena, C: Experimental production of neurofibrillary degeneration. 2. Electron microscopy, phosphatase histochemistry and electron probe analysis. J Neuropathol Exp Neurol 24:200–209, 1965.

324. Terry, RD and Wisniewski, HM: The Ultrastructure of the Neurofibrillary Tangle and the Senile Plaque. In Wolstenholme, GEW and O'Connor, M (eds): CIBA Foundation Symposium on Alzheimer's Disease and Related Conditions. J & A Churchill, London, 1970, p 145.

325. Terry, RD and Wisniewski, HM: Ultrastructure of Senile Dementia and of Experimental Analogs. In Gaitz, CM (ed): Aging and the Brain: The Proceedings of the Fifth Annual Symposium Held at the Texas Research Institute of Mental Sciences in Houston, October 1971. Advances in Behavioral Biology, Vol 3. Plenum Press, New York, 1972, p 89.

326. Terry, RD and Wisniewski, HM: Structural and Chemical Changes of the Aged Human Brain. In Gershon, S and Raskin, A (eds): Genesis and Treatment of Psychologic Disorders in the Elderly. Aging Series, Vol 2. Raven Press, New York, 1975, p 127.

327. Thal, LJ, Fuld, PA, Masur, DM, and Sharpless, NS: Oral physostigmine and lecithin improve memory in Alzheimer's disease. Ann Neurol 13:491–496, 1983.

328. Thal, LJ, Rosen, W, Sharpless, NS, and Crystal, H: Choline chloride

fails to improve cognition in Alzheimer's disease. Neurobiol Aging 2:205–208, 1981.

329. Thomas, L: On the problem of dementia. Discover, August, 1981, pp 34–36.

330. Tomlinson, BE: Morphological Changes and Dementia in Old Age. In Smith, WL and Kinsbourne, M (eds): Aging and Dementia. Spectrum Publications, New York, 1977, p 25.

331. Tomlinson, BE, Blessed, G, and Roth, M: Observations on the brains of demented old people. J Neurol Sci 11:205–242, 1970.

332. Tomlinson, BE and Henderson, G: Some quantitative cerebral findings in normal and demented old people. In Terry, RD and Gershon, S (eds): Neurobiology of Aging. Aging Series, Vol 3. Raven Press, New York, 1976, p 183.

333. Tomlinson, BE, Irving, D, and Blessed, G: Cell loss in the locus coeruleus in senile dementia of Alzheimer type. J Neurol Sci 49:419–429, 1975.

334. Torack, RM: Congophilic angiopathy complicated by surgery and massive hemorrhage: A light and electron microscopic study. Am J Pathol 81:349–359, 1975.

335. Tourtelotte, WG, Van Hoesen, WG, Hyman, BT, Tikoo, RK, and Damasio, AR: Afferents of the thalamic reticular nucleus are pathologically altered in Alzheimer's disease (abstr). J Neuropathol Exp Neurol 48:336, 1989.

336. Traub, R, Gajdusek, DC, and Gibbs, CJ, Jr: Transmissible virus dementia: The relation of transmissible spongiform encephalopathy to Creutzfeldt-Jakob disease. In Smith, WL and Kinsbourne, M (eds): Aging and Dementia. Spectrum Publications, New York, 1977, p 91.

337. Ulrich, J: Alzheimer changes in nondemented patients younger than sixty-five: Possible early stages of Alzheimer's disease and senile dementia of Alzheimer type. Ann Neurol 17:273–277, 1985.

338. Urakami, K, Adachi, Y, and Takahashi, KA: Community-based study of parental age in Alzheimer-type dementia in Western Japan. Arch Neurol 45:375, 1988.

339. U.S. Congress Office of Technology Assessment. Losing a Million Minds: Confronting the Tragedy of Alzheimer's Disease and Other Dementias. OTA-BA-323. Washington, DC, US Government Printing Office, April 1987.

340. Van Broeckhoven, C, Genthe, AM, Vandenberghe, A, Horsthemke, B, Backhovens, H, Raeymaekers, P, Van Hul, W, Wehnert, A, Gheuens, J, Cras, P, Bruyland, M, Martin, JJ, Salbaum, M, Multhaup, G, Masters, CL, Beyreuther, K, Gurling, HMD, Mullan, MJ, Holland, A, Barton, A, Irving, N, Williamson, R, Richards, SJ, and Hardy, JA: Failure of familial Alzheimer's disease to segregate with the A4-amyloid gene in several European families. Nature 329:153–155, 1987.

341. Walford, RL: Immunology and aging. Am J Clin Pathol 74:247–253, 1980.

342. Walker, LC, Kitt, CA, Cork, LC, Struble, RG, Dellovade, TL, and Price, DL: Multiple transmitter systems contribute neurites to individual senile plaques. J Neuropathol Exp Neurol 47:138–144, 1987.

343. Walker, LC, Kitt, CA, Struble, RG, Schechel, DE, Oertel, WH, Cork, LC, and Price, DL: Glutamic acid decarboxylase-like immunoreactive neurites in senile plaques. Neurosci Lett 59:165–169, 1985.

344. Wang, HA and Whanger, A: Brain Impairment and Longevity. In

Palmore, E and Jeffers, FC (eds): Prediction of Life Span. DC Heath, Lexington, MA, 1971, p 95.

345. Whalley, LJ, Carother, AD, Collyer, S, Demey, R, and Frackiewics, A: A study of familial factors in Alzheimer's disease. Br J Psychiatry 140:249–256, 1982.

346. Whalley, LJ, Urbaniak, SJ, Darg, C, Peutherer, JF, and Christie, JE: Histocompatibility antigens and antibodies to viral and other antigens in Alzheimer presenile dementia. Acta Psychiatr Scand 61:1–7, 1980.

347. White, P, Goodhardt, MJ, Keet, JP, Hiley, CR, Carrasco, LH, and Williams, IEI: Neocortical cholinergic neurons in elderly people. Lancet 1:668–670, 1977.

348. Whitehouse, PJ, Martino, AM, Marcus, K, Mayeaux, R, Davis, LE, Price, DL, and Kellar, KJ: Reductions in cortical nicotinic receptors in Parkinson's disease, progressive supranuclear palsy and Alzheimer's disease. Neurology (Suppl 1)36:224, 1986.

349. Whitehouse, PJ, Martino, AM, Marcus, KA, Zweig, RM, Singer, HS, and Price, DL: Reductions in acetylcholine and nicotine binding in several degenerative diseases. Arch Neurol 45:722–724, 1988.

350. Whitehouse, PJ, Price, DL, Struble, RG, Clark, AW, Coyle, JT, and DeLong, MR: Alzheimer's disease and senile dementia: Loss of neurons in the basal forebrain. Science 215:1237–1239, 1982.

351. Whitehouse, PJ, Vale, WW, Zweig, RM, Singer, MD, Mayeux, R, Huhar, MJ, Price, DL, and DeSouza, EB: Reductions in corticotropin releasing factor-like immunoreactivity in cerebral cortex in Alzheimer's disease. Parkinson's disease and progressive supranuclear palsy. Neurology 37:905–909, 1987.

352. Whitson, JS, Selkoe, DJ, and Cotman, W: Amyloid beta protein enhances the survival of hippocampal neurons in vitro. Science 243:1488–1490, 1989.

353. Wilcox, CB, Caspary, EA, and Behan, PO: Histocompatibility antigens and Alzheimer's disease. Eur Neurol 19:262–265, 1980.

354. Williams, LR, Varon, S, Peterson, GM, Wictorin, K, Fischer, W, Bjorklund, A, and Gage, FH: Continuous infusion of nerve growth factor prevents basal forebrain neuronal death after fimbria-fornix transection. Proc Natl Acad Sci USA 83:9231–9235, 1986.

355. Wisniewski, HM, Bruce, ME, and Fraser, H: Infectious etiology of neuritic (senile) plaques in mice. Science 190:1108–1110, 1975.

356. Wisniewski, HM, Moretz, RC, and Lossinsky, AS: Evidence for induction of localized amyloid deposits and neuritic plaques by an infectious agent. Ann Neurol 10:517–522, 1981.

357. Wisniewski, HM, Narang, HK, and Terry, RD: Neurofibrillary tangles of paired helical filaments. J Neurol Sci 27:173–181, 1976.

357a. Wisniewski, HM and Terry, RD: Morphology of the aging brain, human and animal. Prog Brain Res 40:167–186, 1973.

358. Wisniewski, K, Howe, J, Williams, DG, and Wisniewski, HM: Precocious aging and dementia in patients with Down's syndrome. Biol Psychiatry 13:619–627, 1978.

359. Wolozin, B, Scicutella, A, and Davies, P: Reexpression of a developmentally regulated antigen in Down syndrome and Alzheimer disease. Proc Natl Acad Sci USA 85:6202–6206, 1988.

360. Yamaguchi, H, Hirai, S, Morimatsu, M, Shoji, M, and Ihara, Y: A variety of cerebral amyloid deposits in the brains of the Alzheimer-type dementia dem-

onstrated by beta protein immunostaining. Acta Neuropathol 76:541–590, 1988.

361. Yamaguchi, H, Hirai, S, Morimatsu, M, Shoji, M, and Nakazato, Y: Diffuse type of senile plaques in the cerebellum of Alzheimer-type dementia demonstrated by β protein immunostain. Acta Neuropathol 77:314–319, 1988.

362. Yamamoro, T and Hirano, L: A Nucleus raphe dorsalis in Alzheimer's disease: Neurofibrillary tangles and loss of large neurons. Ann Neurol 17:573–577, 1985.

363. Yates, CM, Harmar, AJ, Rosie, R, Sheward, J, Sanchez de Levy, G, Simpson, J, Maloney, AFJ, Gordon, A, and Fink, G: Thyrotropin-releasing hormone, luteinizing hormone-releasing hormone and substance P immunoreactivity in postmortem brain from cases of Alzheimer-type dementia and Down's syndrome. Brain Res 258:45–52, 1983.

364. Yates, CM, Simpson, J, Maloney, AFJ, Gordon, A, and Reid, AH: Alzheimer-like cholinergic deficiency in Down's syndrome. Lancet 2:979, 1980.

365. Zhang, M, Katzman, R, Jin, H, Cai, G, Wang, Z, Qu, G, Grant, I, Yu, E, Levy, P, and Liu, WT: The prevalence of dementia and Alzheimer's disease (AD) in Shanghai, China: Impact of age, gender and education. Ann Neurol 27:428–437, 1990.

Chapter 9

DELIRIUM IN THE ELDERLY

Richard W. Besdine, M.D.,
Robert Dicks, M.D., and
John W. Rowe, M.D.

DETECTION
EPIDEMIOLOGY
COURSE AND OUTCOME
CAUSES
PATHOPHYSIOLOGY
MANAGEMENT

Delirium is among the most important and most common problems encountered in older patients. The frequent occurrence of transient confusion in physically ill old persons makes delirium one of the common denominators of geriatric medicine. Often the first sign of illness, delirium occurs as either a prominent presenting feature of life-threatening disease or as a complication of another disorder and contributes substantially to morbidity and mortality in older patients. Although delirium is a specifically defined syndrome (see below), it has been identified as probably the most common nonspecific presentation of disease in older persons, meaning that its appearance does not help in identifying the disease that provokes it, even in localizing the primary pathology to the central nervous system (CNS). In addition to its morbidity, delirium is emotionally devastating to friends, families, and caregivers of the afflicted; successful medical intervention is as gratifying and desirable as the most heroic technologic "save" in health care.[5] Despite

its widely acknowledged importance, delirium is often neglected in the elderly; studies have shown that two thirds of patients are either misdiagnosed or undiagnosed.[30,31,36,39,43] Failure to systematically evaluate elderly patients is most often identified as the primary reason for inadequate diagnosis. The explanation for this apparent paradox includes both inadequately developed evaluation skills and negative attitudes regarding older persons. One prominent feature of imprecise diagnostic evaluation relates to the frequent coexistence of dementia and delirium in the elderly and the failure to differentiate between them.

There has been considerable discussion as to the reversible nature of delirium, particularly in elderly populations. The perspective of the individual clinician on this issue is often dominated by the particular subsets of delirium the physician encounters most commonly. It is clear that delirium may or may not be reversible depending on the presence of reversible underlying illness or other precipitant. For instance, in nursing home or hospitalized patients, abrupt onset of delirium is usually associated with acute illness. In many, but not all such cases, correction of the underlying process is followed by recovery from delirium. On the other hand, consultant neurologists may be more likely to encounter individuals whose delirium is progressive and un-relenting, leading to death, either with-out an identifiable underlying cause or, if a cause is found, one not amenable to treatment, such as catastrophic neuro-logic event.

DETECTION

Delirium and dementia are both global disturbances of cognitive func-tion, meaning that all modalities of in-tellect are likely disturbed, but not necessarily with equal severity. In ad-dition, delirium is often accompanied by alteration and fluctuation in level of consciousness. Diagnostic criteria for delirium[2] include an attentional disor-der, disorganized thinking, several cor-tical dysfunctions, abrupt onset with fluctuation of severity, and an organic cause or the presumption of one (Table 9–1). Although the 1980 edition of the *Diagnostic and Statistical Manual of Mental Disorders*[1] included "clouding of consciousness" in the definition of delirium, the vagueness of the term has made it of little use and it was omitted in the 1987 revision of the third edition (DSM-III-R).[2]

The patient with cognitive impair-ment who also has an attentional dis-order or diminished level of conscious-ness cannot be said to have dementia regardless of what other clinical fea-tures or mental status impairments are present, because the abnormalities could all be attributable to delirium. Ac-cordingly, it makes sense to evaluate at-tentiveness, alertness, and level of con-sciousness at the beginning of the mental status examination; if any is ab-normal, the rest of the assessment is not useful in determining whether or not dementia is present since the defi-cits could be consistent with delirium alone. Often, a patient with dementia acquires a new illness and delirium is superimposed on dementia.[16] In fact, dementia is a powerful risk factor for delirium, and this sequence of events is quite common. Only in retrospect, when the delirium has cleared and de-

Table 9–1 DIAGNOSTIC CRITERIA FOR DELIRIUM

1. Reduced ability to maintain attention to external stimuli (e.g., questions must be repeated because attention wanders) and to appropriately shift attention to new external stimuli (e.g., perseveres with answer to a previous question).
2. Disorganized thinking, as indicated by rambling, irrelevant, or incoherent speech.
3. At least two of the following:
   a. Reduced level of consciousness, e.g., difficulty keeping awake during examination.
   b. Perceptual disturbances: Misinterpretations, illusions, or hallucinations.
   c. Disturbance of sleep-wake cycle with insomnia or daytime sleepiness.
   d. Increased or decreased psychomotor activity.
   e. Disorientation to time, place, or person.
   f. Memory impairment, e.g., inability to learn new material, such as the names of several unrelated objects after 5 minutes, or to remember events, such as history of current episode of illness.
4. Clinical features develop over a short period of time (usually hours to days) and tend to fluctuate over the course of a day.
5. Either a or b:
   a. Evidence from the history, physical examination, or laboratory tests of a specific organic factor (or factors) judged to be etiologically related to the disturbance.
   b. In the absence of such evidence, an etiologic organic factor can be presumed if the disturbance cannot be accounted for by any nonorganic mental disorder, e.g., manic episode accounting for agitation and sleep disturbance.

Source: Adapted from DSM-III-R,[2] p 103.

mentia remains, can we be confident that both dementia and delirium were present, unless a good history of pre-existing dementia was available at pre-sentation. The DSM-III-R diagnostic criteria for dementia require that delir-ium not be present for a syndrome of dementia to be identified.[2]

Although delirium and dementia are very different disturbances, with nu-merous differential characteristics, hu-mility and an open mind are essential in approaching the evaluation of an older person with disturbed cognition. An accurate history may be the hardest piece of data to obtain during the initial detection and presentation of a cognitively impaired older person. In addition, the hectic, dynamic features of delirium that are common in young patients, such as hallucinations, delusions, paranoia, and hyperactive behavior with autonomic arousal, may be dampened or absent in an older person, who may show only cognitive loss and blunted attention, key components of delirium. Although the definitions are multidimensional and specific, it is crucial to remember that dementia, and delirium as well, are only syndromes, each having a long and diverse list of potential etiologic conditions, which is expanded even further in older persons.[5]

The clinical presentations of delirium and dementia are different, and careful assessment and gathering of the history should produce accurate diagnosis and proper management. Delirium is frequently missed, most often because its clinical picture is mistaken for dementia. Although both dementia and delirium are global disturbances of cognition, the two conditions differ in the changes in alertness and attention that constitute delirium. It is estimated that one third to one half of demented elderly persons who are hospitalized will experience an episode of delirium superimposed on their dementia.[16,44] Demented patients who develop delirium, especially if elderly, often lack agitation and obvious hallucinations and may simply sink quietly into an unresponsive state.[27]

The DSM-III-R definition (see Table 9–1) is widely used. In clinical practice, one can usually assume that a patient is delirious if intellectual function abruptly deteriorates and the patient develops a cognitive-attentional disorder that fluctuates in severity.[20] The active, disoriented, hallucinating patient who is picking at the bed covers (floccillation), or tossing to and fro in bed (jactitation), presents little clinical challenge to the clinician in detecting delirium. The hypoactive, frequently demented patient who has sudden "failure to thrive" or is "less cooperative" presents a more considerable clinical diagnostic challenge, and documentation of delirium in this setting can be more difficult. Although there are, as yet, no sensitive and specific tests for detecting delirium in its more subtle forms, it may be possible (and valuable) through serial testing to detect changes in attention and vigilance that represent the evolution of delirium. A similar approach has been taken in the evaluation and management of patients who have, or are at risk for, metabolic encephalopathy (particularly hepatic), and the information acquired has been of clinical value in making management decisions. Because the presence of impaired attention and impaired vigilance helps to differentiate between delirium and dementia, their quantitative evaluation deserves further comment.

Disturbed attention and alertness characterize delirium and distinguish it from dementia, making it necessary to evaluate and measure attention directly. Unfortunately, commonly used screening tests do not specifically measure attention and vigilance.[26] Brief, bedside mental status examinations do not reliably distinguish between attentional disorders and cognitive deficits.[12,18] The most reliable approach to the clinical detection of delirium currently available combines a series of bedside evaluations, carried out over several hours, along with an electroencephalogram (EEG). In delirium, both evaluations, that is, neuropsychologic and EEG, characteristically demonstrate abnormalities fluctuating over short periods of time.

EPIDEMIOLOGY

Because of methodologic difficulties in the detection of delirium, epidemiologic data remain difficult to interpret. Terms used in earlier studies included *toxic delirious reactions of old age, toxic confusion, acute brain failure, acute organic brain syndrome,* and others[29]; and in some cases, patients with "impaired consciousness" were specifically excluded from evaluation. More recently, there has been an effort to use standardized terminology. Although the DSM-III-R definition is generally accepted, the detection of delirium remains imprecise and problematic. Several recent studies have attempted to employ specific and sensitive diagnostic criteria for delirium, as discussed below.

Prevalence on Hospital Admission

The prevalence of delirium reported among elderly patients at hospital admission has ranged between 10% and 40%.[27] These rates come from studies in numerous and varied clinical settings, including psychiatric hospitals, psychiatric wards in general hospitals, neurologic hospitals, general medical wards, and geriatric units.[27] In a careful prospective evaluation of 2000 patients aged 55 and older admitted to medical wards, 15% were delirious on admission.[13] Further evaluation revealed that 25% of these patients with delirium also had underlying moderate to severe dementia. Delirium was present in 40% of patients with dementia compared to 12% of patients without underlying cognitive loss. Dementia (all ages) had an associated relative risk for delirium of 2.97. Almost half the patients who had coinciding dementia and delirium at admission were over the age of 85. Another study examined all medical ward patients (mean age 73) on admission and found that using bedside mental status measurement tools, 20% had substantial cognitive impairment.[15] Of the patients cognitively impaired on admission, 68% presented with delirium.

Incidence During Hospitalization

Evaluation of all patients admitted to general medical-surgical units, of whom more than 40% were over age 65, revealed that 36% were cognitively impaired on admission.[31] Of those cognitively impaired on admission, 38% experienced delirium during their hospital stays, compared with 9% among patients who were cognitively intact at admission. The mean value for the initial Cognitive Capacity Screening Examination (CCSE) score of those with initial scores greater than 20 (maximum score = 30) and who subsequently developed confusion was relatively low (CCSE of 23), and no one with an initial score greater than 26 developed delirium, suggesting again that diminished cognitive capacity is a risk factor for delirium in the setting of acute illness. Almost 20% of the entire population studied suffered an episode of acute confusion during hospitalization. Previous studies have reported a 25% to 35% incidence of delirium in elderly patients admitted without cognitive impairment,[5] and identify aging and dementia as risk factors for delirium. Parenthetically, most have noted that delirium in the elderly often goes unnoticed in general medical and surgical hospital beds.

Prevalence of Delirium in Geriatric Consultation

The liaison psychiatry consultation experience with organic mental disorders on nonpsychiatric wards found that delirium was the most common psychiatric diagnosis (58%) occurring at a mean age of 59 years.[43] The presence of delirium correlated with the number of medical diagnoses. Patients with two diagnoses had a 49% incidence, and those with three or more diagnoses had a 65% incidence. Dementia and delirium occurred together in 13.5% of patients over the age of 65. The 6-month mortality for patients with delirium was 25%, and two thirds of those deaths occurred during the index admission. Cancer was the most common cause of death among patients who were delirious. Ruskin[39] reported that 2.7% of all elderly patients admitted to medical-surgical wards received psychiatric consult evaluations (2.8% for the entire adult hospital population), and delirium accounted for 22% of the consult diagnoses among the elderly group.

Postoperative Incidence of Confusional States

A prospective study of patients undergoing myocardial revascularization carefully looked for and documented delirium perioperatively with comprehensive neuropsychologic testing.[7] No delirium was noted at postoperative day 6, and transient signs of delirium before day 6 were found in only 7% of both the young and old patient groups. The causes of transient confusion were readily recognized medical complications (such as hypoxemia) in the postoperative period. Although carefully done, these results are in sharp contrast to the previously reported series in which the incidence of delirium following revascularization ranged from 6.5% to 33%, and cardiotomy series where the range was from 13% to 70%.[7] The decreasing rates of delirium in cardiac surgery have been attributed, in part, to improved anesthesia techniques and changes in the intensive care unit (ICU) environment. In contrast, patients undergoing hip fracture repair appear to be extremely vulnerable to postoperative delirium.[17,47] More than half developed confusion postoperatively, and a newer study[17] reported a figure exceeding 60%. In that study, virtually all patients with serious perioperative hypotension developed delirium. The consequences of delirium included a longer length of stay, poor mobility at discharge and after 6 months, an increased need for long-term care, and increased rates of postoperative complications (urinary tract incontinence, pressure sores, feeding problems). Confusion in the ICU is an important and challenging problem,[45] and a comprehensive review of perioperative delirium is suggested.[41]

COURSE AND OUTCOME

The natural history of delirium is not well documented. Kral[24] has suggested that the onset varies, depending on both the severity of the stress and the stress resistance of the patient. During the day, the mildly confused patient may conceal deficits. A common clinical observation is that delirium often first appears at night, and the patient becomes confused about place, often while attempting to get out of bed. As the patient becomes more confused, symptoms are experienced more consistently, and inattention and disorientation are typical. Although the majority of cases of delirium clear within 1 to 2 weeks after the provocative illness is detected and treated, episodes can last longer than 1 month, and some continue to death. Prognosis is good for survivors, as transition from an acute syndrome to dementia has rarely been documented[28] and in truth may indicate patients with undetected pre-existing dementia. Because delirium may signal the onset or exacerbation of life-threatening physical illness, failure to detect and adequately treat the underlying disease can result in death. A British multicenter study attempted to describe the natural history. Within 1 month of admission, 25% of individuals with delirium at admission had died, 35% had been discharged, and 40% remained in the hospital; compared to 12%, 47%, and 41%, respectively, for those mentally normal with similar disease burdens.[19]

CAUSES

A list of the potential causes of delirium in older persons includes most clinical disorders as well as some conditions not within the traditional confines of medicine.[4] By definition, the disorder requires cerebral dysfunction due to (1) systemic or CNS disease, (2) exogenous physical or chemical agents, or (3) withdrawal from certain substances of abuse.[28] Little is known, however, about the mechanisms producing delirium. Etiologic conditions enumerated by a National Institute on Aging Task Force[35] are listed in Table 9–2. Intoxication with drugs, particularly those with anticholinergic properties, is perhaps the single most frequent cause of delirium. Age-related changes in the metabolism, distribution, and clearance of drugs, coupled with high drug consumption and polypharmacy in the elderly, are clearly related to the high incidence of drug-related delirium.[5,21] Some of the drugs most often implicated among older persons are listed in Table 9–3.

Stroke

Although for several decades acute stroke has been generally recognized as causing delirium, the incidence due to stroke is debated and the clinical manifestations incompletely defined. Reviews on delirium have reported an incidence between 0% and 30% as a result of acute stroke. Studies quoted, however, were performed prior to the availabilty of sophisticated computed tomography (CT) scanning, and usually relied on clinical examination and isotopic brain scanning. A report on CT scan diagnosis of stroke has demonstrated right hemispheric lesions in more than half of patients presenting with delirium but did not indicate whether the stroke was acute or a preexisting lesion.[34] Another study carefully evaluated consecutive patients admitted to a psychogeriatric ward for delirium and found that one third of the cases were ''caused by'' an acute stroke.[23] Here again, no clear indication of whether the CT abnormality was truly acute is provided. Although the studies available do not define the incidence of acute stroke presenting as de-

Table 9–2 CAUSES OF DELIRIUM IN THE ELDERLY

THERAPEUTIC DRUG INTOXICATION
Metabolic disorders
Azotemia–renal failure (dehydration, diuretics, obstruction, hypokalemia)
Hyponatremia (diuretics, excess ADH, salt wasting, IV fluids)
Volume depletion (diuretics, bleeding, inadequate fluids)
Hypoglycemia (insulin, oral hypoglycemics, starvation)
Hepatic failure
Hyperthyroidism
Hypercalcemia
Cushing syndrome
Any infection and/or fever

CARDIOVASCULAR
Congestive heart failure
Arrhythmia
Acute myocardial infarction

BRAIN DISORDERS
Stroke
Trauma
   Subdural hematoma
   Postconcussion syndrome
Infection
   Meningitis
   Subdural empyema
   Brain abscess
Tumors
   Metastatic to brain
   Primary in brain
Pain, especially fecal impaction or urinary retention
Sensory deprivation states, such as blindness or deafness

HOSPITALIZATION
Anesthesia or surgery
Environmental change and isolation
Alcohol toxicity
Anemia
Tumor—systemic effects of nonmetastatic malignancy
Chronic lung disease with hypoxia or hypercapnia

CHEMICAL INTOXICATIONS
Heavy metals such as arsenic, lead, or mercury
Consciousness altering agents
Carbon monoxide
Accidental hypothermia

Source: Modified from National Institute on Aging Task Force,[35] pp 244, 259–263, 1980.

lirium, there is reason to suspect that stroke has been overlooked in the past. With the improvement in diagnostic capacity of newer generation CT scan-

Table 9–3 DRUGS ASSOCIATED WITH DELIRIUM IN THE ELDERLY

1. Any anticholinergic (psychoactive or medical)
2. Psychoactive
   a. Sedatives and hypnotics
      (1) Long-acting benzodiazepines (flurazepam [Dalmane], diazepam [Valium])
      (2) Short-acting benzodiazepines (less often a problem)
      (3) Barbiturates
      (4) Chloral hydrate, methyprylon, others
   b. Antidepressants
      (1) Sedating heterocyclics (amitriptyline [Elavil], doxepin [Sineguan], trazodone [Desyrel])
      (2) Lithium
   c. Neuroleptics
   d. Anticonvulsants
      (1) Phenytoin (Dilantin) especially
      (2) Carbamazepine (Tegretol), especially high dose
   e. Antiparkinsonian agents
      (1) Amantidine
      (2) Levodopa
      (3) Bromocriptine
3. Medical agents
   a. Cardiac
      (1) Digitalis glycosides
      (2) Diuretics
      (3) Antiarrhythmics (most)
      (4) Calcium channel blockers
      (5) Antihypertensives
         (a) β-blockers
         (b) Central-acting agents (α-methyldopa)
   b. Gastrointestinal
      (1) H_2 receptor antagonists (cimetidine, ranitidine)
      (2) Metaclopramide (Reglan)
   c. Bronchodilator agents
      (1) Theophylline
      (2) β-agonists
      (3) Atropine
   d. Analgesics, especially narcotics and derivatives
   e. Anti-inflammatory
      (1) Corticosteroids
      (2) Nonsteroidal anti-inflammatory drugs (NSAIDs)
   f. Topical ophthalmologic anticholinergic agents
4. Over-the-counter drugs
   a. Cold remedies (antihistamines, pseudoephedrine)
   b. Sedatives (antihistamines)
   c. NSAIDs
   d. Stimulants for appetite reduction or to stay awake
   e. Antinauseants
   f. Alcohol

ners, it is now possible to acquire high-resolution images rapidly enough to gain diagnostic information on acutely confused uncooperative patients.

The clinical diagnosis of stroke presenting as delirium remains difficult, however, as it may be obscured by the confusional state; the peripheral neurologic findings of these strokes may be very subtle and unreliably assessed. Few motor and sensory neurologic findings occur when stroke presents as delirium because of the infarct location. Most strokes complicated by delirium appear to be in the right middle cerebral artery (RMCA) territory, dominant for global attention, perhaps accounting for the occurrence of delirium in right-sided lesions. Features of the RMCA stroke include distractibility, impersistence, increased susceptibility to intrusion, and neglect. Depending on the presence or absence of lesions in the basal ganglia, inferior parietal lobe, or temporal lobes, other disturbances may also be present. The difficulty of clinical diagnosis is nicely illustrated in the case studies presented by Mesulam.[33] Because obvious neurologic deficits appear to be often either absent or untestable in delirium caused by RMCA stroke, special attention should be given to testing for unilateral neglect in vision and visual-spatial domains. Posterior cerebral artery territory strokes causing delirium occur predominantly on the left side and may produce delirium by interruption of limbic and neocortical interconnections or disruption of occipital attentional centers.[10] Visual field testing demonstrating hemianopsia is the major reproducible neurologic finding reported. The diagnosis of acute stroke as the cause of delirium can be difficult and cannot be made reliably from clinical examination alone. It is therefore reasonable to consider CT scanning of the head in the evaluation of delirium in appropriate settings.

PATHOPHYSIOLOGY

Because delirium is a clinical syndrome of multifactorial etiology, it may well be that there is not a single physiologic or chemical mechanism to account for the variety of confusional states seen in the elderly. However, there are shared features in all acute confusional states that suggest a final common pathway for the elaboration of symptoms.[11,40] The cardinal features of (1) global cognitive dysfunction and (2) disturbances of attention and of the sleep-wake cycle may be produced either through a disturbance in arousal mechanisms or diffuse neocortical dysfunction, or both. As suggested decades ago by Engel and Romano,[11] reduction in cerebral oxidative metabolism could account for the EEG abnormalities they noted as well as the clinical features of delirium.

Study of the neurologic correlates of arousal and attention (central features of consciousness) continues, and neurologic systems responsible for alertness and awakeness have been further defined.[40] The afferent activating pathways are diffuse cholinergic projections to the neocortex and arise primarily from the nucleus basalis of Meynert (nbM) in the basal forebrain, receiving input from the rostral pons and posterolateral hypothalamus. These (and other direct) projection pathways are believed to be responsible for regulation of hippocampal and neocortical activation in humans.[40] Acute disruption of these activating pathways produces a decrease in the levels of consciousness and arousal that, after a recovery period, return to normal.

In addition to changes in level of consciousness, lesions in the cholinergic cortical projection decrease the general activation of the forebrain and produce cognitive deficits. It is surprising that slow development of small lesions in the same area does not produce a decrease in level of consciousness, but does create cognitive deficits; a process perhaps analogous to the pathophysiology of AD or other progressive neurodegenerative dementias. Diffuse neocortical (forebrain) injury or dysfunction has similar clinical features of impaired consciousness and cognition.

To summarize, altered consciousness seems to occur as a result of deficits in or damage to neocortical processing, arising from insufficient afferent activation, or from disorders of the cortex itself, or both. The spectrum of disease includes cortical malfunction (e.g., dementia), cortical hypofunction (e.g., stupor, coma), and mixtures of both (delirium).[40]

Substantial research supports an important, perhaps central, role for dysfunction of the afferent cholinergic projection system in the development of both attentional and cognitive deficits. Central muscarinic cholinergic blockade depresses the level of consciousness and produces confusion, emotional lability, and memory impairment, as well as other features of delirium.[37] Drugs are common offending agents, and older persons are most sensitive to adverse drug effects in general, and to drug-induced delirium in particular,[5] especially those with underlying cognitive deficits. The prevalent view is that normal aging is associated with a progressive decline in brain levels of acetylcholine, presumably due to degeneration of cholinergic projection neurons, which, by producing a relative cholinergic deficit, could make the elderly more sensitive to CNS side effects of anticholinergic agents.[9,22,37] With their cholinergic depletion, AD patients would be expected to be particularly prone to delirium caused by any anticholinergic drug or simply to stress provoked by illness; and many studies confirm their vulnerability.[13,27,31]

Improvement of delirium with physostigmine, an acetylcholinesterase inhibitor, has been observed in several settings. In addition to the reversal of anticholinergic drug-induced delirium, physostigmine has been shown to reverse or improve delirium associated with nonanticholinergic drugs, including benzodiazepines, cimetidine and ranitidine, quinidine, inhalational anesthetics, amantadine, and fentanyl citrate (Innovar). Patients suffering from delirium tremens also have improved with physostigmine administration. Oversedation secondary to benzodiazepine administration also improves with physostigmine, but not through an obvious cholinergic repletion effect or interaction with CNS benzodiazepine receptors. Instead, physostigmine appears to reverse benzodiazepine effects on CBF and cerebral oxygen consumption and produce an objective increase in both.[20] Whether the ability of physostigmine to improve delirium is due to its enhancement of CBF and oxygen consumption or is mediated directly through cholinergic cortical innervation, or both, is uncertain. Abnormalities in the function of the cerebral cortex and the EEG probably result from changes in CBF and metabolic rate, but whether these measured differences represent primary disturbances or are consequences of a disorder of another system (e.g., arousal pathways) is not yet determined.[40]

Preliminary investigations into a possible role for β-endorphin (endogenous opiate peptide) in the development of delirium have shown that surgical stress and disturbed circadian neurohumeral patterns are associated with both increased β-endorphin levels and delirium in postoperative patients.[32] Cause and effect have not yet been established, however. Another interesting recent hypothesis suggests a possible role for interleukin-1 (IL-1, endogenous pyrogen) in the delirium of febrile illnesses and possibly other inflammatory diseases in which pyrogen is released.[8] IL-1 is produced in response to a variety of toxic, infectious, and inflammatory stimuli. Among the many actions of IL-1, in addition to producing hypothalamically mediated fever by resetting the body's thermostat upward, is its ability to increase slow-wave sleep in experimental animals. The slow-wave EEG pattern is exactly the one seen in delirium, and it seems plausible that IL-1 contributes to delirium by a direct effect on the cortex.

Although earlier studies indicated that nearly a quarter of elderly patients with delirium have no identifiable organic cause for the disturbance, our broader understanding of precipitants of delirium and more vigorous diagnostic evaluation now commonly employed often reveal several concurrent potential causes, including sleep deprivation and sensory isolation or overload.

MANAGEMENT

Successful management of the acutely confused patient depends first on the correct identification of the clinical picture and, second, on the correct diagnosis of its specific etiology. Once delirium is detected, it is imperative to look for all possible causes, as more than one etiologic factor may be implicated. A mnemonic, *SUNDOWNERS*, identifies factors that may contribute to the risk for delirium.

Use of the SUNDOWNERS mnemonic does not imply that all delirium begins at night. It has been suggested that reduced lighting and activity, combined with nadirs of several circadian hormones, make the aged brain vulnerable to a misinterpretation of reality, but sundowning, or onset of delirium at night, refers to only one subset of all cases of delirium. One early observation reported reproducing the sundowning syndrome by placing an older person with dementia in a dark room during the day.[8] It was first noted that interference with visual input could produce delirium in older persons of normal baseline cognitive function when half a dozen postoperative cataract patients developed "black-patch delirium."[46] Although questions have occasionally been raised concerning whether sundowning is different from "ordinary" delirium, current majority opinion suggests that it is simply a variant of delirium provoked by sensory deprivation.

One study of sundowning in the nursing home attempted to define the syndrome and identify associated factors.[14] Eleven of 89, predominantly black, female, nursing home residents, observed morning and evening on two consecutive days, developed confusion accompanied by increased restlessness and noisiness during late afternoon or evening. Associated factors were poorer cognitive function, being awakened more frequently for care during the night, and shorter stay in room of residence. Although not generalizable for a number of reasons, additional investigations of sundowning are important because of its prevalence and close relationship, if not identity, with delirium.

A second use of the mnemonic is to enumerate potentially remediable risk factors that if addressed promptly in older persons, may allow prevention or amelioration of an impending delirium. Thus, the mnemonic becomes a checklist for clinicians, suggesting that to prevent delirium, it may be useful to (1) treat Sickness, (2) rule out or relieve Urinary retention or fecal impaction, (3) be sensitive to the psychic needs of the Newly admitted elder in a new environment, (4) promptly identify the patient with pre-existing Dementia and reduce confusing stimulation, (5) realize that the very Old patient is at high risk, (6) be particularly attentive to analgesics for the patient Writhing in pain, (7) recognize that patients Not adequately worked up can have discoverable conditions whose treatment may prevent delirium, (8) supply adequate sensory inputs to those with impairments in Eye or ear function, (9) be aware of the great potential of many therapeutic drugs (Rx) for producing or contributing to delirium, and (10) prevent Sleep deprivation. A third value for the mnemonic is to alert the clinical team to those patients who have risk factors for delirium that although identified, are not remediable and therefore mark those individuals as especially likely to become acutely confused. Whether delirium can be prevented is not known and is an important issue for further investigation.

Identification and treatment of the underlying pathology is most important in management of delirium. A principle of geriatric medicine is that the usual presentations of disease are often absent or muted, and instead nonspecific problems or functional losses appear. Delirium is a common manifestation of illness in or outside of the CNS among older persons. Whenever an older individual presents with confusion, the search for physical illness, either acute or chronic with acute flare, should begin immediately. Many acutely confused patients with reversible disorders go untreated because they are not properly worked up. The misidentification of the clinical picture of delirium as chronic dementia aborts the search for and treatment of an underlying reversible physical illness. Misdiagnosis of causation, such as the attribution of confusion to a psychosis brought on by a recent life event or psychosocial stress, can be disastrous in provoking the wrong treatment or preventing further evaluation.

Drug toxicity is one of the most common preventable causes of acute confusion. Identification and careful scrutiny of all drugs taken by the patient are critical, and those drugs that can produce delirium should be eliminated to the extent possible. When one or another agent is considered essential, a reduction in the dosage may be sufficient to eliminate adverse effects. A useful strategy in the delirious old patient is to stop all drugs and resume those for which a clinical indication emerges, and then only at lower doses. Or, as Sir Ferguson Anderson has said, "When coming across a fuddled old person, it is often better to stop a drug than start one."[3] Additionally, an episode of delirium may have a multifactorial etiology; for example, a psychoactive drug given to quiet the early delirium of pneumonia produces urinary retention and infection, all of which summate to produce major delirium whose management requires careful identification and treatment of all contributing elements. Maintenance of fluid and electrolyte balance and attention to hematocrit and sound nutrition are important general principles that can potentially reduce the risk for delirium.

While identifying and treating the underlying cause or causes of delirium, symptomatic supportive measures must be given equal attention; it often takes days to weeks for treatment of the underlying cause to relieve delirium. Measures should be instituted to avoid the extremes of sensory input, including deficient or excessive stimulation, since either is likely to exacerbate delirium and both are potentially preventable.[42] Eyeglasses and hearing aids, often left at home or in the nursing home during the hectic transfer to the acute hospital, should be retrieved and provided to the patient as quickly as possible. Loud, disruptive noise should be eliminated when possible, but manageable sensory stimulation can help. Hospital staff should assume a calm and consistent approach toward confused patients, providing frequent reorientation and reassurance. Family members and friends should be encouraged to visit.

The physical environment of the patient also merits special attention. Abrupt relocation to a new and unfamiliar location, especially at night, should be avoided. The hospitalized patient with delirium should be placed in a safe and ordered environment with familiar personal objects, such as toiletries, bedclothes, photographs, and family mementos. The patient should rest in a quiet, well-lighted, private room during the day, and a night light sufficient to allow visual orientation at night is essential. Minimizing demands on impaired function can be achieved through the use of orienting devices, such as written signs, clocks, and calendars that give the place, date, time, and identify important objects and locations. Staff should attempt to make the immediate environment as constant as possible, avoiding room changes and providing labels for the bathroom, the patient's closet, and even such items as the bed. Nursing routines and personnel should be ad-

justed to make them as consistent as possible. Safety precautions such as siderails and close observation are imperative during periods of confusion. In some cases, restraints may be unavoidable to protect the patient; when considered necessary, they should be padded and accompanied by frequent explanations as to their purpose and by close monitoring.[6,38]

Drug therapy is an important aspect of the management of the delirious agitated patient, and several different classes of drugs are commonly employed. But it should be emphasized from the outset than any psychoactive drug will likely prolong some of the mental status abnormalities present in the delirious patient, although ameliorating the agitation, paranoia, and adrenergic hyperactivity. Thus, starting any agent for the delirium is a trade-off of better manageability in exchange for prolonged mental blunting. Benzodiazepines should only be used for minor degrees of agitation or anxiety because they themselves may cause excessive drowsiness or paradoxic agitation. Shorter acting agents, including lorazepam and oxazepam, are preferred when a benzodiazepine is indicated.[45]

The neuroleptics are sometimes used in delirious patients because they may help diminish hallucinations and delusions. Individual agents can be selected for varying degrees of sedation, as required by the patient's condition. These drugs have a prolonged clearance time in the aged, and elderly individuals show earlier and greater sensitivity to adverse effects, necessitating lower doses than used in younger individuals. The aged are more susceptible to the side effects of neuroleptics, perhaps in part because of reduced CNS levels of acetylcholine and dopamine. The choice of drug depends on the side effects that are most important to minimize and the degree to which certain side effects are desirable. Some agents have higher anticholinergic potential and sedation, and may cause orthostatic hypotension. Other drugs, with low anticholinergic potential, have serious extrapyramidal side effects, including akathisia, parkinsonism, dystonia, and tardive dyskinesia. Akathisia in particular is troublesome because it tends to occur early in treatment and mimic the agitation and restlessness for which the drug was started, potentially provoking increasing doses.

For the elderly patient with underlying dementia who becomes acutely confused, a sedating neuroleptic is generally desirable because of the high degree of agitation usually accompanying delirium; thioridazine (Mellaril) is a reasonable choice. Concern over an anticholinergic effect should not be excessive when using thioridazine. Although thioridazine is the most anticholinergic of the commonly used neuroleptics, its atropine equivalence is only 0.003 mg/mg; thus, each 10-mg dose of thioridazine yields 0.03 mg atropine effect. For comparison, the least anticholinergic agent among the tricyclic antidepressant drugs, desipramine, is used with enthusiasm in elderly patients, in part because of its modest anticholinergic side effects, yet its atropine equivalence is identical with thioridazine, 0.003 mg/mg. Accordingly, it seems reasonable to use thioridazine if its sedating effects are indicated, especially in the agitated, delirious, and already demented elderly patient.

Several general principles are useful in administering neuroleptic drugs to elderly delirious patients:

1. Target symptoms should be identified at the outset, and when goals are achieved, drugs should be reduced and later withdrawn unless symptoms persist or recur.

2. The initial dose should be half the smallest dose supplied by the manufacturer, followed by careful continuing assessment of the effect.

3. Expect that the effective dose, if administered for more than a few days consecutively, will likely lead to side effects, especially excess sedation, and will need to be reduced.

4. The beneficial effect on behavior is limited to the period during which delirium is present, and, thus, the neuroleptic should usually be reduced and then withdrawn as delirium abates.

5. Oversedation from drugs may be mistaken for continuing hypoactive delirium and result in permanent drug administration and continuing stupor.

6. Neuroleptic agents, especially low-potency phenothiazines, should probably not be used in delirium related to alcohol or sedative-hypnotic withdrawal because of the risk of inducing seizures.

Thus, a variety of management strategies may be useful for the acutely confused patient, both during evaluation and after treatment of the underlying cause is begun. Supportive and symptomatic measures should be given at least as much attention as drug therapy. Only when all measures are employed in a coordinated and sensible way can success be anticipated in managing these most challenging and vulnerable elderly patients.

CONCLUSION

The diagnosis of delirium is an important but often neglected responsibility of the physician. Delirium is frequently reversible but may also coexist with dementia, leading to imprecise diagnosis. To distinguish delirium from dementia, the physician must evaluate and measure attention directly, usually through a series of bedside neuropsychologic evaluations and an EEG. Delirium is quite common among hospitalized elderly patients and even more prevalent among those who are also cognitively impaired. Its presence correlates strongly with the number of medical diagnoses, and delirium is also common postoperatively, especially among patients with perioperative hypotension.

There is a large number of potential causes of delirium in the elderly, including various diseases, drug intoxication, and drug withdrawal, but there is as yet no consensus regarding the actual physiologic mechanism behind delirium. The mnemonic SUNDOWNERS not only identifies risk factors for delirium but also serves as a checklist for preventing or ameliorating delirium. Supportive and symptomatic interventions, particularly with regard to the patient's physical environment, are crucial in the management of delirium. Although drug therapy is also an important aspect of management of agitated delirious patients, the physician must be aware of the older patient's greater sensitivity to such drugs, the trade-off of better manageability for prolonged mental blunting, and the potentially serious side effects.

REFERENCES

1. American Psychiatric Association: Diagnostic and Statistical Manual of Mental Disorders, ed 3. American Psychiatric Association, Washington, DC, 1980.
2. American Psychiatric Association: Diagnostic and Statistical Manual of Mental Disorders, ed 3, revised. American Psychiatric Association, Washington, DC, 1987.
3. Anderson, WF: Personal communication, 1971.
4. Arie, T: Confusion in old age. Age Ageing 7:72–76, 1978.
5. Besdine, RW: Dementia and Delirium. In Rowe, JW and Besdine, RW (eds): Geriatric Medicine, ed 2. Little Brown, Boston, 1988, pp 375–401.
6. Boss, OJ: Acute mood and behavior disturbances of neurological origin: Acute confusional states. Neurosurg Nurs 14:61–78, 1982.
7. Calabrese, JR, Skwerer, RG, and Gulledge, AD: Incidence of postoperative delirium following myocardial revascularization. Clev Clin J Med 54:29–32, 1987.
8. Cameron, O: Studies in senile nocturnal delirium. Psychiatr Q 15:47–53, 1941.
9. Davies, P: Neurotransmitter-related enzymes in senile dementia of the Alzheimer type. Brain Res 171:319–327, 1979.
10. Devinsky, O: Confusional states following PCA infarction. Arch Neurol 45:160–163, 1988.
11. Engel, GL and Romano, J: Delirium, a syndrome of cerebral insufficiency. J Chron Dis 9:260–277, 1959.
12. Erkinjuntti, T, Sulkava, A, Wikstrom, J, and Autio, L: Short portable mental status questionnaire as a screening test for dementia and delirium among the elderly. J Am Geriatr Soc 35:412–416, 1987.
13. Erkinjuntti, T, Wikstrom, J, Palo, J, and Autio, L: Dementia among medical inpatients. Arch Intern Med 146:1923–1926, 1986.
14. Evans, LK: Sundown syndrome in institutionalized elderly. J Am Geriatr Soc 35:101–108, 1987.
15. Fields, SD, MacKenzie, CR, Charlson, ME, and Perry, SW: Reversibility of cognitive impairment in medical inpatients. Arch Intern Med 146:1593–1596, 1986.
16. Gillick, MR, Serrel, NA, and Gillick, LS: Adverse consequences of hospitalization in the elderly. Soc Sci Med 16:1033–1038, 1982.
17. Gustafson, Y, Berggren, D, Brannstrom, B, Bucht, G, Norberg, A, Hansson, L-I, and Winblad, B: Acute confusional states in elderly patients treated for femoral neck fracture. J Am Geriatr Soc 36:525–530, 1988.
18. Haddad, LB and Coffman, TL: A brief neuropsychological screening exam for psychiatric-geriatric patients. Clin Gerontol 6:3–10, 1987.
19. Hodkinson, HM: Mental impairment in the elderly. J R Coll Physicians Lond 7:305–317, 1973.
20. Hoffman, WE, Albrecht, RF, Miletich, DJ, Hagen, TJ, and Cook, JM: Cerebrovascular and cerebral metabolic effects of physostigmine, midozolam, and a benzodiazepine antagonist. Anesth Analg 65:639–644, 1986.
21. Hollister, LE: Drug induced psychiatric disorders and their management. Med Toxicol 1:428–448, 1986.

22. Karp, HR and Mirra, SS: Dementia in Adults. In Baker, AB and Joynt, RJ (eds): Clinical Neurology, Vol 3. JB Lippincott, Philadelphia, 1986, pp 1–60.

23. Koponen, H: Acute confusional states in the elderly: A radiological evaluation. Acta Psychiatr Scand 76: 726–731, 1987.

24. Kral, VA: Confusional States: Description and Management. In Howells, JG (ed): Perspectives in the Psychiatry of Old Age. Brunner Mazel, New York, 1975, pp 356–362.

25. Krueger, JM, Walter, J, Dinarello, C, Dinarello, CA, Wolff, S, and Chedid, L: Sleep-promoting effects of endogenous pyrogen (interleukin-1). Am J Physiol 246:994, 1984.

26. Levin, HS and Benton, AL: Neuropsychologic Assessment. In Baker, AB and Joynt, RJ (eds): Clinical Neurology, Vol 2. JB Lippincott, Philadelphia, 1984, pp 8–9.

27. Levkoff, SE, Besdine, RW, and Wetle, T: Acute confusional states (delirium) in the hospitalized elderly. Annu Rev Gerontol Geriatr 6:1–26, 1986.

28. Lipowski, ZJ: Transient cognitive disorders (delirium, acute confusional states) in the elderly. Am J Psychiatry 140:1426–1436, 1983.

29. Liston, EH: Delirium in the aged. Psychiatr Clin North Am 5:49–66, 1982.

30. McCartney, JR: Physicians' assessment of cognitive capacity. Arch Intern Med 146:177–178, 1986.

31. McCartney, JR and Palmateer, LM: Assessment of cognitive deficit in geriatric patients. J Am Geriatr Soc 33:467–471, 1985.

32. McIntosh, TK, Bush, HL, Yeston, NS, Grasberger, R, Palter, M, Aun, F, and Egdahl, RH: Beta-endorphin, cortisol and postoperative delirium: A preliminary report. Psychoneuroendocrinology 10:303–313, 1985.

33. Mesulam, A: Acute confusional states with RMCA infarctions. J Neurol Neurosurg Psychiatry 39:84–89, 1976.

34. Mullally, W: Frequency of acute confusional states with lesions of the right hemisphere. Ann Neurol 12:113A, 1982.

35. National Institute on Aging Task Force: Senility reconsidered: Treatment possibilities for mental impairment in the elderly. JAMA 244:259–263, 1980.

36. Perez, EL and Silverman, M: Delirium: The often overlooked diagnosis. Int J Psychiatry Med 14:181–189, 1984.

37. Richardson, JS, Miller, PS, Lemay, JS, Jyu, CA, Neil, SG, Kilduff, CJ, and Keegan, DL: Mental dysfunction and the blockade of muscarinic receptors in the brains of the normal elderly. Prog Neuropsychol Biol Psychiatry 9:651–654, 1985.

38. Richeimer, SH: Psychological intervention in delirium. Postgrad Med 81:173–180, 1987.

39. Ruskin, FE: Geropsychiatric consultation in a university hospital: A report on 67 referrals. Am J Psychiatry 142:333–336, 1985.

40. Saper, CB and Plum, F: Disorders of Consciousness: Handbook of Clinical Neurology, Vol. 1 (45). Clinical Neuropsychology. Elsevier Scientific, Amsterdam, 1985, pp 107–128.

41. Seibert, CP: Recognition, management, and prevention of neuropsychological dysfunction after operation. Int Anesthesiol Clin 24:39–58, 1986.

42. Trockman, G: Caring for the confused or delirious patient. Am J Nurs 78:1495–1499, 1978.

43. Trzepacz, PT, Teague, GB, and Lipowski, ZJ: Delirium and other organic mental disorders in a general hospital. Gen Hosp Psychiatry 7:101–106, 1985.

44. Warshaw, GA, Moore, JT, Friedman, SW, Currie, CT, Kennie, DC, Kane, WJ, and Mears, PA: Functional disability in the hospitalized elderly. JAMA 248:847–850, 1982.

45. Weber, RJ, Oszko, MA, Bolender, BJ, and Grysiak, DL: The intensive care unit syndrome: Causes, treatment, and prevention. Drug Intell Clin Pharm 19:13–20, 1985.

46. Weisman, AD and Hackett, TP: Establishment of a specific doctor-patient relationship in the prevention and treatment of "black-patch delirium." N Engl J Med 258:1284–1289, 1958.

47. Williams, MA, Campbell, EB, Raynor, WJ, Musholt, MA, Mlynarczyk, SM, and Crane, LF: Predictors of acute confusional states in hospitalized elderly patients. Res Nurs Health 8:31–40, 1985.

Chapter 10

FALLS AND GAIT

Leslie Wolfson, M.D.

THE ANATOMY AND PHYSIOLOGY OF
  NEUROMUSCULAR CONTROL OF
  GAIT AND BALANCE
THE EFFECTS OF AGE ON MOTOR
  FUNCTION
EVALUATION OF THE PATIENT WITH
  IMPAIRED MOBILITY OR A
  HISTORY OF FALLS
THE SYNDROMES OF GAIT AND
  BALANCE DYSFUNCTION
DEFINING "SENILE" GAIT AND
  BALANCE DISORDERS

Impaired mobility and falls are important causes of morbidity, mortality, and limited function in older people. They produce serious loss in the quality of life of older people and when severe are a major factor causing institutionalization. Although the vast majority of falls produce only minor cuts and bruises, one half of all accidental injuries in the elderly are the result of falls.[1] Two hundred thousand hip fractures per year as well as other injuries incurred by falls produce a large amount of morbidity and nearly 10,000 deaths per year in this population.[56,78] The majority of studies suggest that in the course of 1 year, one third of elderly living at home will report a fall,[7] while long-term care facilities report 0.67 to 2 falls per bed per year.[29,65] The prevalence of falls increases with age and is greater among women than among men.[35] Factors underlying these falls include vision and hearing deficits, arthritis, cardiovascular disease, medication, and impaired neuromus-

cular function related to diseases of the nervous system. Moderate to severe dementia is an important element in producing falls, especially among institutionalized elderly. Impaired judgment and memory make it difficult for a demented individual to assess environmental hazards, plan corrective action, and benefit from prior mistakes. In addition, dementing illnesses are often associated with impaired neuromuscular control. This dual effect of dementia on falls is a major reason for their frequent occurrence in long-term facilities despite the presence of relatively few environmental hazards. By contrast, dementia is not a factor in the vast majority of home-dwelling elderly who fall.

In some individuals with limited mobility, the cause of falling is apparent after history and examination (e.g., Parkinson disease [PD]). In the majority of elderly patients with impaired mobility, however, even after neurologic evaluation the etiology is not determined despite the presence of impaired neuromuscular control of the lower extremities in the form of poor gait and balance. In one series of 37 patients referred to the author because of failing gait and balance, after initial evaluation and appropriate imaging procedures, about one third had demonstrable neurologic diagnoses. Although the majority had varying degrees of impaired gait and balance, they did not fit into traditional diagnostic patterns. In these healthy elderly living at home, only rarely do secondary factors such as debility, impaired aerobic work capacity, or skeletal abnormalities (e.g., osteoarthritis) contribute significantly to the compromised function. The nervous system dysfunction underlying this "idiopathic" impairment of neuromuscular control of the lower extremities is unknown. In the first portion of this chapter we will review the anatomy and physiology of neuromuscular control of gait and balance. This is included to provide the background necessary for the reader to think of the motor system in pathoanatomic terms. We will then look at the effects of aging and previously defined disease on this mechanism to understand the unique nature of this critically important problem.

THE ANATOMY AND PHYSIOLOGY OF NEUROMUSCULAR CONTROL OF GAIT AND BALANCE

Sensorimotor Function Underlying Gait and Balance

Using environmental cues (sensory information) the motor system transforms our needs into neural output that results in the coordinated movement of muscles, joints, and extremities, thereby allowing us to interact with our surroundings. Gait and postural mechanisms use motor control structures to provide these functions. The following are some of the structures and functions central to the motor control of gait and balance.

The pyramidal cells of the motor cortex, with contributions from both premotor and parietal cortex, provide the cells of origin for the corticospinal tract, which controls contralateral voluntary movement of distal extremity musculature. The premotor and supplementary motor cortex provide the programming of motor sequences and the control of the axial and proximal limb musculature among other functions.

The basal ganglia consist of two upper brainstem nuclei (i.e., the substantia nigra [SN] and subthalamic nu-

cleus), which connect to three nuclear groups deep within the hemisphere: the caudate nucleus, putamen, and globus pallidus. The large pigmented neurons of the dorsal portion of the SN ascend to the caudate and putamen (i.e., striatum), providing presynaptic dopamine innervation. A second important striatal input originates in the frontal cortex. Major striatal output projects to the ventrolateral nuclei of the thalamus, which in turn project to the prefrontal cortex and cerebellum, thereby tying output from the basal ganglia into the remainder of the motor system. Major functions of these nuclei include the suppression of unintended movement (e.g., tremor and chorea) and the facilitation of planned and reflex movement, including posture and gait.

The cerebellum is a somatotopically organized structure receiving input from all sensory modalities. The output of the cerebellum consists primarily of projections of neurons to spinal cord, thalamus, and cortex. The medial cerebellum (vermis) is responsible for the control of axial and proximal musculature, while the intermediate portion controls distal limb muscles. Sensory feedback, in the form of vestibular, visual, auditory, and tactile-proprioceptive input (through vestibulocerebellar and spinocerebellar pathways), is related to intended movement and corrections of execution are made. Lesions within the cerebellum or its connections produce abnormalities in the order of muscle contraction during movement resulting in a wide-based unsteady gait, poor postural control, intention tremor, and an inability to perform skilled or sequenced movement.

Spinal Cord and Somatosensory Function

The corticospinal pathways descend in both the lateral (limb muscles) and anteromedial (axial muscles) funiculi of the spinal cord. At the appropriate levels they synapse with motor neurons and interneurons, which control voluntary movement and segmental reflexes, respectively. The axon of the motor neuron extends out through the ventral root as a large myelinated motor nerve fiber to innervate a motor unit (several muscle fibers).

Tactile and pain sensations are mediated by a variety of skin receptors that respond selectively to specific kinds of stimuli. Proprioception is accomplished primarily through muscle-spindle afferents, which become large, myelinated, rapidly conducting nerve fibers mediating segmental and long-loop reflexes as well as our perception of limb position. Collaterals of ascending fibers have a segmental spinal cord distribution, which mediates local reflexes (e.g., knee or ankle jerk) as well as ascending spinocerebellar components. Sensory information is integrated within the ventral posterior nuclei of the thalamus, which in turn projects to the parietal cortex, where sensation becomes conscious. Sensory information from the parietal cortex projects to motor and premotor cortex, the basal ganglia, and the cerebellum.

The two vestibular receptors, the semicircular canals and otoliths, consist of specialized sensory epithelium, called hair cells, housed in interconnected endolymph-filled cavities within the petrous bone. The three semicircular canals are directionally arrayed to detect angular acceleration of the head in any plane, while the two otoliths detect linear acceleration as well as fixing the head position with respect to the vertical. Displacement of the projections of the hair cells by movement of the endolymph, as well as the effects of gravity, produces the input carried by the eighth nerve to the four pontine vestibular nuclei. These nuclei project to the cerebellum and serve as the origin for descending spinal tracts as well as the vestibular input to oculomotor nuclei for oculovestibular reflexes.

Gait and Balance

As the prototype of a motor activity, gait uses all aspects of motor system feedback and control just discussed.

Animal studies suggest the presence of preprogrammed neurons within the lumbosacral cord that automatically generate the rhythmic components of gait. These programmed responses are modulated both by ascending sensory input and by descending control from the midbrain reticular system. At this time, however, there is no evidence for a spinal cord gait generator in humans. Similarly, the neural mechanisms subserving balance have not been explicitly defined, although it is assumed that they also use the motor pathways. Postural responses (or balance) are often defined as the automatic response to perturbations of body position that disturb our normal equilibrium, thereby putting us at risk for falls. Utilizing tactile-proprioceptive, visual, and vestibular input, the postural response provides for the automatic adjustments of limbs, torso, and head to maintain the center of body mass above its base of support (the feet). This is accomplished by a series of overlapping reflexes collectively termed "the balance response." Although there may be some segmental (short-latency) spinal contribution to this response, the vast majority of the response is suprasegmental through brainstem and cortical connections that are called long-loop reflexes. As one would expect, impulses utilizing cortical loops involving volition have the greatest latency, while those using subcortical structures involving reflex-evoked patterned muscle responses have intermediate latency. By contrast with spinal reflexes, long-loop reflexes are heavily influenced by prior experience, motor set, and volition. Balance is therefore mediated through portions of the peripheral nervous system (PNS) and central nervous system (CNS) that support other aspects of motor control.

THE EFFECTS OF AGE ON MOTOR FUNCTION

It has been widely accepted that in childhood our cognitive and motor faculties wax, while senescence is associated with the waning of these same abilities. In the course of the last 30 years, critical analysis of this thesis has revealed that the vast majority of cognitive changes previously attributed to aging occur as a result of the effects of disease. It is now accepted that relatively modest changes in memory are associated with age. In the section that follows we will examine the effects of age on neuromuscular function to determine if this adequately explains the impaired mobility and balance so common among the elderly.

Sensory Function

Quantitative testing of the perception of joint movement and position (proprioception) at the knee reveals a deterioration with age.[72] Proprioceptive testing at the toe and ankle reveals higher thresholds in the toes but not the fingers of 61- to 84-year-olds as compared with younger subjects.[38] Quantitative testing of vibratory sensibility[81] has demonstrated a significant decrease after age 50,[74] involving primarily the lower extremities,[37] resulting in a more than twofold increase in the perceptual threshold.[59,62,63] Tactile sensitivity also decreases with age.[5,22] Clinically demonstrable abnormalities of proprioception are revealed in 13% to 20% of "normal" elderly during neurologic testing.[37] The studies indicate modest but consistent decreases in both clinical and quantitative sensory testing, suggesting a real loss of sensory function with age. The clinical significance of these changes as well as the underlying mechanism (e.g., age effects on receptor(s) and/or peripheral nerve, etc.) remain to be determined, although it is likely that they represent a mild peripheral neuropathy often noted with age but do not explain functional motoric deterioration.

Motor Function

Isometric strength (constant muscle length) peaks in the mid-20s, decreases slowly until after age 50, and then declines rapidly.[41] Healthy 60- to 80-year-olds experience a 20% to 40% decrease in isometric strength in all muscle groups tested relative to young adults.[42] In routine walking and balance activities, muscle torque is generated during limb movement (i.e., during muscle contraction); power is therefore most appropriately measured during muscle contraction (using an isokinetic dynamometer).[51] Measured in this way, there is a 38% decrement of strength in the third through seventh decades that is most prominent at higher speeds of muscle contraction.[42] Selective type II (fast-twitch muscle fibers) loss has also been demonstrated in the elderly. Loss of these fast-twitch fibers may play a role in the prominent loss of power during high-speed muscle contraction.[42] Loss of anterior horn cells in aging has been demonstrated both by neurophysiologic[12] and autopsy[36] studies in both cervical[12] and lumbar spinal[36] cord. Both neuronal loss and disuse atrophy (due to inactivity) may be related to type-selective muscle atrophy observed in the elderly.

In addition to this modest loss of power with age, there is a slowing of motor reaction times. The times required for tasks using simple responses (e.g., tapping) increases modestly from the third through seventh decades, while the time necessary for more complex responses increases to a greater extent.[80] The role of synaptic dysfunction in slowing of these complex tasks is difficult to evaluate although studies in aged rats suggest slowed impulse transmission in multisynaptic pathways.[17]

Electrophysiology

Electrophysiologic findings are consistent with modest but progressive decrease in the velocity of peripheral nerve sensory conduction (−16%) as well as in the amplitude of the action potential (−50%) from age 20 through age 80. The velocities of peripheral nerve motor impulses decrease simi-

Table 10–1 RELATIONSHIP OF NORMAL AGING AND
FALLS TO STRIDE LENGTH AND SPEED

	Stride Length, m	Walking Speed, m/s
NORMATIVE DATA		
Healthy men[52]		
Age 20–25	1.54	1.50
50–55	1.60	1.57
81–87	1.26	1.18
Age 20–87	1.39±0.23	1.46±0.16
Healthy women[53]		
Age 20–70	1.33±0.23	1.30±0.15
EFFECT OF FALLS		
Unselected elderly in the community[33]		
No falls (× Age* = 77)	1.01±0.29	0.83±0.24
Hx falls (× Age = 78)	0.83±0.28	0.66±0.27
Residents of long-term care facility[85]		
No falls (× Age = 82)	0.82±0.22	0.64±0.21
Hx falls (× Age = 84)	0.53±0.21	0.37±0.17

*Mean age.

larly.[68] The extent of this decline does not imply significant peripheral nerve dysfunction. Finally, the conduction velocity of afferent impulses within the dorsal column of the spinal cord decreases modestly (during somatosensory evoked potentials), but only after age 60.[13,14,20]

Effects of Age on Gait and Balance

Aerobic work capacity and cardiovascular conditioning, as well as the aforementioned indices of neuromuscular function, decrease with age. It is therefore not surprising that gait and balance, which are complex interactions of these functions, also decline. In healthy elderly of both sexes, stride length and walking speed, two components that describe the quality of gait, decline modestly by comparison with young adults (Table 10–1).[32,52] In elderly individuals with increasingly limited activity levels, there is a decrease in stride length and walking speed when compared with vigorous elderly (Table 10–1).[32,85] The posture of "normal" older men during walking has been described as flexed forward at both the head and torso, with increased flexion of both the elbows and knees in associ-

ation with diminished arm swing.[52] By contrast, the gait of elderly women has been characterized as narrow-based with a waddling quality.[6,24] It has been our experience that, even though these patterns are present in the gait of healthy elderly, the variation between individuals precludes a general characterization of walking patterns.[85]

Postural stability (static balance) is readily determined by a variety of techniques that measure body sway during standing. Body sway increases with age, particularly in women.[32,58] Balance, which utilizes the segmental and long-loop reflexes discussed earlier, maintains body equilibrium during movement, allowing us to correct for encounters with environmental hazards.[55] Using these accepted definitions, it is clear that dynamic balance is most directly related to the maintenance of effective balance during daily activities. Dynamic balance also declines with age, although normal elderly still retain effective balance reflexes.[83,84] During testing on a balance platform, elderly subjects demonstrated significantly greater sway and tendency to fall when visual and/or lower extremity somatosensory input was experimentally decreased. Sudden perturbation of the platform resulted in an increased latency of the balance response as well as diminished compensatory hip and ankle movement. Both controls and older subjects showed a significant capacity to adapt to serial presentations of the destabilizing forces.[83] EMG recording during postural perturbations in the elderly suggests a disorganization of the muscle synergies used for balance.[86] In compensating for moderate perturbations of their equilibrium, elderly subjects respond with one or more steps that vertically align body mass and the base of support. Under similar circumstances, younger subjects utilize muscle synergies that are a more adaptive series of movements of the extremities and torso, producing vertical alignment without resorting to stepping.[84]

Structural and Chemical Changes within the Nervous System

As in other portions of the nervous system, the structures subserving motor control are affected by aging. The results of prior studies as well as problems with the interpretation of this data were detailed in an earlier chapter. Neuronal counts in the motor cortex[11,31,69] and SN[45,48] have been reported to decrease from 20% to 50% from young childhood to retirement age. A loss of one quarter of cerebellar Purkinje cells, but not granule cells, from birth to old age has also been reported.[30] In addition, large pyramidal neurons serving as projection neurons from the motor cortex of aged individuals lose elements of their dendritic tree, which subserve neuronal interconnections.[54] No clear-cut loss of cells has been reported within the motor or sensory components of the PNS, although numerous structural changes have been noted.[68] It is difficult to interpret the meaning of these structural changes within the PNS.

Postmortem studies reveal a decline in striatal dopamine in normal elderly compared with young adults.[16] There is a significant loss (approximately 50%) of tyrosine hydroxylase, the rate-limiting enzyme of dopamine synthesis, from young adulthood to old age.[47] By comparison, individuals with PD have at least an 80% decrease in their striatal dopamine.[9] Motor function of elderly individuals often has parkinsonian features.[67,76] Such individuals are often bradykinetic, and they may walk with a forward stoop, with small steps, demonstrating poor dynamic balance. This has prompted some investigators to suggest that the gait and balance changes in the elderly are due to the loss of striatal dopamine discussed earlier. The absence of other features of the disease, but most importantly a lack of response to replacement with L-dopa,[57] strongly suggests the contrary.

Are these age-related changes in structure and chemistry the underlying mechanism for the functional changes in motor function noted earlier? The decrements in both are in the order of 20% to 50%. Until direct evidence indicates otherwise, logic suggests a clinical relationship between these parallel changes in structure and function. Most importantly, however, the magnitude of these changes serves as a guideline for what can be accepted as changes in function attributable to aging as contrasted with those that should be attributed to age-related disease processes.

The decrement of the components of motor control associated with disease are superimposed on those seen with aging and often lead to severe compromise of the measurable components of functional motor status. By contrast, based on the magnitude of the changes in normal elderly, it will be our thesis that age-associated decrements weaken and slow motor responses, but reserves are adequate to support motor function (e.g., balance, gait).

Our experience with quantitative measures of gait,[85] balance,[84] and strength[82] in elderly nursing home residents with no demonstrable neurologic disease support our thesis. Isokinetic strength determinations (i.e., during muscle contraction) in the lower extremities of 17 subjects with a history of one or more unexplained falls in the prior year (fallers) as compared with 17 controls, indicate that the power output in the foot dorsiflexors of fallers was less than 10% of that of the controls. Despite the absence of a readily demonstrable cause, the magnitude of this deficit vis-à-vis the controls suggests disease-related rather than age-related etiology. The use of quantitative measures of neuromuscular function, such as those noted above, allows for cross-sectional comparisons (e.g., above) as well as longitudinal studies. Healthy adults often continue their lifelong activity patterns into their old age. Active elderly are likely to have more functional motor reserves than their sedentary counterparts and thereby may be less susceptible to the effects of both age and disuse. Consistent with this, there are reports that active elderly have faster reaction and movement times[73] and walk faster[32] than their sedentary counterparts (among other functions). Furthermore, conditioning, even among elderly, can improve strength[4] and balance.[83] Despite this, the role of activity and conditioning in augmenting motor functioning and thereby combatting frailty remains to be defined.

EVALUATION OF THE PATIENT WITH IMPAIRED MOBILITY OR A HISTORY OF FALLS

Although abnormalities of gait and balance predispose one to fall, there are many other causes of falls among elderly individuals. The history is central in determining the etiology of a fall. The causes of falls are listed from two series previously reported.[58,70] The antecedent occurrence of light-headedness, vertigo, or altered consciousness is suggestive of cardiovascular etiology, transient ischemic attach (TIA), or seizure. In the absence of symptoms suggestive of brainstem ischemia or manifestations of epilepsy, a diagnosis of TIA or

seizure is not realistic. Furthermore, our experience and that of prior reported series[58,70] indicate that both TIAs and seizures are rarely the cause of falls. Light-headedness leading to a blackout of vision and/or loss of consciousness is suggestive of transient global brain ischemia secondary to a cardiovascular etiology.

Orthostatic hypotension is common among the elderly (see Chapter 13) and is responsible for a small although significant number of falls. These falls are especially important in that they are often remediable. It may be produced by autonomic dysfunction within the central (e.g., Shy-Drager syndrome) or peripheral autonomic (e.g., diabetic neuropathy) nervous systems but is most frequently idiopathic in the elderly. Its prevalence is compounded by the widespread use of medication, especially antihypertensives. Most often, orthostatic hypotension produces light-headedness relieved by sitting, but occasionally even in the absence of a loss of consciousness, a fall ensues. The symptoms occur on the assumption of a standing position or after one has been standing for a while and can be diagnosed with measurements of lying and standing pulse and blood pressure. To document the diagnosis, the symptoms are elicited in association with a significant drop in blood pressure (20 mm Hg), which is usually unaccompanied by a change in pulse rate. Multiple determinations may be necessary to demonstrate this. Syncope associated with an associated arrhythmia or valvular heart disease occurs more often lying or sitting than standing. It may be suspected after clinical examination and confirmed by ECG, Holter, or echocardiographic monitoring.

A drop attack is a fall that occurs without warning associated with a transient inability of postural muscles to bear weight. It is not related to head movement, postural changes, altered consciousness, or other focal neurologic signs or symptoms. Frequently the patient is unable to arise immediately after a fall, although the inability to support oneself disappears rapidly. Drop attacks almost exclusively affect women (of all ages).[75] Although these repetitive falls have been reported to account for 12% to 25% of falls,[58,70] we have considered this diagnosis a possibility in only two patients over the past 10 years, suggesting that it may be less common than previously indicated. A clear relationship between these episodes and vertebrobasilar ischemia has not been demonstrated.

It is reported that 4% to 5% of all falls in the elderly are related either to lateral head turning or to flexion-extension movements.[58,70] The falls occur in association with head movement and may be accompanied by light-headedness, vertigo, or occasionally, loss of consciousness, but rarely in association with symptoms of vertebrobasilar ischemia.[10] Possible factors in these falls include carotid sinus hypersensitivity,[64] labyrinthine dysfunction, or vertebrobasilar ischemia. Vertebrobasilar ischemia may be produced by a combination of atherosclerosis and bony impingement on the vertebral arteries during head turning.[10] In our experience, head movements may induce light-headedness or even vertigo but rarely falls. Evaluation of these patients should include an attempt to reproduce the symptoms with head turning. Positional vertigo accompanied by nausea and gaze evoked nystagmus is often induced by vestibular-labyrinthine dysfunction[66] and is usually self-limited, lasting several days. If these symptoms do not disappear, evaluation of hearing and vestibular function is warranted. In the absence of symptoms referable to the brainstem, it is not possible to make a diagnosis of vertebrobasilar ischemia. Empiric treatment with a neck collar and the use of daily aspirin are sometimes successful. A small percentage of falls occur because of light-headedness. This symptom, which may be episodic or continual, is especially common among elderly patients. In light-headed, elderly patients, the syndrome of multiple sensory deficits, hyperventilation, and cardiovascular etiologies should be considered.[21]

Once it is determined that the fall was *not* preceded by altered sensorium, it is necessary to ascertain if it was precipitated by environmental hazards. In the series reported, environmental factors account for almost half the falls. Stairs, poor illumination, and slippery or uneven surfaces were the major factors. It is obvious that an isolated slip on ice or stairs has far different implications from multiple spontaneous falls occurring on well-lit, nonslip surfaces. Environmental factors often implicated in falls include slippery or uneven surfaces, lighting, distractions, obstacles, clothing, stairs, and curbs. Elderly individuals rarely seek medical attention for an isolated fall unless they sustain significant injuries or there is fear of additional falls. To avoid the risk of falls, cognitively normal elderly often severely restrict their activities. Thus, mobility is often the casualty of the fear of falling, and, by limiting activities, elderly may avoid falls. Therefore, it is important to determine the scope of these activities during the course of the history. A mobility scale adapted from other investigators[34] is presented for guidance in history taking (Fig. 10–1). Impaired mobility should suggest the presence of dysfunction within the motor control system. The history should suggest the presence of dysfunction within the motor control system. The history should delineate the time course and extent of the disability as well as the presence (or absence) of relevant neurologic symptoms. These symptoms aid the neurologist in localizing the neurologic dysfunction and include dementia, brainstem and cerebellar symptoms, urinary symptoms, weakness, and sensory abnormalities.

Falls and impaired mobility often have multifactorial etiology. Other factors contributing to diminished motor function include arthritis, which produces pain and compromises the mechanical efficiency of joints, and debility, which may affect aerobic work

Mobility/Life Space Index

	Daily	= 4	Monthly	= 1
Frequency:	3–4x/week	= 3	Never	= 0
	Weekly	= 2		

Life Space   Frequency

1.   Bedroom to bathroom   ____

2.   Rest of apartment (or floor)   ____

3.   Within building   ____

4.   Immediate exterior—25 yards

      (e.g., garden, porch)   ____

5.   Block (including crossing street)   ____

6.   Neighborhood   ____

7.   Unrestricted local travel (i.e., public

      transportation and/or car)   ____

Figure 10–1. A mobility scale based on the Life Space/Mobility Diary developed by Dr. Bernard Isaacs for guidance in history taking. (Adapted from Issacs.[34])

Total Score   ____

capacity and produce generalized weakness. Medication may produce falls either by inducing orthostatic hypotension (e.g., tricyclic antidepressants) or by impairing balance and/or coordination (e.g., sedative-tranquilizers or alcohol).

The clinical approach to multiple falls is summarized in Table 10–2. In view of the many potential loci of neurologic abnormalities underlying balance and gait dysfunction, the examination must be complete with emphasis on the functional characteristics of gait, turning, balance, and arising from a chair. Walking should be a series of synchronous, fluid movements of the torso and upper and lower extremities. In the swing phase, one foot is lifted and propelled forward while the other, still on the ground, has started to shift weight from heel to toes. The shifting of

the weight is completed in the stance phase (in preparation for the next step) while the swing foot has struck the ground heel first and starts to roll forward.[32] The gait pattern of even healthy elderly lacks the vigorous quality of younger individuals (see Fig. 4–1). Turning is accomplished by a healthy older person with a fluid pivoting motion, while turning by an impaired elderly person becomes a series of small steps. Arising from a low stool is an excellent test of both proximal muscle strength of the lower extremities and balance (while arising, the reflex shifting of one's center of gravity forward is an excellent test of postural control). Balance is tested by using forward- or backward-directed pushes. Healthy elderly people are capable of easily checking small pushes with muscle synergies without resorting to stepping

Table 10–2 A CLINICAL APPROACH TO MULTIPLE FALLS

I. History
  A. Episodes of impaired consciousness
    1. The absence of associated symptoms suggests syncope
    2. Focal neurologic symptoms suggest a focal seizure (e.g., partial complex seizure) or a TIA
  B. Mobility (evaluated by history, confirmed by examination of gait aid balance)
    1. Normal mobility is often associated with falls due to
      (a) Medication
      (b) Dementia
      (c) Environment
    2. Impaired mobility may be due to either/both II-A, II-B.
II. Physical Examination
  A. Musculoskeletal function
    1. Abnormalities may impair lower extremity function (e.g., joint deformity or pain due to arthritis) or alignment of the body mass and base of support (e.g., severe kyphoscoliosis).
    2. Limitations are additive to motor dysfunction or other etiologies of falls.
  B. Neuromuscular control as determined by neurologic evaluation
    1. Abnormalities may suggest syndromes that are associated with impaired motor function (e.g., bifrontal syndrome, spastic paraparesis, PD).
    2. A "nonlocalizing" examination associated with impaired gait and balance may have multifactorial etiology or suggest motor dysfunction due to inadequately described disease mechanisms (e.g., multiple infarcts in the subfrontal white matter[46]). Impaired mobility is not a result of the effects of "normal" aging.

or loss of balance. During balance testing, examiners must position themselves to prevent a fall if the subject cannot check the small postural perturbation.

THE SYNDROMES OF GAIT AND BALANCE DYSFUNCTION

Clinically distinct syndromes of gait and balance impairment are related to lesions at different sites within the nervous system. They can be separated by the characteristics of the gait and balance impairment as well as the associated neurologic signs and symptoms.

The Frontal Lobe Syndrome

The disorder, often termed "gait apraxia," is caused by bilateral frontal lobe dysfunction, which is described as a slow, sliding gait in which the patient's feet seem to adhere to the floor. Walking is difficult to initiate and obstacles hard to overcome.[8,19,50] Balance is impaired and often the patients cannot check a small push. Sometimes the disability is so severe that, while standing, the subjects are leaning backward so that their weight is concentrated at the rear of their base of support. In such individuals, small shifts in weight can result in spontaneous retropulsion or falls. From this, one may infer that transcortical long-loop reflexes using the frontal lobes are important for postural control. The clinical features of this balance disorder are similar to those of PD although the pathophysiology may be quite different. Perhaps the basal ganglia facilitate the rapid, efficient use of these same transcortical reflexes, thereby producing similarities in their clinical manifestations.

Other bifrontal symptoms often reported by patients or relatives are a mild dementia in which the answers, although slow, are often correct; emotional lability or absence of affect; and urinary complaints (which include incontinence, frequency, and urgency). Neurologic abnormalities often elicited include frontal lobe release signs (e.g., palmar and plantar grasp), increased tone in the lower extremities, as well as Babinski signs. The causes of this syndrome are multiple cerebral infarcts, hemorrhages (caused by hypertension, cerebral trauma, or a ruptured anterior communicating artery aneurysm), intra-axial tumors (e.g., butterfly glioma), extra-axial tumors (e.g., olfactory nerve meningioma), chronic communicating hydrocephalus (i.e., normal pressure hydrocephalus [NPH]), and

AD, but only in the late stages. MRI makes it possible to visualize mass lesions as well as small subcortical infarcts involving primarily white matter (i.e., lacunes).

The most controversial element of the bifrontal syndrome has been an overenthusiasm for the diagnosis of NPH. Following a description of three patients with a bifrontal syndrome due to NPH who improved following CSF shunting procedures,[2] there was liberal interpretation of the diagnostic criteria. Patients with prominent dementia and enlarged ventricles were shunted with variable, often unsatisfactory results. For the diagnosis of NPH, important elements of the history may include a history of meningitis or cerebral trauma. Ventricular dilatation should be well out of proportion to any cortical atrophy that may be present. Laboratory confirmation of the diagnosis of NPH is difficult. In our experience infusion tests, which stress the CSF absorptive mechanism, and isotope cisternography (IC), which documents the circulation of CSF, are not diagnostic by themselves. More recently, documentation of abnormal fluctuations of intracranial pressure[43] with intracranial pressure monitoring, as well as the clinical response to the removal of CSF,[25] have been used to predict the response to shunting procedures although many clinicians rely solely on the clinical and imaging features. Patients with recent progressive gait abnormalities and mild dementia as well as severe hydrocephalus with no cortical atrophy are the most likely to improve after shunting procedures.[49]

Autopsy studies indicate that there is a high frequency of lacunar infarcts in patients with the bifrontal gait syndrome and evidence of enlarged ventricles.[39] Even in patients with autopsy-proved lacunes, shunting or the removal of CSF may lead to a transient improvement.[39] Although the reason for this improvement is unclear, it may well explain the high incidence of NPH reported in some series and difficulties predicting those who will respond to shunts. Furthermore, it is possible that the loss of periventricular white matter due to lacunar infarction may produce the appearance of hydrocephalus (i.e., *ex-vacuo*) without concomitant cortical atrophy.

Parkinson Disease

PD is a common illness occurring in approximately 0.1% of the population.[61] It is an age-related disease that rarely occurs under age 40, with a peak incidence in the seventh and eighth decades,[40] making it a common cause of gait and balance dysfunction among the elderly. Walking is characterized by an anteroflexed posture, with diminished arm swing and torso movement as well as small shuffling steps. Turning is accomplished with multiple unsteady steps that, en bloc, turn a stiff unmoving torso. Arising from a stool may be slow or even impossible because of an inability to shift the weight forward over a new base of support. Both static and dynamic balance are from mildly to severely impaired, thereby producing falls and/or limited mobility. The gait and balance dysfunction frequently account for a significant portion of the disability.

The other primary signs and symptoms of PD include a slowness and decrease in the amount of movement (e.g., gestures or facial expression), termed bradykinesia; a characteristic 3- to 8-Hz resting tremor that is usually most prominent in the hands; and a ratchet-like resistance to passive stretch called cogwheel rigidity. Although there are other causes of parkinsonian signs and symptoms, in elderly patients not receiving neuroleptics, idiopathic PD is overwhelmingly likely. In patients medicated with neuroleptics, a diagnosis of PD cannot be made unless the medication is discontinued and the signs and symptoms persist. Often the clinician encounters elderly patients with some of the gait and balance dysfunction associated with parkinsonism but none of the other cardinal features of the disease. It has been our experience, and that of others,[57] that these elderly patients do not have PD and do not respond to a therapeutic trial of L-dopa–carbidopa, which we frequently attempt. The anatomic site of dysfunction for this disorder is unclear, although the gait and balance impairment is reminiscent of that of the bifrontal syndrome.

During the ensuing 2 to 20 years after a diagnosis of PD is made, the slow worsening of the signs and symptoms is likely to be primarily related to a continued loss of dopaminergic neurons. Problems produced by the long-term use of L-dopa and other dopamine agonists may compound the morbidity.[23,26] Although important functions such as speech and handwriting are often impaired, loss of mobility is the primary motoric disability. The loss of efficacy of dopamine agonists and rapid fluctuations of the symptoms (e.g., on-off phenomena), in addition to the emergence of dyskinesias, make the treatment of advanced PD difficult for even the most experienced clinicians. Treatment with low-dose L-dopa–carbidopa (Sinemet) (220 to 400 mg) is indicated for significantly symptomatic illness. For advanced disease, optimal therapeutic regimens include the use of maximally tolerated dosages of L-dopa–carbidopa at 2-hour intervals or a controlled-release L-dopa–carbidopa as well as other dopamine agonists (e.g., Pergolide, bromocriptine). Other drugs of some value include centrally acting anticholinergics and amantidine. L-Deprenyl (Eldepryl), a selective MAO-B inhibitor, may slow the course of early PD.[71,77] A low-protein diet may facilitate absorption of L-dopa from the gastrointestinal tract as well as passage across the blood-brain barrier. Therefore, low-protein daytime meals have been used as a means of lowering L-dopa dose and decreasing symptom fluctuation.[60] Surgical treatment, particularly the implantation of fetal nigral cells into the putamen, may be a new therapeutic approach with promise for advanced PD.[44]

Diseases Involving the Corticospinal Tracts

Diseases impairing corticospinal tract function result in upper extremity weakness and clumsiness as well as weak, stiff lower extremities that are circumducted, everted, and plantar flexed during walking. The involvement of both corticospinal tracts results in a characteristic stiff gait with hyperadduction of both lower extremities called scissoring (i.e., spastic paraparesis). In the elderly, hemiparesis is usually caused by cerebral infarction, with tumors (glioma or metastases) being relatively unusual. Despite this, the recent onset of hemiparesis warrants evaluation, which should include a CT scan or MRI. Spastic paraparesis may be produced by multiple small infarcts (lacunes), bony overgrowth within the cervical spinal canal (i.e., cervical spondylosis), ALS, or, occasionally, spinal tumors or metastases. Even in the very old who are ambulatory, a progressive spastic paraparesis should be evaluated and an etiology established. The availability of MRI and CT scanning supplemented by myelography has made delineation of the lesion(s) relatively simple. In otherwise healthy, symptomatic elderly who have cervical spondylosis with bony lesions at a single level we have recommended surgery, most often with gratifying results.

Ataxia

An ataxic, unsteady gait with interjected staggering and poor turns is most suggestive of cerebellar dysfunction but can be seen with acute vestibular-brainstem lesions and in elderly patients with both impaired vision and proprioception. Age-related loss of cerebellar Purkinje cells[30] may produce minor unsteadiness, although a progressive syndrome resulting in moderate or severe ataxia should be assumed to be related to disease processes. The availability of MRI makes delineation of both intra-axial and extra-axial posterior fossa masses as well as brainstem-cerebellar infarction possible. The differentiation of acute end organ vestibular dysfunction from brainstem-cerebellar ischemia can be made by the presence of prominent positional vertigo accompanied by nausea, vomiting, and gaze-evoked nystagmus in the absence of associated neurologic signs and symptoms. Other causes of ataxia include alcoholism, vitamin E deficiency, hypothyroidism, and cortical cerebellar and olivopontocerebellar atrophies. Ataxia sometimes results from cancer as well. Proprioceptive loss results in a tendency to watch the ground while walking and difficulty in walking on uneven surfaces, especially in the dark. A minor degree of tactile proprioceptive impairment occurs in some elderly and has been presumed to be related to aging changes in primary sensory nerves. Such a loss, in association with visual impairment due to cataracts or glaucoma, may lead to mild ataxia and unsteadiness.

In an earlier section, we discussed the changes in peripheral nerve function that were attributable to aging. Sensory thresholds were increased and conduction velocity slowed albeit functional capacity was not compromised. We have observed patients with hereditary sensorimotor neuropathy who became functionally impaired in their mid-70s presumably due to the progression of their illness superimposed on changes due to age. The unsteadiness due to weakness and depressed sensation was considerable, although it did not fit into a characteristic gait pattern.

Gait Abnormalities Produced by Neuropathic and Myopathic Diseases

Often, however, weakness due to neuromuscular dysfunction results in characteristic abnormalities of gait that are related to the site involved. For example, bilateral proximal weakness due to an inflammatory myopathy or hypothyroidism may result in a characteristic waddling gait, while weakness of the dorsiflexors of the foot result in a foot-slapping, high-stepped gait. The clinician should be able to readily identify these and the other gait patterns noted earlier.

Progressive Supranuclear Palsy and Other Diseases Associated with Dementia

Progressive supranuclear palsy (PSP) is an uncommon disease (1% of PD prevalence)[18] that may be difficult to distinguish from PD because of similar motoric manifestations. The disease is more rapidly progressive than PD (median survival 6 years) with dysarthria, dysphagia, dementia, and prominent gait-balance disorder.[27] The gait pattern has many features of the bifrontal syndrome and balance may be severely impaired. There is a pronounced extensor rigidity of axial muscles, as well as bradykinesia and mild dementia. The dementia is characterized by slowness of cognitive processing and difficulty with complex conceptual tasks. Affect is blunted and the appearance of depression common. The unique feature of PSP is the abnormality of eye movement, which may vary from slow incomplete vertical gaze to a disappearance of voluntary eye movements. Treatment with antiparkinsonian agents is ineffective. The pathology of PSP is distinct from PD and includes neuronal loss and the occurrence of NFTs in the basal ganglia and other central neuronal structures. Parkinsonian features may be associated with other neurologic manifestations (e.g., multiple systems or olivopontocerebellar atrophies) or autonomic failure (i.e., Shy-Drager syndrome).

In the early and middle stages, AD has little apparent effect on the motor system. Patients are often demented with no obvious change in their gait or balance. A comparison of the indices of gait quality in nine patients with moderately advanced AD and nine controls demonstrates both impaired gait quality (e.g., diminished step size and walking speed) and static balance (increased total sway path).[79] Another study reports a correlation between the Blessed Information Memory Concentration Test (a measure of the severity of AD) and the Postural Stress Test (a measure of dynamic balance).[84] The studies suggest an impairment of transcortical long-loop reflexes in AD, although obviously the motor deficits are not as prominent as the cognitive loss. In other progressive dementias, motor function may be compromised comparably with, or more severely than, cognitive function (e.g., MID or PSP).

DEFINING "SENILE" GAIT AND BALANCE DISORDERS

The widespread use of terminology that implies that gait and balance dysfunction are a natural part of aging (e.g., senile gait) presents an obstacle to progress in that it suggests an inevitability that is unalterable by remediation. If one accepts that age-associated changes in both gait and balance modestly alter function but do not compromise it, then the next step is to define the underlying disease processes. Given that the accepted diseases of the motor system discussed earlier are not present in the majority of patients with impaired balance and gait, what remains to define this disorder is to separate the groups that may represent individual disease. This was attempted in a recent report of 40 elderly subjects (20 multiple fallers and 20 controls).[46] The study related the history of falls, cognitive status, and quantitative measures of gait and dynamic balance to CT scan indices of brain structure "blindly" rated by two neuroradiologists. The group of fallers had impaired gait and dynamic balance by comparison with the controls as well as significantly diminished density within their

hemispheric white matter. This hypodensity of the white matter was significantly correlated with both gait and dynamic balance but not with cognitive status.[46] Disruption of ascending and descending transcortical long-loop reflexes at this level could explain these deficits. In two subjects from the above series with severely compromised gait and balance and CT evidence of white matter hypodensity, the autopsy demonstrated prominent ischemic changes in the hemispheric white matter. Prior autopsy series have also demonstrated gait abnormalities in patients with ischemic subcortical white matter lesions.[15,28] The relative importance of vascular disease as a pathophysiologic mechanism in these patients is insignificant, although we feel it is likely to be significant. The importance of mobility to the well being of our elderly population dictates that these and other tentative "steps" be followed by a sustained commitment to define the causes and underlying mechanisms of this problem. Only then can specific, disease-oriented interventions be attempted.

In the short term, however, it will be worthwhile to consider the use of interventions directed toward augmenting gait and balance as well as the underlying deficits of neuromuscular function in impaired elderly. We have recently measured the response to postural stresses of normal elderly in sequential trials on a balance platform (EquiTest, Neurocom, Clackamas, Oregon). Under conditions of mild stress, elderly subjects did about as well as young subjects. With more difficult postural stresses, the elderly subjects had almost twice as much sway as younger subjects. By the third trial, however, the sway was almost one half of the initial value, suggesting the possibility of significant improvement with training.[83] A concerted program of balance conditioning might well significantly improve impaired balance. Furthermore, the underlying weakness in the lower extremities of individuals with a history of falls (and impaired balance) is also likely to improve with conditioning. Older individuals have responded to training with increased strength and a higher proportion of fast-twitch fibers.[3,4] Effective remediation of this as yet unexplained weakness might well improve balance in that rapid, vigorous ankle movements are a vital, initial portion of many of the muscle synergies used in postural reflexes. Empiric testing of these and other functionally oriented strategies is indicated at this time.

Short of comprehensive rehabilitative programs, what does the practitioner have to offer an elderly individual with impaired balance? Appropriate shoes may be of value. Individuals with the inability to check a backward displacement (retropulse) should be given shoes with a heel lift that counteracts this, whereas flat shoes should be used for those with a tendency to anteropulse. Comfortable neutral shoes (minimal lift) with nonslip soles should be used for the elderly with impaired balance. A cane appropriately sized to contact the floor with approximately 15° of elbow flexion will broaden the base of support without interfering unduly with gait. Other assistive devices (e.g., a walker) provide more support but are very disruptive to gait patterns and increase the effort required to walk.

Visual cues may be important for balance especially in the elderly with impairment of tactile proprioceptive or vestibular input. Correction for vision should be specifically attempted to optimize visual input necessary for balance. The risks of environmental hazards are compounded by the elderly who may well have varying degrees of impaired vision and balance. The positive effects of appropriate lighting and the removal of obvious hazards can be amplified by user-friendly environmental aids (e.g., rails or grab bars). Environmental manipulations can decrease the risk of falls. For this risk to be minimized there must be an accompanying education regarding the avoidance of dangerous activity (e.g., tall step stools or icy sidewalks).

There is an emerging realization of the importance of motor dysfunction in the elderly. This, in conjunction with the increasing use of quantitative measures of neuromuscular and balance function and the availability of sophisticated electrophysiologic and imaging techniques, suggests that the future may hold rapid progress in this area. The problem warrants nothing less.

REFERENCES

1. Accident Facts and Figures, 1978 ed. Chicago National Safety Council, 1978.
2. Adams, RD, Fisher, CM, Hakim, S, Ojeman, RG, and Sweet, WH: Symptomatic occult hydrocephalus with "normal" cerebrospinal fluid pressure. N Engl J Med 273:117–126, 1965.
3. Aniansson, A, Grimby, G, and Rundgren, A: Isometric and isokinetic quadriceps muscles strength in 70 year old men and women. Scand J Rehab Med 12:161–168, 1980.
4. Aniansson, A, Grimby, G, Rundgren, A, Svanborg, A, and Orlander, J: Physical training in old men. Age Ageing 9:186–187, 1980.
5. Axelrod, S and Cohen, LD: Senescence and embedded figure performance in vision and touch. Percept Psychophys 12:283–287, 1961.
6. Azar, GJ and Lawton, AH: Gait and stepping as a factor in the frequent falls of elderly women. Gerontologist 4:83–84, 103, 1964.
7. Baker, SP and Harvey, AH: Fall Injuries in the Elderly. In Radebaugh, TS, Hadley, E, and Suzman, R (eds): Clinics in Geriatric Medicine, Vol I, No 3. (Symposium on Falls in the Elderly: Biologic and Behavioral Aspect). WB Saunders, Philadelphia, 1985.
8. Barron, RE: Disorders of gait related to the aging nervous system. Geriatrics 22:113–119, 1967.
9. Bernheimer, H, Birkmayer, W, Hornykiewicz, O, Jellinger, K, and Seitelberger, F: Brain dopamine and the

syndromes of Parkinson and Huntington: Clinical morphological and neurocorrelations. J Neurol Sci 20:415–455, 1973.

10. Brain, RW: Some unsolved problems of cervical spondylosis. Br Med J 1:771–777, 1963.

11. Brody, H: Organization of the cerebral cortex. III. A study of aging in the human cerebral cortex. J Comp Neurol 102:511–556, 1955.

12. Brown, WF: A method for estimating the number of motor units in the-nar muscles and the changes in motor unit count with aging. J Neurol Neurosurg Psychiatry 35:845–852, 1972.

13. Buchthal, F and Rosenfalck, A: Evoked action potentials and conduction velocity in human sensory nerves. Brain Res 3:1–22, 1966.

14. Buchthal, F, Rosenfalck, A, and Behse, F: Sensory Potentials of Normal and Diseased Nerve. In Dyck, PJ, Thomas, PK, and Lamber, EH (eds): Peripheral Neuropathy. WB Saunders, Philadelphia, 1975, p 442.

15. Caplan, LR and Schoene, WC: Clinical features of subcortical arteriosclerotic encephalopathy (Binswanger's disease). Neurology 28:1206–1215, 1978.

16. Carlsson, A and Winblad, B: Influence of age and time interval between death and autopsy on dopamine and 3-methoxy tyramine levels in human' basal ganglia. J Neural Transm 38:271–276, 1976.

17. Chambers, WP, Donihue, PN, Smith, CJ, Blanchard, RR, Taylor, CH, and Hill, DB: Effect of vasopressin and adrenal steroids on cortical responses evoked at midbrain level in aged rats. Gerontologia 12:65–73, 1966.

18. Davis, PH, Golbe, LI, Duvoisin, RC, and Schoenberg, BS: The natural history and prevalence of progressive supranuclear palsy (abstr). Neurology (Suppl 1)37:121, 1987.

19. Denny-Brown, D: The nature of apraxia. J Nerv Ment Dis 126:9–32, 1958.

20. Dorfman, LJ and Bosley, TM: Age-re-lated changes in peripheral and central nerve conduction in man. Neurology 29:38–44, 1979.

21. Drachman, NA and Hart, CW: An approach to the dizzy patient. Neurology 4:323–334, 1972.

22. Dyck, PJ, Shultz, PW, and O'Brien, PC: Quantification of touch pressure sensation. Arch Neurol 26:465–473, 1972.

23. Fahn, S and Bressman, SB: Should levodopa therapy for Parkinson's disease be started only of late. Evidence against early treatment. Can J Neurol Sci 11:2000–2006, 1984.

24. Finley, FR, Cody, KA, and Finzie, RV: Locomotion patterns in elderly women. Arch Phys Med Rehab 50:140–146, 1969.

25. Fisher, CM: Hydrocephalus as a cause of gait disturbance in the elderly. Neurology 32:1358–1363, 1982.

26. Goetz, C, Tanner, CM, and Shannon, K: Progression of Parkinson's disease without L-dopa. Neurology 37:695–698, 1987.

27. Golbe, LI and Davis, PH: Progressive Supranuclear Palsy: Recent Advances. In Jankovic, J and Tolusa, E (eds): Parkinson's Disease and Movement Disorders. Urban and Schwarzenberg, Baltimore, 1988.

28. Gray, F, Dubas, F, Roullet, G, and Escourolle, R: Leukoencephalopathy in diffuse hemorrhagic cerebral amyloid angioplasty. Ann Neurol 18:54–59, 1985.

29. Gryfe, CL, Amies, A, and Ashley, MJ: A longitudinal study of falls in an elderly population. I. Incidence and morbidity. Age Ageing 6, 201–210, 1977.

30. Hall, TC, Mill, AKH, and Corsellis, JHN: Variations in the human Purkinje cell population according to age and sex. Neuropathol Appl Neurobiol I:267–292, 1975.

31. Henderson, GB, Tomlinson, BE, and Gibson, PH: Cell counts in human cerebral cortex in normal adults throughout life using an image analysing computer. J Neurol Sci 46:113–136, 1980.

32. Imms, FJ and Edholm, OG: The assess-

ment of gait and mobility in the elderly. Age Ageing 8(Suppl):261–267, 1979.

33. Imms, FJ and Edholm, OG: Studies of gait and mobility in the elderly. Age Ageing 10:147–156, 1981.

34. Isaacs, B: Clinical and laboratory studies of falls in old people. Clin Geriatr Med 1:513–525, 1985.

35. Kalenthaler, T, Bascon, R, and Quintus, V: Falls in the institutionalized elderly. J Am Geriatr Soc 26:425–428, 1978.

36. Kawamura, Y, O'Brien, P, Okazak, H, and Dyck, P: Lumbar motor neurons of man: The number and diameter distribution of large- and intermediate-diameter cytons in "motorneuron columns" of spinal cord of man. J Neuropathol Exp Neurol 36:861–874, 1977.

37. Klawans, HL, Tufo, HM, and Ostfeld, AM: Neurologic examination in an elderly population. Dis Nerv Syst 32:274–279, 1971.

38. Kokmen, E, Bossemeyer, RW, and Williams, W: Quantitative evaluation of joint motion sensation in an aging population. J Gerontol 33:62–67, 1978.

39. Koto, A, Rosenberg, G, Zingesser, LH, Houroupian, D, and Katzman, R: Syndrome of normal pressure hydrocephalus: Possible relation to hypertensive and arteriosclerotic vasculopathy. J Neurol Neurosurg Psychiatry 40:73–79, 1977.

40. Kurland, LT, Hauser, WA, Okazake, H, and Nobrega, FT: Epidemiologic Studies of Parkinsonism with Special Reference to the Cohort Hypothesis. In Gillingham, FJ and Donaldson, IML (eds): Third Symposium on Parkinson's Disease. E & S Livingstone, Edinburgh, Scotland, 1969.

41. Larsson, L: Aging in Mammalian Skeletal Muscle. In Mortimer, JA, Pirazzolo, FJ, and Maletta, GJ (eds): The Aging Motor System. Praeger, New York, p 60, 1982.

42. Larsson, L, Grimley, G, and Karlsson, J: Muscle strength and speed of movement in relation to age and muscle morphology. J Appl Physiol 46:451–456, 1979.

43. Launas, E and Lobata, RD: Intraventricular pressure and CSF dynamics in chronic adult hydrocephalus. Surg Neurol 12:287–295, 1979.

44. Lindvall, O, Brundin, P, Widner, H, Renncrona, S, Gustavii, B, Frackowiak, R, Leenders, KL, Sawle, G, Rathwell, JC, Marsden, CD, Bjorklund, A: Grafts of fetal dopamine neuron survive and improve function in Parkinson's disease. Science 297:574–577, 1990.

45. Mann, DM, Yates, PO, and Marcyniuk, B: Monoaminergic neurotransmitter systems in presenile Alzheimer's disease and in senile dementia of Alzheimer type. Clin Neuropathol 3:199–205, 1984.

46. Masdeu, JC, Wolfson, LI, Lantos, G, Tobin, JN, Grober, E, Whipple, R, and Amerman P: Brain white matter disease in elderly prone to falling. Arch Neurol 46:1292–1296, 1989.

47. McGeer, EG: Aging and Neurotransmitter Metabolism in the Human Brain. In Katzman, R, Terry, RD, and Bick, KL (eds): Alzheimer's Disease, Senile Dementia and Related Disorders, Aging Series, Vol 7, Raven Press, New York, 1976, p 427.

48. McGeer, PL, McGeer, EG, and Suzuki, JS: Aging and extrapyramidal function. Arch Neurol 34:33–35, 1977.

49. Messert, B and Wannamaker, BB: Reappraisal of the occult hydrocephalus syndrome. Neurology 24:224–231, 1974.

50. Meyer, JS and Barron, DW: Apraxia of gait: A clinicophysiological study. Brain 83:261–284, 1960.

51. Moffroid, M, Whipple, R, Hofkosh, J, Lowman, E, and Thistle, H: A study of isokinetic exercise. Phys Ther 49:735–747, 1969.

52. Murray, MP, Kory, RC, and Clarkson, BH: Walking patterns in healthy old men. J Gerontol 24:169–178, 1969.

53. Murray, MP, Kory, RC, and Sepic, SB:

Walking patterns of normal women. Arch Phys Med Rehab 51:637–650, 1970.

54. Nakamura, SI, Akiguchi, M, Kamegama, M, and Mizuno, W: Age related changes to pyramidal cell basal dendrites in layers III and V of human motor cortex: A quantitative Golgi study. Acta Neuropathol (Berl) 65:281–284, 1985.

55. Nashner, LM: Strategies for Organization of Human Posture. In Igarashi, M and Black, FO (eds): Vestibular and Visual Control on Posture and Locomotor Equilibrium. 7th Int. Symposium Int Soc Posturography, Houston, Texas, 1983 Karger, Basel, p 1, 1985.

56. National Center for Health Statistics, 1986.

57. Newman, RP, LeWitt, PA, Jaffe, M, Colne, DB, and Larsen, TA: Motor function in the normal aging population: Treatment with levodopa. Neurology 35:571–573, 1985.

58. Overstall, PW, Exton-Smith, AN, Imms, FJ, and Johnson, AL: Falls in the elderly related to postural imbalance. Br Med J 1:261–264, 1977.

59. Perret, E and Reglis, F: Age and the perceptual threshold for vibratory stimuli. Eur Neurol 4:65–76, 1970.

60. Pincus, JH and Barry, K: Influence of dietary protein on motor fluctuations in Parkinson's disease. Arch Neurol 44:270–272, 1987.

61. Pollock, M and Hornabrook, RW: The prevalence, natural history and dementia of Parkinson's disease. Brain 89:429–488, 1966.

62. Potvin, AR, Syndulko, K, Tourtellotte, WW, Goldberg, Z, Potvin, JH, and Hansch, EC: Quantitative Evaluation of Normal Age-Related Changes in Neurologic Function. In Pirozzolo, FJ and Maletta, GJ (eds): Advances in Neurogerontology, Vol 2. Praeger, New York, 1980.

63. Potvin, AR, Syndulko, K, Tourtellotte, WW, Lemmon, JA, and Potvin, JH: Human neurologic function and the aging process. J Am Geriatr Soc 28:1–9, 1980.

64. Ritch, AE: The significance of carotid sinus hypersensitivity in the elderly. Gerontol Clin 17:146, 1975.

65. Rubenstein, LZ, Robbins, AS, Schulman, BC, Rosada, T, Osterweil, D, and Josephson, KR: Falls and instability in the elderly. J Am Geriatr Soc 36:266–268, 1988.

66. Rudge, P: Clinical Neuro-otology. Churchill Livingstone, New York, 1983.

67. Sabin, TD: Biologic aspects of falls and mobility in the elderly. J Am Geriatr Soc 30:51–58, 1982.

68. Schaumburg, HH, Spencer, PS, and Ochoa, J: The Aging Human Peripheral Nervous System. In Katzman, R and Terry, RD (eds): The Neurology of Aging. FA Davis Co, Philadelphia, p 111, 1983.

69. Shefer, UF: Absolute number of neurons and thickness of the cerebral cortex during aging, senile and vascular dementia and Pick's and Alzheimer's disease. Neurosci Behav Physiol 6:319–324, 1973.

70. Sheldon, JH: On the natural occurrence of falls in old age. Br Med J 2:1685, 1960.

71. Shoulson, I, et al (The Parkinson Study Group): The effect of deprenyl on the progression of disability in early Parkinson's disease. N Engl J Med 321:1365–1371, 1989.

72. Skinner, HB, Barrack, RL, and Cook, SD: Age-related decline in proprioception. Clin Orthop 184:208–211, 1984.

73. Spirduso, WW and Clifford, P: Replication of age and physical activity effects on reaction and movement time. J Gerontol 33:26–30, 1978.

74. Steiness, I: Vibratory perception in normal subjects. Acta Scand 58:315–325, 1957.

75. Stevens, DC and Matthews, WB: Autogenic drop attacks in affliction of women. Br Med J 1:439–442, 1973.

76. Teravainen, H and Calne, DB: Motor System in Normal Aging and Parkinson's Disease. In Katzman, R and Terry, RD (eds): The Neurology of Aging. FA Davis, Philadelphia, 1983, p 85.

77. Tetrud, JW and Langston, JW: The effect of deprenyl (seligiline) on the natural history of Parkinson's disease. Science 245:519–522, 1989.

78. United States Bureau of the Census, 1985.

79. Visser, H: Gait and balance in senile dementia of the Alzheimer's type. Age Ageing 12:296–301, 1983.

80. Welford, AT: Sensory perceptual and motor processes in older adults. In Birren, JE and Swane, RB (eds): Handbook of Mental Health and Aging. Prentice Hall, Englewood Cliffs, New Jersey, p 192, 1980.

81. Whipple, R and Wolfson, LI: Increased vibration threshold in patient with a history of falls. 1990, submitted.

82. Whipple, R, Wolfson, LI, and Amerman, P: The relationship of knee and ankle weakness to falls in nursing home residents. An Isokinetic study. Am Geriatr Soc 35:13–20, 1987.

83. Whipple, R, Wolfson, L, Singh, D, Derby, C, and Tobin, JN: Postural mechanisms in community-residing elderly compared to controls: A balance platform study. 1990, submitted.

84. Wolfson, LI, Whipple, R, Amerman, P, and Kleinberg, A: Stressing the postural response: A quantitative method for testing balance. J Am Geriatr Soc 34:845–850, 1986.

85. Wolfson, LI, Whipple, R, Amerman, P, and Tobin, JN: Gait assessment in the elderly: A gait abnormality rating scale and its relation to falls. J Gerontol 45:M12–M19, 1990.

86. Woollacott, MH, Shumway-Cook, A, and Nashner, L: Postural Reflexes and Aging. In Wolfson, LI, Whipple, R, Amerman, P, and Tobin, JN: Gait assessment in the elderly: A gait abnormality rating scale and its relation to falls. J Gerontol 45:M12–M19, 1990.

86. Woollacott, MH, Shumway-Cook, A and Nashner, L: Postural Reflexes and Aging. In Mortimer, JA, Pirozzolo, FJ, and Maletta, GJ (eds): The Aging Motor System. Praeger, New York, p 98, 1982.

Chapter 11

TRANSIENT LOSS OF CONSCIOUSNESS

Lewis A. Lipsitz, M.D., and
Palmi V. Jonsson, M.D.

EPIDEMIOLOGY
PATHOPHYSIOLOGY
AGE- AND DISEASE-RELATED
  CHANGES PREDISPOSING TO
  SYNCOPE IN THE ELDERLY
ETIOLOGY
EVALUATION
THERAPEUTIC ISSUES

Transient loss of consciousness is a common neurologic symptom in the elderly, generally referred to as *syncope.* Syncope is defined as transient loss of consciousness accompanied by loss of postural tone, with spontaneous recovery, not requiring resuscitation. This common symptom has multiple underlying causes and suggests an increased risk of sudden death when the etiology is cardiac. Syncope of all causes has potential adverse consequences, such as falls, fractures, subdural hematomas, soft-tissue injuries, and loss of independent function.

EPIDEMIOLOGY

There is little information on the incidence and prevalence of syncope in the elderly. Studies of young people show a prevalence of syncope as high as 47%, which is primarily due to benign causes such as vasovagal reac-

tions.[65] Data from the Framingham Study show an increase in prevalence of syncope with age.[56] One percent of emergency ward visits and up to 3% of admissions to hospitals are for the evaluation of syncope. Most of these hospital visits are by elderly patients. A study of very elderly nursing home residents revealed a 10-year prevalence of 23% and 1-year incidence of 6%. The recurrence rate for syncope is about 30%.[43] Community-dwelling patients with cardiac causes for syncope are at the highest risk for death, having a 40% 2-year mortality. Patients with noncardiac causes for syncope have a 20% 2-year mortality, similar to that of syncope of unknown cause.[6,30] Although syncope is associated with a high mortality, this is probably due to the underlying diseases that cause it, rather than to an independent relationship between syncope and death. Recurrent syncope that is unexplained after thorough initial evaluation is not associated with excess mortality.[29,42]

PATHOPHYSIOLOGY

Syncope results from inadequate energy delivery to the brain. The major energy substrates are oxygen and glucose. Significant hypoglycemia tends to result in coma rather than syncope and a prolonged cessation of oxygen delivery results in death. Transient cerebral hypoxia from decreased cerebral blood flow is the final common pathway in most cases of syncope. Thus, hypoxemia from cardiac or pulmonary diseases and decreased oxygen carrying capacity of the blood from anemia are risk factors for syncope, but rarely the sole cause. Infrequently, focal stenosis of arteries supplying critical areas of the brain causes syncope.

Blood pressure is determined by the product of cardiac output and peripheral arterial resistance. A reduction in either variable without an increase in the other will lower blood pressure and potentially result in syncope. Cardiac output may fall because of a reduction in stroke volume or because of bradyarrythmias or tachyarrhythmias. Reduced stroke volume may result from an obstruction to flow within the heart or pulmonary vasculature, myocardial pump failure, or a reduction in venous return. Venous return may decrease as a result of venous blood pooling or hypovolemia. A reduction in arterial resistance can result from autonomic failure, medication effects, or abnormal cardiovascular reflexes.

AGE- AND DISEASE-RELATED CHANGES PREDISPOSING TO SYNCOPE IN THE ELDERLY

One of the characteristics of elderly persons that predisposes them to syncope is the presence of multiple clinical abnormalities.[40] Accumulation of age- and disease-related conditions that threaten cerebral blood flow or reduce oxygen content in the blood may bring oxygen delivery close to the threshold needed to maintain consciousness. A situational stress that further reduces blood pressure, such as posture change or a Valsalva maneuver during voiding, may reduce cerebral oxygen delivery below the critical threshold and result in syncope.

Several homeostatic mechanisms that normally preserve blood pressure and cerebral oxygen delivery in the face of such stresses become impaired with age. These mechanisms include cerebral autoregulation,[32] baroreflexes,[60] myocardial diastolic relaxation,[22] and renal sodium conservation.[12]

Cerebral blood flow declines with normal aging.[32] In hypertension, which often accompanies advancing age, the threshold for cerebral autoregulation is shifted to higher levels of blood pressure, making hypertensive elderly more vulnerable to cerebral ischemia from relatively small degrees of hypotension.[62] Baroreflex sensitivity is also impaired with advanced age. This can be demonstrated by a blunted bradycardic response to hypertensive stimuli and diminished tachycardic response to blood pressure reduction. At the bedside, this is evident in the absent or modest cardioacceleration associated with posture change in the elderly patient.

The elderly are particularly vulnerable to the hypotensive effects of a rapid heart rate. Because of progressive myocardial stiffness, impaired diastolic relaxation, and reduced early diastolic ventricular filling with advancing age, the aged heart becomes more dependent on atrial contraction to fill the ventricle and maintain cardiac output. A rapid heart rate further reduces the opportunity to adequately fill the ventricle with blood and therefore threatens cardiac output. During atrial fibrillation, the loss of atrial contraction further reduces cardiac output, independent of heart rate. This makes rapid atrial fibrillation particularly dangerous in the elderly patient.

Declines in basal and stimulated plasma renin and aldosterone concentrations,[12] as well as elevations in atrial natriuretic peptide[19] with advancing age predispose to volume depletion. Furthermore, many elderly persons have an impaired thirst response to hyperosmolality and therefore may not consume enough fluids to prevent dehydration.[52]

ETIOLOGY

Multiple studies have shown that 20% to 30% of syncopal episodes have cardiac causes, 10% to 20% have noncardiac causes, and 30% to 50% remain *unexplained* despite extensive evaluation.[26,61] Table 11–1 shows the common causes of syncope in the elderly.

Structural Heart Disease

The three main structural heart diseases that cause syncope in the elderly are aortic stenosis, hypertrophic cardiomyopathy, and mitral regurgitation. They all feature systolic murmurs that need to be distinguished from the more prevalent but benign aortic sclerosis. About 30% of patients over 65 years of age and 60% of people over 80 years of age have systolic murmurs.[55] The distinguishing features of these murmurs are often absent, making their clinical assessment difficult in the elderly.

AORTIC VALVE DISEASE

Hemodynamically significant aortic stenosis (AS) is present in approximately 5% of elderly patients with a systolic murmur. Congenitally bicuspid valves are the principal cause in the 60- to 70-year-old age group, whereas degenerative calcification of an otherwise normal tricuspid aortic valve is the most frequent cause of AS in the very elderly.[54] Rheumatic heart disease is now an infrequent cause of AS in the elderly. Most often AS will present insidiously as congestive heart failure, but

---

Table 11–1 CAUSES OF SYNCOPE

1. *Cardiac disease* (decreased cardiac output)
   a. *Structural* (mechanical obstruction to flow)
      Aortic stenosis
      Mitral stenosis
      Atrial myxoma
      Cardiomyopathy
      Pulmonary embolism
   b. *Myocardial*
      Acute myocardial infarction (MI)
   c. *Electrical*
      Tachyarrhythmias
      Bradyarrhythmias (conduction disturbance, sinus node dysfunction)
2. *Hypotension* (decreased volume or peripheral vascular resistance)
   a. *Orthostatic hypotension*
      Prolonged inactivity
      Medications (vasodilator, antihypertensives, antidepressants, neuroleptics, diuretics)
      Central nervous system (Shy-Drager, Parkinson disease)
      Peripheral autonomic neuropathies (diabetic, alcoholic, amyloid)
      Idiopathic
   b. *Postprandial hypotension*
   c. *Volume depletion*
      Fluid or blood loss
3. *Reflex* (decreased cardiac output or peripheral vascular resistance)
   Vasovagal
   Defecation
   Micturition
   Cough
   Swallowing
   Carotid sinus syndrome
4. Abnormal blood composition (reduced energy substrates)
   Hypoxemia
   Hypoglycemia
   Acute anemia
5. Central nervous system disease
   Seizures
   Cerebrovascular insufficiency

---

angina and syncope are still frequent manifestations.[43] The mechanism of syncope may be arrhythmia or reflex vasodilatation secondary to stimulation of ventricular vagal afferent fibers by a powerful ventricular contraction.[46]

HYPERTROPHIC CARDIOMYOPATHY

Hypertrophic cardiomyopathy (HCM) is commonly overlooked in elderly patients, despite the fact that as many as 33% of patients with idiopathic HCM are over 60 years of age.[33] Hypertensive HCM has recently been described in the elderly and appears to be most common in black women.[64] HCM can present with angina, dyspnea, or syncope. Syncope is either due to left ventricular outflow obstruction or tachyarrhythmias. Most patients with HCM have diastolic dysfunction characterized by impaired isovolumic relaxation, slow filling during the rapid filling phase of diastole, and an excessive dependence on atrial systole to optimize ventricular volume.[47] Echocardiography is the diagnostic test of choice. It is important to think of HCM because it is exacerbated by commonly used inotrophic and vasodilating medications.

MITRAL REGURGITATION

Mitral valve prolapse, papillary dysfunction, idiopathic calcification of the mitral valve anulus, and rheumatic disease are the common causes of mitral regurgitation (MR). It usually presents with congestive heart failure, but can cause syncope.

Electrical Heart Disease

Syncope may result from asystole, bradycardia, or tachycardia. Myocardial infarction may produce syncope via any of these mechanisms and accounts for about 6% of cases of syncope in the elderly.[40] Because arrhythmias are common in elderly people, their presence between attacks in a patient with syncope may be coincidental and noncontributory to the syncopal event. Routine 24-hour ambulatory monitoring rarely shows correlations between symptoms and rhythm disturbances.[18] A syncopal episode can be attributed to an arrhythmia only if the arrhythmia is found on an electrocardiogram at the time of the event or if it is associated with symptoms of dizziness, near syncope, or syncope during ambulatory monitoring under the same conditions in which the syncopal episode occurred.

RHYTHM ABNORMALITIES

Ventricular and supraventricular tachyarrhythmias or bradyarrhythmias may produce syncope, but they are also common in asymptomatic elderly persons.[1] In the Baltimore Longitudinal Study on Aging, 13% of healthy people 60 to 85 years of age showed asymptomatic paroxysmal atrial tachycardia and 50% showed complex ventricular arrhythmias, including multiform ventricular premature contractions (VPCs) in 35%, couplets in 11%, and ventricular tachycardia in 4%.[15] Seriousness of ventricular ectopy correlates closely with the degree of impaired left ventricular function, persistent ST-segment elevation, and with the extent of obstructive coronary artery disease.[21] Thus, ventricular ectopic activity in the absence of structural or ischemic heart disease is associated with a good prognosis.[31]

Conduction Disturbances

Conduction disturbances are common in the elderly and are thought to be markers for transient heart block and associated syncope. First-degree heart block is never causally related to syncope.[50] On the other hand, second- and third-degree atrioventricular (AV) block are often seen in the elderly and may be associated with syncope, either directly through progression to complete heart block, or through their close association with coexistent ventricular arrhythmias. Complete heart block is most commonly due to degenerative sclerosis of the conduction system rather than coronary artery disease.[36] The development of syncope in a patient with complete heart block (Stokes-Adams attack) is associated with increased mortality and should be treated with cardiac pacing.[9]

The prevalence of left bundle-branch block ranges from 0.6% to 2.5%, and of right bundle-branch block from 1.9% to 3.5%.[48] In the absence of symptoms, these alone do not have predictive value for syncope. Bifascicular or trifascicular conduction disease in association with syncope is of more concern.[14] Several large studies[7,48] have shown that in asymptomatic patients with this finding, the risk of progression to high-degree AV block is low. However, in patients with transient, unexplained, neurologic symptoms and bifascicular or trifascicular block, the finding of an AV interval greater than 70 milliseconds on an electrophysiologic study was associated with significantly greater progression to second- or third-degree AV block on follow-up. Therefore, prophylactic pacemaker implantation has been recommended in such patients for control of symptoms.[57] But syncope in patients with bifascicular block is often due to causes other than heart block and does not predict sudden death. Pacemaker insertion does not prevent sudden death, which presumably is due to ventricular arrhythmias, but may prevent serious morbidity associated with syncopal falls, if heart block is the cause of syncope.

SINUS NODE DISEASE

Sinus bradycardia alone in an elderly patient may be a normal finding that does not imply cardiac disease and has no effect on mortality.[1,17] However, sinus node disease, or the *sick sinus syndrome,* characterized by sinus bradycardia in association with paroxysmal supraventricular tachyarrhyth-

mias, is a common cause of syncope in old people. Conduction disturbances are also common in the sick sinus syndrome, occurring in approximately 50% of patients.[49,51] One of the major causes of syncope in sick sinus syndrome is prolonged asystole after abrupt cessation of an associated supraventricular tachycardia. Although there is potential morbidity from dizziness, falls, and syncope, the mortality of sick sinus syndrome is quite low; in one study an 80% 5-year survival was found, similar to that for a normal age- and sex-matched population.[59] Pacemaker implantation is indicated for control of symptoms, not prolongation of life.

Hypotension

Due to age-related abnormalities in blood pressure homeostasis, as well as superimposed conditions that reduce intravascular volume and/or peripheral vascular resistance, hypotensive syndromes are common in elderly patients.

ORTHOSTATIC HYPOTENSION

Orthostatic hypotension, defined as a systolic blood pressure decline of 20 mm Hg or more on assumption of upright posture, has been reported to occur in 20% to 30% of community-dwelling elderly.[4,23] However, recent studies suggest that this may be due to age-associated medical conditions such as hypertension, rather than age per se.[45] Many elderly patients have marked variability in orthostatic blood pressure, which may be due to impaired baroreflex function.[41] These elderly patients have normal elevations in plasma norepinephrine in response to posture change.

The major pathologic causes of orthostatic hypotension are shown in Table 11–1. Autonomic dysfunction is commonly accompanied by a fixed heart rate, visual difficulty, incontinence, constipation, inability to sweat, heat intolerance, impotence, and fatigability.[68]

Central and peripheral autonomic insufficiency can be differentiated on the basis of plasma norepinephrine levels. Patients with the peripheral condition, idiopathic orthostatic hypotension, have lower basal plasma norepinephrine levels while supine, no increase in norepinephrine level with standing, a lower threshold for the pressor response to infused norepinephrine, and lower plasma norepinephrine levels in response to tyramine despite a greater pressor response to the drug.[69] These findings suggest that in idiopathic orthostatic hypotension there is depletion of norepinephrine from sympathetic nerve endings with resultant postsynaptic denervation supersensitivity. In central autonomic insufficiency, such as occurs with multiple cerebral infarctions or multiple system atrophy (the Shy-Drager syndrome), circulating norepinephrine and the response to infused norepinephrine and tyramine are normal, but plasma norepinephrine levels also fail to increase with standing.[53] This syndrome is associated with degeneration of neurons in the central nervous system (CNS).

POSTPRANDIAL HYPOTENSION

Postprandial hypotension is a recently identified abnormality in blood pressure homeostasis.[38] Institutionalized and healthy community-dwelling elderly have an average 11-mm Hg decline in blood pressure by 1 hour after a meal. Whereas in most elders this is an asymptomatic age-related abnormality, individuals with postprandial syncope have more profound declines in blood pressure, which are probably responsible for fainting episodes.[39] Postprandial hypotension may be related to an inability to compensate for splanchnic blood pooling during digestion.

VOLUME DEPLETION

The elderly are at increased risk for dehydration and associated orthostatic hypotension caused by an age-related impairment in renal salt and water conservation (see above), and any disease that threatens access to fluids or results in volume loss.

Abnormal Cardiovascular Reflexes

VASOVAGAL SYNCOPE

Vasovagal syncope, the most common cause of syncope in a younger population, is seen in the elderly, but appears to be less common. Syncope without an apparent cause is often inappropriately labeled vasovagal. The exact prevalence is unknown. There is often a precipitant such as a painful or unpleasant experience, surgical manipulation, or trauma, commonly associated with hunger, fatigue, crowding, or warmth. There are premonitory signs and symptoms of intense autonomic nervous system (ANS) stimulation, such as marked weakness, sweating, pallor, epigastric discomfort, nausea, yawning, sighing, hyperventilation, blurred vision, impaired hearing, a feeling of unawareness, and mydriasis. Most often these symptoms occur while standing and are aborted by lying down. The circulatory changes preceding vasovagal syncope are biphasic, with an initial increase in heart rate, blood pressure, total systemic resistance, and cardiac output, followed by peripheral vasodilatation, an increase in muscle blood flow, and a decrease in venous return to the heart.[11] The prognosis is good in true vasovagal syncope.

CAROTID SINUS SYNDROME

Carotid sinus hypersensitivity is a common abnormality of reflex blood pressure regulation that in its pathologic extreme may result in syncope. A hypersensitive carotid sinus reflex, defined by a greater than 50% sinus slowing (cardioinhibitory) or systolic blood pressure decline (vasodepressor) of over 50 mm Hg or to hypotensive levels during carotid sinus massage, may identify a predisposition for syncope but does not prove that it is responsible for a given episode. When carotid sinus hypersensitivity is associated with syncope, it is designated the *carotid sinus syndrome*.[44] A number of patients with undiagnosed syncope may have the carotid sinus syndrome. Unfortunately, many physicians may overlook the carotid sinus syndrome by not doing carotid sinus massage on patients with syncope.

DEFECATION,[28] MICTURITION,[27] SWALLOWING,[24,37] AND COUGH SYNCOPE[58,63]

Syncope may occur in response to any of these activities. The mechanism of syncope may be decreased venous return during the activities, an intermittent conduction disturbance or arrhythmia, or reflexly induced vasodilatation. Patients with syncope during these activities may develop syncope later under different conditions. The prognosis depends on the underlying pathophysiologic mechanism.

Abnormal Blood Constitution

The maintenance of consciousness depends not only on delivery of blood to the brain, but also on adequate levels of glucose and oxygen in the blood to support oxidative cerebral metabolism. Thus, hypoxemia, anemia, and hypoglycemia may predispose to syncope.

CNS Disease

Syncope can be attributed to cerebrovascular insufficiency only if transient, focal, neurologic deficits are associated with the episode. The new onset of a seizure disorder may present as syncope. Conversely, syncope from other causes may be associated with seizure activity.[2]

EVALUATION

The history is the most important part of the evaluation, providing a diagnosis in up to 50% of cases where a cause is found. The physical examination makes the diagnosis in another 20% of cases.[35]

The *history* includes four key questions. First, was there an obvious *precipitant?* Emotional stress, pain, cough, micturition, defecation, swallowing, exertion (AS), neck turning (carotid sinus syndrome), change in position, and recent meal or medication are all important clues. Second, were there any *associated symptoms?* For example, hunger, fatigue, abdominal discomfort, and autonomic symptoms may precede vasovagal syncope. Flushing on recovery can suggest a Stokes-Adams attack. Palpitations, dyspnea, or chest pain may suggest pulmonary embolism, angina pectoris, or myocardial infarction. Focal neurologic symptoms suggest a neurologic disorder. Third, could *medications* have been responsible? Various antihypertensive and antianginal medications can cause hypotension. Nitrates and psychotropic medications have been found to be the most common drug-related causes of syncope in institutionalized elderly.[40] Digoxin and various antiarrhythmic medications can paradoxically cause arrhythmias. Fourth, *how long did the symptoms last?* If symptoms last for more than 15 minutes, one should consider TIA, seizure, hypoglycemia, or hysteria.

The *physical examination* should focus on postural vital signs, cardiovascular and neurologic systems, and a search for trauma. Blood pressure and heart rate are measured after at least a 5-minute rest in the supine position, then after 1 and 3 minutes of standing. If the patient cannot stand, sitting will suffice but may lead to failure to diagnose orthostatic hypotension. A symptomatic blood pressure drop focuses further evaluation on the causes of orthostatic hypotension. In the young patient, excessive acceleration of the pulse in response to a posture change suggests that volume depletion may be the cause of orthostatic hypotension. However, this finding is often absent in the dehydrated elderly patient because of baroreflex impairment. If pulse rate does not accelerate, autonomic dysfunction may also be the cause.

Careful evaluation of the carotid pulsations for their contour, amplitude, and sound is important. Although the carotid upstroke is characteristically delayed in aortic stenosis, a normal upstroke does not rule out the diagnosis of aortic stenosis in the elderly patient because of an age-related increase in vascular rigidity that increases the rate of rise of the carotid pulse. When aortic stenosis develops, the rate of rise falls, but to an amplitude that may feel normal for a younger patient.[16] Also a diminished carotid pulse or bruit may be suggestive of cerebrovascular disease, but its absence does not rule out a diagnosis of cerebral ischemia. In patients with severe AS, simultaneous palpation of the carotid and apical impulses yields a palpable lag time between the two, which may suggest severe AS.[5]

Cardiopulmonary examination focuses on detection of obstructive cardiovascular disorders such as aortic stenosis, hypertrophic cardiomyopathy and pulmonary embolism. Unfortunately, cardiac murmurs become exceedingly common with advanced age and significant murmurs in the elderly may be atypical in character or location.[10] Thus, associated clinical symptoms, such as congestive heart failure or angina pectoris, or signs, such as a diminished second aortic sound or left ventricular hypertrophy, should heighten the suspicion of hemodynamically significant conditions and stimulate further studies, such as Doppler echocardiography of the heart. Stools should be checked for blood, and a careful neurologic examination should include a search for focal deficits that suggest cerebral infarction, hemorrhage, or tumor.

Carotid sinus massage is an important test in the evaluation of syncope if cerebrovascular disease or cardiac conduction disturbances are not present. With the electrocardiogram (ECG) running and the head slightly extended and rotated to the opposite side, the carotid sinus is massaged for 5 seconds. The blood pressure is taken before and immediately after the procedure. Two to 3 minutes later the procedure is repeated on the other side. Only symptomatic bradycardia or hypotension can be considered truly positive responses indicating carotid sinus hypersensitivity. However, there is general agreement that a systolic blood pressure decline of more than 50 mm Hg (or an absolute value less than 90 mm Hg) or a sinus pause of 3 seconds or longer is sufficient to produce syncope, particularly if the patient was in an upright position at the time of the syncopal event.

An *ECG* is indicated in all patients presenting with syncope, since it can provide diagnostic clues for myocardial infarction, ischemia, or transient tachyarrhythmias or bradyarrhythmias. Multifocal and frequent atrial and ventricular ectopic beats are an indication for prolonged cardiac monitoring. A short PR interval may indicate an accessory pathway. QT prolongation is associated with ventricular tachycardia and fibrillation. Sinoatrial pauses or inappropriate sinus bradycardia may indicate a sinus node disorder. The presence of AV conduction abnormalities or bundle branch block hints at transient heart block as the etiology of syncope.

Tests for autonomic function are indicated in any patient with orthostatic or postprandial hypotension. The simplest tests are deep breathing and the Valsalva maneuver.[20] The cold pressor and pharmacologic tests are poorly tolerated, potentially dangerous, and usually unnecessary in elderly patients.

Since electrical cardiac disease is so common in elderly patients, in-hospital cardiac monitoring (telemetry) is usually indicated, even without clues from the ECG, unless noncardiac causes are positively identified. *Ambulatory cardiac monitoring* is only indicated in those syncope patients who are still suspected, after initial evaluation and/or telemetry monitoring, to have a symptomatic and safely treatable arrhythmia or conduction disturbance. Ambulatory monitoring should be performed during the patient's usual daily activities to increase the diagnostic yield. When monitored for 24 to 48 hours, 10% to 40% of patients will have transient symptoms. Of these patients, an arrhythmic etiology can be confirmed or excluded in half to three quarters.[25]

Laboratory tests are generally of low yield but useful in the geriatric syncope patient without apparent etiology on history and physical examination, because syncope may be the atypical presentation of several conditions evident only on laboratory testing. Cardiac enzymes should be obtained if there is any associated chest pain or ECG change, raising the suspicion of myocardial infarction. Electrolytes, blood urea nitrogen, and creatinine are important to evaluate volume status and identify abnormalities that predispose to arrhythmias. Arterial blood gases are indicated if there are pulmonary symptoms. A hematocrit is helpful to rule out anemia. Blood sugar should be obtained to look for hypoglycemia and marked hyperglycemia, both of which usually produce prolonged loss of consciousness but may manifest as syncope in the elderly patient. Drug levels of anticonvulsants, antiarrhythmics, digoxin, or bronchodilators are useful to detect drug toxicity or undertreatment of a prior condition known to produce syncope.

Echocardiography is an invaluable study when structural heart disease is suspected. Recently, doppler echocardiography has been shown to identify patients with significant aortic valve gradients. Doppler echocardiography correlates well with invasive cardiac catheterization, particularly when combined with two-dimensional echo.[67,70]

The electroencephalograph (EEG) and a computed tomography (CT) scan of the head should be obtained in the presence of focal neurologic abnormalities on physical examination or signs and symptoms of seizures. More invasive studies such as cerebral or coronary angiography are only indicated to confirm specific clinical diagnoses.

Electrophysiologic studies of the heart are indicated in patients with cardiovascular disease and *recurrent syncope* in whom there is a high suspicion of sinus node dysfunction, conduction disease, or life-threatening arrhythmias. The overall incidence of findings (sinus node dysfunction, complete AV block, ventricular tachycardia) considered to be positively related to syncope ranges from 18% to 69%. Most investigators find plausible cause in approximately 50%, with the lower numbers in patients without structural heart disease and the higher numbers in patients with heart disease.[8] During follow-up, usually between 70% and 90% of those patients who received therapy on the basis of positive electrophysiologic findings remained asymptomatic. Although the results are impressive, it should also be noted that an average of 50% of patients not specifically treated also remained free of recurrent syncope.

Predictors for a positive electrophysiologic study include[34] a left ventricular ejection fraction less than 0.40, the presence of bundle branch block, coronary artery disease, remote myocardial infarction, use of type I antiarrhythmic drugs, injury related to loss of consciousness, and male sex. Predictors for a negative study were an ejection fraction greater than 0.40, the absence of structural heart disease, a normal ECG, and normal ambulatory electrocardiographic monitoring. The benefits

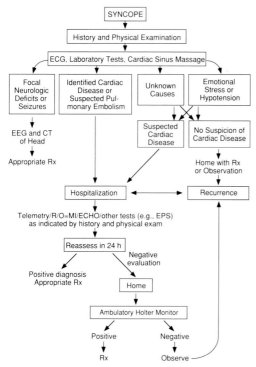

Figure 11–1. Algorithm for the diagnostic evaluation of the elderly syncope patient. (From Hazzard, WR, Andres, R, Bierman, EL, and Blass, JP, [eds]: Principles of Geriatric Medicine and Gerontology. McGraw-Hill, New York, 1985, p 1075, with permission.)

of any invasive procedure should be balanced against the risk of the procedure and the potential adverse effects of therapy (including surgery and medications). The diagnostic approach to the elderly syncope patient is summarized in Figure 11–1.

THERAPEUTIC ISSUES

The purpose of treating an elderly patient with syncope is to prevent the morbidity and mortality associated with recurrent episodes. When the cause of a syncopal episode is readily apparent, specific therapy can be planned if potential morbidity of the treatment is less than that of recurrent syncope. Because therapeutic interventions may be toxic to elderly patients, they should be instituted with cautious

attention to age- and disease-related physiologic changes that may effect response and side effects of treatment. No person should be denied therapy on the basis of age alone.

When the cause of a syncopal episode is not clear, the therapy should be directed toward minimizing the risk of recurrent syncope by correcting predisposing conditions and eliminating drugs that may contribute to a syncopal event. For example, the risk of syncope in an older person may be substantially reduced by treating anemia with a blood transfusion, correcting hypoxia with supplemental oxygen, improving cardiac ischemia with calcium channel blockers (observe for orthostatic hypotension), or preventing orthostatic hypotension with a high salt intake (observe for congestive heart failure) and support stockings. The mainstay of therapy for autonomic insufficiency is fludrocortisone and salt loading, but new pharmacologic approaches are being investigated, for example the use of caffeine, ergotamine, and somatostatin.

Before prescribing pharmacologic or surgical therapy for a diagnosed condition, the safe, simple, commonsense treatments should be implemented. Such treatments include discontinuation of potentially harmful drugs such as digoxin, propranolol, or α-methyldopa, which may predispose to carotid sinus hypersensitivity or suppress the sinus node; avoidance of extreme neck rotation and tight collars when there is evidence of carotid sinus hypersensitivity; slow arising from the supine position and dorsiflexing the feet a few minutes before standing, in persons prone to postural hypotension; maintaining adequate intravascular volume through regular fluid intake in cognitively impaired or acutely ill patients; and urinating while sitting down in men with micturition syncope. Often a simple behavior change or drug elimination is the only therapy necessary to prevent recurrent syncopal episodes.

Antiarrhythmic medications should be prescribed only for *symptomatic* rhythm disturbances and initially at one half the usual dose, due to their prolonged half-life and increased toxicity in elderly patients.[13] Clinically significant adverse reactions are seen in up to half of the young patients treated, with major reactions noted in one third.[66] Proarrhythmic effects (i.e., worsening of arrhythmia as a result of therapy) are now appreciated complications of antiarrhythmic medications in up to one third of patients. When the high incidence of serious side effects is coupled with the fact that no controlled studies have conclusively proved that elderly patients with arrhythmias benefit from antiarrhythmic drug therapy, a high threshold for initiating therapy is fully justifiable in the older patient.

Basic monitoring of medication levels, electrolytes, the electrocardiographic QT interval, and arrhythmia frequency on the ambulatory cardiac monitor is important when antiarrhythmic medications are prescribed.

Pacemakers are generally indicated for the amelioration of symptoms due to bradyarrhythmias. Only in Stokes-Adams attacks do pacemakers improve longevity.[9] The most common indications are third-degree AV block and sick sinus syndrome. Symptomatic second-degree AV block and carotid sinus syndrome are also indications for a permanent pacemaker. A single-chamber ventricular pacemaker is generally adequate, but in the elderly patient who is dependent on atrial contraction to generate an adequate cardiac output, a dual-chamber pacemaker should be considered. Indications for antiarrhythmic medications, pacemakers, and electrophysiologic studies are continually being reassessed, and the latest consensus should be sought and carefully considered prior to prescription in the elderly.

Invasive therapy such as aortic valve repair, balloon valvuloplasty, coronary angioplasty, and coronary artery bypass surgery have been shown to be feasible and effective in the elderly patient with an acceptable, relatively low mortality in patients who are otherwise well. Recent experience with balloon valvuloplasty for aortic stenosis suggests that this procedure may be of particular benefit to the symptomatic elderly patient who is a high surgical risk.[3]

CONCLUSION

Age-related physiologic changes and disease-related abnormalities predispose the geriatric patient to syncope. Syncope may be the atypical manifestation of diseases or situational stresses not expected to produce it. Attention to situational stresses, such as posture change, meals, or drug ingestion, is likely to increase the diagnostic yield and lead to simple therapy that can reduce the morbidity and potential mortality of recurrent episodes. Therapy should be directed toward minimizing multiple risks for syncope, avoiding toxic interventions, and treating specific *symptomatic* diseases, using underlying disease rather than age as the criterion for invasive treatment.

REFERENCES

1. Agruss, NS, Rosin, EY, Adolph, RJ, and Fowler, NO: Significance of chronic sinus bradycardia in elderly people. Circulation 46:924–930, 1972.

2. Aminoff, NJ, Scheinman, MM, Griffin, JC, and Herre, JM: Electrocerebral accompaniments of syncope associated with malignant ventricular arrhythmias. Ann Intern Med 108:791–796, 1988.

3. Brady, ST, Davis, CA, Kussmaul, WG, Laskey, WK, Hirshfeld, JW, and Herrmann, HC: Percutaneous aortic balloon valvuloplasty in octogenarians: Morbidity and mortality. Ann Intern Med 110:761–766, 1989.

4. Caird, FI, Andrews, GR, and Kennedy, RD: Effect of posture on blood pres-

sure in the elderly. Br Heart J 35:527–530, 1973.

5. Chun, PKC and Dunn, BE: Clinical clues of severe aortic stenosis. Simultaneous palpation of the carotid and apical impulses. Arch Intern Med 142:2284, 1982.

6. Day, SC, Cook, EP, Funkenstein, H, and Goldman, L: Evaluation and outcome of emergency room patients with transient loss of consciousness. Am J Med 73:15–23, 1982.

7. Dhingra, RC, Denes, P, and Wu, DI: Syncope in patients with chronic bifascicular block: Significance, causative mechanisms, and clinical implications. Ann Intern Med 81:302–306, 1974.

8. DiMarco, JP: Electrophysiologic studies in patients with unexplained syncope. Circulation (Suppl III)75:140, 1987.

9. Dunst, N: Cardiac pacemakers. Med Clin North Am 57:1515, 1973.

10. Duthie, EH, Gambert, SR, and Tresch, D: Evaluation of the systolic murmur in the elderly. J Am Geriatr Soc 29:498–502, 1981.

11. Engel, GL: Psychologic stress, vasodepressor (vasovagal) syncope, and sudden death. Ann Intern Med 89:403–412, 1978.

12. Epstein, N and Hollenberg, NH: Age as a determinant of renal sodium conservation in normal man. J Lab Clin Med 87:411–417, 1976.

13. Everitt, DE and Avorn, J: Drug prescribing for the elderly. Arch Intern Med 146:2393, 1986.

14. Ezri, M, Lerman, BB, Marchlinski, FE, Buxton, AE, and Josephson, ME: Electrophysiologic evaluation of syncope in patients with bifascicular block. Am Heart J 106:693–697, 1983.

15. Fleg, JL and Kennedy, HL: Cardiac arrhythmias in a healthy elderly population: Detection by 24 hour ambulatory electrocardiography. Chest 81:302–307, 1982.

16. Flohr, KH, Weir, EK, and Chesler, E: Diagnosis of aortic stenosis in older age groups using external carotid

pulse recording and phonocardiography. Br Heart J 45:577–582, 1981.

17. Gann, D, Tolentino, A, and Samet, P: Electrophysiologic evaluation of elderly patients with sinus bradycardia: A long-term follow-up study. Ann Intern Med 90:24–29, 1979.

18. Gibson, TC and Hertzman, MR: Diagnostic efficacy of 24-hour electrocardiographic monitoring for syncope. Am J Cardiol 5:398, 1984.

19. Haller, BGD, Zust, H, Shaw, S, Gnadinger, MP, Uehlinger, DE, and Weidmann, P: Effects of posture and ageing on circulating atrial natriuretic peptide levels in man. J Hypertension 5:551–556, 1987.

20. Henrich, WL: Autonomic insufficiency. Arch Intern Med 142:339, 1982.

21. Horan, MJ and Kennedy, HL: Ventricular ectopy: History, epidemiology and clinical implications. JAMA 251:380, 1984.

22. Iskandrian, AS and Hakki, AH: Age-related changes in left ventricular diastolic performance. Am Heart J 112:75, 1986.

23. Johnson, RH, Smith, AC, Spalding, JMK, and Wollner, J: Effect of posture on blood pressure in elderly patients. Lancet 1:731–733, 1965.

24. Kadish, AH, Wechsler, L, and Marchlinski, F: Swallowing syncope: Observations in the absence of conduction system or esophageal disease. Am J Med 81:1098–1100, 1986.

25. Kapoor, WN: Evaluation of syncope in the elderly. J Am Geriatr Soc 35:826, 1987.

26. Kapoor, WN, Karpf, M, Maher, Y, Miller, RA, and Levey, GS: Syncope of unknown origin: The need for a more cost-effective approach to its diagnostic evaluation. JAMA 247:2687–2691, 1982.

27. Kapoor, WN, Peterson, JR, and Karpf, M: Micturition syncope: A reappraisal. JAMA 253:796–798, 1985.

28. Kapoor, WN, Peterson, JR, Karpf, M: Defecation syncope: A symptom

with multiple etiologies. Arch Intern Med 146:2377–2379, 1986.

29. Kapoor, WN, Peterson, J, Wieand, H, and Karpf, M: Diagnostic and prognostic implications of recurrences in patients with syncope. Am J Med 83:700–708, 1987.

30. Kapoor, WN, Snustad, D, Peterson, J, Wieand, H, Cha, R, and Karpf, M: Syncope in the elderly. Am J Med 80:419–428, 1986.

31. Kennedy, HL, Whitlock, JA, Sprague, NH, Kennedy, LJ, Buckingham, TA, and Goldberg, RJ: Long-term follow-up of asymptomatic healthy subjects with frequent and complex ventricular ectopy. N Engl J Med 312:193–197, 1985.

32. Kety, SS: Human cerebral blood flow and oxygen consumption as related to aging. J Chronic Dis 3:478–486, 1956.

33. Krasnow, N and Stein, RA: Hypertrophic cardiomyopathy in the aged. Am Heart J 96:326–336, 1978.

34. Krol, RB, Morady, F, Flaker, GC, DiCarlo, LA, Jr, Baerman, JM, Hewett J, and DeBuitleir, M: Electrophysiologic testing in patients with unexplained syncope: Clinical and noninvasive predictors of outcome. J Am Coll Cardiol 10:358–363, 1987.

35. Kudenchuk, PJ and McAnulty, JH: Syncope: Evaluation and treatment. Mod Conc Cardiovasc Dis 54:25; 1985.

36. Leu, M: Anatomic basis for atrioventricular block. Am J Med 37:742, 1964.

37. Levin, B and Posner, JB: Swallow syncope. Report of a case and review of the literature. Neurology 22:1086–1093, 1972.

38. Lipsitz, LA, Nyquist, RP, Wei, JY, and Rowe, JW: Postprandial reduction in blood pressure in the elderly. N Engl J Med 309:81–83, 1983.

39. Lipsitz, LA, Pluchino, FC, Wei, JY, Minaker, KL, and Rowe, JW: Cardiovascular and norepinephrine responses after meal consumption in elderly (older than 75 years) persons with postprandial hypoten-

sion and syncope. Am J Cardiol 58:810–815, 1986.

40. Lipsitz, LA, Pluchino, FC, Wei, JY, and Rowe, JW: Syncope in institutionalized elderly: The impact of multiple pathological conditions and situational stress. J Chronic Dis 39:619–630, 1986.

41. Lipsitz, LA, Storch, HA, Minaker, KL, and Rowe, JR: Intraindividual variability in postural blood pressure in the elderly. Clin Sci 69:3377–3341, 1985.

42. Lipsitz, LA, Wei, JY, and Rowe, JW: Syncope in an elderly, institutionalized population: Prevalence, incidence, and associated risk. Q J Med 216:45–54, 1985.

43. Lombard, JT and Selzer, A: Valvular aortic stenosis. Ann Intern Med 106:292–298, 1987.

44. Lown, B and Levine, SA: The carotid sinus: Clinical value of its stimulation. Circulation 23:766–786, 1961.

45. Mader, SL, Josephson, KR, and Rubenstein, LZ: Low prevalence of postural hypotension among community-dwelling elderly. JAMA 258:1511–1514, 1987.

46. Mark, AL: The Bezold-Jarisch reflex revisited: Clinical implications of inhibitory reflexes originating in the heart. J Am Coll Cardiol 1:90, 1983.

47. Maron, BJ, Bonow, RO, Cannon, RO, III, Leon, MB, and Epstein, SE: Hypertrophic cardiomyopathy. N Engl J Med 316:780–786, 1987.

48. McAnulty, JH, Rahimtoola, SH, Murphy, E, DeMots, H, Ritzmann, L, Kanarek, P, and Kauffman, S: Natural history of "high-risk" bundle-branch block: Final report of a prospective study. N Engl J Med 307:137–143, 1982.

49. Moss, AJ and Davis, RJ: Brady-tachy syndrome. Prog Cardiovasc Dis 16:439–454, 1974.

50. Mymin, D, Mathewson, FAL, Tate RB, and Manfreda, J: The natural history of primary first-degree heart block. N Engl J Med 315:1183–1187, 1986.

51. Obel, IWP, Cohen, E, and Millar, RN: Chronic symptomatic sinoatrial block: A review of 34 patients and their treatment. Chest 65:397–402, 1974.

52. Phillips, PA, Rolls, BJ, and Ledingham, JGG: Reduced thirst after water deprivation in healthy elderly men. N Engl J Med 311:753–759, 1984.

53. Polinsky, RJ, Kopin, IJ, Ebert, MH, and Weise, V: Pharmacologic distinction of different orthostatic hypotension syndromes. Neurology 31:1–7, 1981.

54. Pomerance, A: Pathogenesis of aortic stenosis and its relation to age. Br Heart J 34:569, 1972.

55. Pomerance, A: Cardiac Pathology in the Elderly. In Noble, RJ and Rothbaum, DA (eds): Geriatric Cardiology. FA Davis, Philadelphia, 1981, pp 28–29.

56. Savage, DD, Corwin, L, McGee, DL, Kannel, WB, and Wolf, PA: Epidemiologic features of isolated syncope: The Framingham Study. Stroke 16:626–629, 1985.

57. Scheinman, MM, Peters, RW, Modin, G, Brennan, M, Mies, C, and O'Young, J: Prognostic value of infranodal conduction time in patients with chronic bundle branch block. Circulation 56:240–244, 1977.

58. Sharpey-Schafer, EP: The mechanism of syncope after coughing. Br Med J 2:860, 1953.

59. Shaw, DB, Holman, RR, and Gowers, JI: Survival in sinoatrial disorder (sick-sinus syndrome). Br Med J 280:139–141, 1980.

60. Shimada, K, Kitazumi, T, Ogura, H, Sadakane, N, and Ozawa, T: Differences in age-independent effects of blood pressure on baroreflex sensitivity between normal and hypertensive subjects. Clin Sci 70:489–494, 1986.

61. Silverstein, MD, Singer, DE, Mulley, AG, Thibault, GE, and Barnett, GO: Patients with syncope admitted to medical intensive care units. JAMA 248:1185–1189, 1982.

62. Strandgaard, S: Autoregulation of cerebral blood flow in hypertensive patients: The modifying influence of prolonged antihypertensive treatment on the tolerance to acute, drug-induced hypotension. Circulation 53:720–727, 1976.

63. Strauss, MJ, Longstreth, WT, and Thiele, BL: Case report: Atypical cough syncope. JAMA 251:1731, 1984.

64. Topol, EJ, Traill, TA, and Fortuin, NJ: Hypertensive hypertrophic cardiomyopathy of the elderly. N Engl J Med 312:277–283, 1985.

65. Wayne, HH. Syncope: Physiological considerations and an analysis of the clinical characteristics in 510 patients. Am J Med 30:418–438, 1961.

66. Woosley, RL: Risk/benefit considerations in antiarrhythmic therapy. JAMA 256:82–84, 1986.

67. Yaeger, M, Yock, PG, and Popp, RL: Comparison of doppler-derived pressure gradient to that determined at cardiac catheterization in adults with aortic valve stenosis: Implications for management. Am J Cardiol 57:644–648, 1986.

68. Ziegler, MG: Postural hypotension. Annu Rev Med 31:239–245, 1980.

69. Ziegler, MG, Lake, R, and Kopin, IJ: The sympathetic nervous system defect in primary orthostatic hypotension. N Engl J Med 296:293–297, 1977.

70. Zoghbi, WA, Farmer, KL, Soto, JG, Nelson, JG, and Quinones, MA: Accurate noninvasive quantification of stenotic aortic valve area by doppler echocardiography. Circulation 73:452–459, 1986.

Chapter 12

VOIDING DYSFUNCTION AND URINARY INCONTINENCE*

Neil M. Resnick, M.D.

LOWER URINARY TRACT ANATOMY
 AND PHYSIOLOGY
THE IMPACT OF AGE ON
 INCONTINENCE
THE DIAGNOSTIC APPROACH
THERAPY

Urinary incontinence affects 15% to 30% of community-dwelling elderly,[25,46] one third of older individuals in acute-care settings,[45,59] and roughly half of the institutionalized elderly.[37] Its burden is substantial and must be measured in medical, psychosocial, and economic terms.[47] Medically, individuals are predisposed to perineal rashes, pressure sores, urinary tract infections, urosepsis, falls, and fractures. Another unappreciated complication is recurrent lower limb cellulitis. This occurs when incontinent individuals' shoes are chronically soaked by urine, become hardened, and abrade their feet; it is especially apt to occur in individuals with impaired peripheral sensation.

The psychosocial concomitants of incontinence are also significant. Individuals are frequently embarrassed, iso-lated, stigmatized, depressed, and regressed; they are also predisposed to institutionalization, although the extent remains undefined.[25,36] Economically, the costs of incontinence are startling. In America, over $8 billion was devoted to incontinence in 1984.[26] This figure exceeds the annual amount devoted to dialysis and coronary artery bypass surgery combined.[47]

Despite its considerable prevalence, morbidity, and expense, however, incontinence remains a largely neglected problem. Only the minority of incontinent individuals consult a health care provider; and sadly—when they do—the physician who initiates even the most rudimentary evaluation is the exception.[47] This is unfortunate because incontinence is no more a part of normal aging than is chest pain; and, like chest pain, it is a symptom of a variety of underlying conditions. Moreover, several studies have documented that, regardless of the context in which it is found, incontinence is a highly treatable and even curable disorder.[12,19,39,40,43,45,47,57,70,73]

This chapter will review the basics of urinary incontinence in the elderly. This will entail a brief review of the anatomy and physiology of the lower urinary tract, an examination of the impact that normal aging has on the system, a theoretical consideration of

---

*Modified from Cassel, CK, Riesenberg, DE, Sorensen, LB, and Walsh, JR, (eds): Geriatric Medicine, ed 2. Springer-Verlag, New York, 1990, pp 501–518, with permission.

what can go wrong, and a review of what does go wrong. This knowledge will be used to formulate a targeted clinical evaluation to the incontinent individual and to propose a logical diagnostic and therapeutic approach.[44]

LOWER URINARY TRACT ANATOMY AND PHYSIOLOGY

Details of the anatomy and physiology of normal micturition remain controversial and are reviewed elsewhere.[65] For the present purposes, however, we can simplify both. The lower urinary tract includes the urethral outlet, and a muscular storage and contractile portion known as the detrusor. The proximal portion of the urethra comprises a sphincter (internal urethral sphincter), which is located in the region of the bladder neck, is predominantly smooth muscle, and is autonomically innervated. A few centimeters distal to this is the external sphincter, which is composed of striated muscle and lies at the level of the urogenital diaphragm.

The innervation of the lower urinary tract is derived from three sources: the parasympathetic (from S-2 to S-4), the sympathetic (from T-10 to L-2), and the somatic (voluntary) nervous systems (from S-2 to S-4). The parasympathetic nervous system innervates the detrusor; increased cholinergic activity increases the force and frequency of detrusor contraction, while reduced activity has the opposite effect. The sympathetic nervous system innervates both the bladder and the urethra, with its effect determined by local receptors. Although adrenergic receptors are sparse in the bladder body, those normally present are β receptors; their stimulation relaxes the bladder. Receptors at the base of the bladder and in the proximal urethra, on the other hand, are α receptors; their stimulation contracts the internal sphincter. Thus, activation of the sympathetic nervous system facilitates storage of urine in a coordinated manner. The somatic nervous system innervates the urogenital diaphragm and the external sphincter, although the external sphincter probably receives other innervation as well.[65] The central nervous system (CNS) integrates control of the urinary tract. The pontine micturition center mediates synchronous sphincter relaxation and detrusor contraction, while higher centers in the frontal lobe, basal ganglia, and cerebellum (among others) exert inhibitory and facilitatory effects.

Storage of urine is mediated by detrusor relaxation and closure of the sphincters. Detrusor relaxation is accomplished by CNS inhibition of parasympathetic tone, while sphincter closure is mediated by a reflex increase in α-adrenergic and somatic activity. Voiding occurs when detrusor contraction, mediated by the parasympathetic nervous system, is coordinated with sphincter relaxation.

THE IMPACT OF AGE ON INCONTINENCE

Normal aging affects the lower urinary tract in a variety of ways, but incontinence is not one of them. Although there is still a dearth of data and no longitudinal studies, several points emerge from cross-sectional studies. Bladder capacity, the ability to postpone voiding, and urinary flow rate probably decline in both sexes, while maximum urethral closure pressure and urethral length probably decline in women.[43] The prevalence of uninhibited contractions probably increases with age, but there are few studies of younger individuals available for comparison.[14,43] Postvoiding residual volume may increase, but probably to no more than 50 to 100 mL.[43] Another important age-related change is an alteration in the pattern of fluid excretion. While younger individuals excrete the bulk of their daily ingested fluid before bedtime, many healthy elderly excrete the bulk of theirs during the night. This is true even for those without peripheral venous insufficiency, renal disease, heart failure, or prostatism. Thus, one to two episodes of nocturia per night may be normal, especially if the pattern is long-standing, unchanged, and other conditions have been excluded.[43] Finally, virtually all men experience an age-related increase in prostatic size.

None of these age-related changes causes incontinence, since each has been documented in studies of either asymptomatic or continent individuals. Nonetheless, each predisposes to incontinence. This predisposition, coupled with the increased likelihood that an older person will be subjected to an additional pathologic, physiologic, or pharmacologic insult, underlies the higher incidence of incontinence in the elderly. The corollary is equally important. The new onset or exacerbation of incontinence in an older person is likely to be due to a precipitant outside the lower urinary tract that is amenable to medical intervention. Treatment of the precipitant alone may be sufficient to restore continence. These principles provide a rationale for dividing the causes of incontinence in the elderly into categories of transient and established incontinence.

Transient Incontinence

Transient incontinence is common in the elderly, affecting up to one third of community-dwelling incontinent individuals and up to half of hospitalized incontinent patients.[43] The causes can be recalled easily using the mnemonic "DIAPPERS" (misspelled with an extra "P"; Table 12–1).[42]

Table 12–1 CAUSES OF TRANSIENT INCONTINENCE

Delirium/confusional state
Infection–urinary (symptomatic)
Atrophic urethritis-vaginitis
Pharmaceuticals
Psychological, especially depression
Excess urinary output (e.g., CHF, hyperglycemia)
Restricted mobility
Stool impaction

Source: Adapted from Resnick,[42] p 284.

In the setting of *delirium,* incontinence is merely an associated symptom that will abate once the underlying cause of confusion is identified and treated. The patient needs medical rather than bladder management.

Symptomatic *urinary tract infection* causes transient incontinence when dysuria and urgency defeat the older person's ability to reach the toilet. On the other hand, asymptomatic infection, which is more common in the elderly, is usually not a cause of incontinence.[7,43]

Atrophic vaginitis only occasionally causes transient incontinence, but it commonly contributes.[55] It can present as urethral "scalding," dysuria, dyspareunia, urinary urgency, or urge or stress urinary incontinence. In demented individuals, vaginitis may present as agitation. The symptoms are readily responsive to treatment with a low dose of estrogen, administered either orally (0.3 mg conjugated estrogen per day) or topically. The optimal route is unclear. Orally administered, estrogen has adverse hepatic-mediated effects but beneficial effects on blood lipids[13] and costs approximately 10 cents per day. Applied intravaginally, estrogen is considerably more expensive and inconvenient; additionally, systemic levels are attained equivalent to orally administered estrogen and the hepatic effect is not eliminated. More recently, estrogen has been given transcutaneously, but studies of its impact on atrophic vaginitis are not yet available. The transcutaneous route seems promising, however, because it requires application only twice weekly and preliminary data suggest that it may have beneficial effects on lipids without adverse hepatic effects.[27] Whichever route is chosen, symptoms respond in a few days to 6 weeks, although the intracellular biochemical response may take much longer.[58] Although the duration of therapy has not been well established, we administer a low dose of estrogen on a daily basis for 1 to 2 months and then start to taper it. Eventually, most patients can probably be weaned to a dose given as infrequently as two to four times per month; after 6 months, estrogen can be discontinued entirely in some patients, although recrudescence is common. Since the estrogen dose is low and given briefly, its carcinogenic effect is likely slight, if present at all. In fact, the only adverse effect we have seen is mild and irregular vaginal bleeding in a small percentage of patients. However, if long-term treatment with estrogen is required, a progestin should probably be added if the patient still has a uterus. In addition, because estrogen-responsive breast cancer is common in older women, mammography should probably be performed prior to initiating hormone therapy. Of note, the dose of estrogen employed for the treatment of atrophic vaginitis is substantially lower than the dose required to prevent bone loss.

Pharmaceuticals are one of the most common causes of voiding dysfunction (Table 12–2). Long-acting sedative hypnotics, such as diazepam and flurazepam, have longer half-lives in the elderly and thus may accumulate, inducing confusion and secondary incontinence.[43] Another sedative used by patients is alcohol, which both induces a diuresis and clouds the sensorium. "Loop" diuretics induce a brisk diuresis, which may overwhelm bladder capacity and result in incontinence. Vincristine can cause a partially reversible neuropathy associated with urinary retention.[69]

Drugs with anticholinergic properties are in common use. Older patients often take several nonprescribed preparations for conditions such as insomnia, coryza, pruritis, and vertigo. Because three quarters of the elderly use nonprescription agents,[20] and because many do not regard them as "medicines" worth mentioning to their physicians, it is worth inquiring about such drugs directly. If the agents have anticholinergic effects, urinary retention and overflow incontinence may result.

Adrenergic agents also affect the lower urinary tract. Because the proximal urethra contains primarily alpha

Table 12–2 COMMON MEDICATIONS THAT CAN CAUSE INCONTINENCE

SEDATIVE HYPNOTICS
  Flurazepam
  Diazepam
  Ethanol
DIURETICS
  Furosemide
  Ethacrynic acid
  Bumetanide
ANTICHOLINERGIC AGENTS
  Antipsychotic agents
  Antidepressants
  Drugs for PD (trihexyphenidyl and benztropine mesylate, not L-dopa or deprenyl)
  Disopyramide
  Antispasmodic agents
  Antihistamines
  Opiates
ADRENERGIC AGENTS
  Sympathomimetics
  Sympatholytics
  Vincristine

Source: Adapted from Resnick,[42] p 285.

adrenoceptors, its tone can be decreased by alpha antagonists and increased by alpha-agonists. Alpha antagonists are contained in many antihypertensive medications. When taken by an older woman, whose urethra has shortened and weakened with age, these drugs may precipitate stress incontinence.[29] On the other hand, nonprescribed preparations containing alpha agonists (such as decongestants) may provoke acute retention in a man with otherwise asymptomatic prostatic enlargement—especially if the preparation additionally contains an antihistamine (anticholinergic). It is apparent that many nonprescription cold remedies are effectively, albeit inadvertently, formulated to cause lower urinary tract dysfunction in older men. In fact, a not uncommon cause of urinary retention occurs when an older man medicates himself with a multicomponent "cold" capsule, long-acting nose drops, and a hypnotic (usually an antihistamine).[43] How commonly this scenario results in an unnecessary or premature prostatectomy is unknown.

Calcium channel blockers reduce smooth muscle contractility throughout the body, including the bladder; they not infrequently induce urinary retention which is occasionally significant.[43]

Psychologic causes of incontinence have not been well studied in the elderly, but are probably much less common than in younger individuals. Intervention is properly directed at the psychologic disturbance, usually depression or life-long neurosis. However, once the psychologic disturbance has been treated, persistent incontinence warrants further evaluation. *Excessive urine output* commonly contributes to or even causes geriatric incontinence. Causes include excessive fluid intake: disorders associated with fluid retention (e.g., CHF); metabolic disorders (e.g., hyperglycemia or hypercalcemia); and medications (in addition to diuretics [drugs that cause peripheral edema] such as nifedipine and indomethacin).

Restricted mobility commonly contributes to incontinence in the elderly. It can result from arthritis, hip deformity, poor eyesight, inability to ambulate, fear of falling, a stroke,[9] or simply being restrained in a bed or a chair. A careful search will often identify correctable causes. If not, a urinal or bedside commode may still improve or resolve the incontinence.

Stool impaction has been implicated as a cause of urinary incontinence in up to 10% of patients referred to incontinence clinics[43]; the mechanism may involve stimulation of opioid receptors.[24] Patients usually present with either urge or overflow incontinence and typically have associated fecal incontinence as well. Disimpaction restores continence.

These eight reversible causes of incontinence should be assiduously sought in every elderly patient. In our series of hospitalized patients, when these causes were identified, continence was regained by most of those who became incontinent in the context of acute illness.[45] Regardless of their frequency, however, their identifica-

tion is important in all settings because they are easily treatable. A case presentation may illustrate these points more effectively.[48]

An 80-year-old man was referred for evaluation of urinary incontinence. He had been healthy until a year earlier, when he noted progressive generalized stiffness and trouble walking. He then fell, was hospitalized for a hip fracture, and subsequently developed pneumonia and confusion. The confusion was treated with haloperidol and the pneumonia with antibiotics. He was noted to be newly incontinent, and this persisted even after the pneumonia cleared. A urologist thought the prostate was palpably enlarged and suggested a prostatectomy, but the family refused. Awaiting placement in a nursing home, the patient remained on haloperidol. Physical examination revealed confusion, congestive heart failure, parkinsonism, a distended bladder, an enlarged prostate, and fecal impaction.

The etiology of his incontinence was multifactorial. During the prior year he had developed Parkinson disease (PD), which limited his mobility, was the cause of his fall, and was exacerbated by haloperidol. The anticholinergic effect of haloperidol also contributed to fecal impaction and urinary retention. Congestive heart failure, as well as the discomfort of urinary retention and fecal impaction, and the anticholinergic effect of haloperidol, all led to his becoming confused. Obviously, the role played by his prostate could not yet be determined, especially since the size of the prostate as palpated rectally correlates poorly with the presence of outlet obstruction.[34,43] Therefore, he was disimpacted and diuresed, haloperidol was discontinued, the bladder was drained, physical therapy was begun, and fiber was added to his diet. L-Dopa/carbidopa (Sinemet) was initiated because moderately severe PD had preceded treatment with haloperidol. Within 2 weeks, stigmata of PD subsided, bowel movements became regular, exercise tolerance increased, ambulation improved, and incontinence resolved; the postvoid residual was 10 mL, and prostatectomy was deferred. He remained dry and asymptomatic a year later.

Established Incontinence

LOWER URINARY TRACT
CAUSES (TABLE 12–3)

If leakage persists after transient causes of incontinence have been addressed, the lower urinary tract causes of established incontinence must be considered. These are due to dysfunction of the bladder, the outlet, or both.

The lower urinary tract can malfunction in only four ways. Two involve the bladder and two involve the outlet: The bladder either contracts when it should not (detrusor overactivity) or fails to contract when or as well as it should (detrusor underactivity); alternatively, outlet resistance is high when it should be low (obstruction) or low when it should be high (outlet incompetence). Because incontinence in older individuals is frequently due to a cause other than the classic types of "neurogenic bladder,"[53] it is probably better to think of the causes of incontinence in terms of the four pathophysiologic mechanisms just mentioned and to realize that each mechanism has a set of "neurogenic" as well as "nonneurogenic" causes (Table 12–3). This section provides an overview of the four basic

mechanisms and their causes; a later section provides more clinical details and treatment strategies for each.

Detrusor Overactivity. The most common cause of geriatric incontinence,[43,53] detrusor overactivity is a condition in which the bladder contracts precipitantly, usually emptying itself completely. Recently, however, detrusor overactivity has been found to exist as two physiologic subsets—one in which contractile function is preserved and one in which it is impaired. The latter condition has been termed detrusor hyperactivity with impaired contractility (DHIC).[49] DHIC is the most common cause of established incontinence in frail elderly,[53] and it has several implications. First, since the bladder is weak, urinary retention develops commonly in these patients, and DHIC must be added to outlet obstruction and detrusor underactivity as a cause of retention. Second, DHIC mimics virtually every other lower urinary tract cause of incontinence. For instance, if the uninhibited contraction is triggered by or occurs coincident with a stress maneuver and the weak bladder contraction (often only 2 to 6 cmH$_2$O) is not detected, the condition will be misdiag-

Table 12–3 LOWER URINARY TRACT CAUSES OF ESTABLISHED INCONTINENCE

Urodynamic Diagnosis	Some Neurogenic Causes	Some Nonneurogenic Causes
Detrusor overactivity	Stroke, Parkinson disease, Alzheimer disease	Urethral obstruction or incompetence, cystitis, bladder carcinoma, bladder stone, idiopathic
Detrusor underactivity	Disk compression, plexopathy, surgical damage (e.g., anterior-posterior resection), autonomic neuropathy (e.g., diabetes mellitus, alcoholism, vitamin B$_{12}$ deficiency)	Chronic outlet obstruction, idiopathic (common in women)
Outlet incompetence	Surgical lesion (rare), lower motor neuron lesion (rare)	Urethral hypermobility (type 1 and 2 SUI),* sphincter damage (type 3 SUI),* postprostatectomy
Outlet obstruction	Spinal cord lesion with detrusor-sphincter dyssynergia	Prostatic enlargement, urethral stricture, large cystourethocele

*SUI = stress urinary incontinence.

nosed as stress incontinence. Alternatively, since DHIC is associated with urinary urgency, frequency, weak flow rate, significant residual urine, and bladder trabeculation, it commonly mimics prostatism in men.[7a] Third, bladder weakness often frustrates anticholinergic therapy of DHIC since urinary retention is induced so easily. Thus, alternative therapeutic approaches are often required.

Whether the bladder is weak or strong, detrusor overactivity presents clinically as urge incontinence. It may result from disease such as stroke, Alzheimer disease (AD), or PD, which damage the CNS inhibitory centers. Alternatively, the etiology may be in the urinary tract itself, where a source of irritation—such as cystitis (interstitial, radiation, or chemotherapy-induced), a bladder tumor, or a stone—overwhelms the brain's ability to inhibit bladder contraction. Two other important local causes are outlet obstruction and outlet incompetence, both of which may lead to secondary detrusor overactivity.[2,32]

Traditionally, detrusor overactivity has been thought to be the primary cause of incontinence in demented geriatric patients. Although this is true, it is also the most common cause in nondemented geriatric patients and a recent study found no definite association between cognitive status and detrusor overactivity. Thus, it is no longer tenable to ascribe incontinence in demented individuals merely to detrusor overactivity.[43,53]

Detrusor Underactivity. The least common cause of geriatric incontinence, detrusor underactivity may be caused by mechanical injury to the nerves supplying the bladder (e.g., disk compression or tumor involvement) or to the autonomic neuropathy of diabetes, pernicious anemia, PD, alcoholism, Guillain-Barré syndrome, or tabes dorsalis. Alternatively, the detrusor may be replaced by fibrosis and connective tissue, as occurs in men with chronic outlet obstruction, so that even when the obstruction is removed, the bladder fails to empty normally. Detrusor replacement by fibrosis may also occur in women, but the cause is unknown.

Outlet Incompetence. Outlet incompetence is the second most common cause of incontinence in older women,[43,53] and is associated most often with pelvic floor laxity. This results in "urethral hypermobility" and allows the proximal urethra and bladder neck to "herniate" through the urogenital diaphragm when abdominal pressure increases. Such herniation results in unequal transmission of abdominal pressure to the bladder and urethra and consequent stress incontinence (Fig. 12–1). A less common cause of stress incontinence is "sphincter incompetence," in which the sphincter is so weak that merely the hydrostatic weight of a full bladder overcomes outlet resistance. This condition is also known as type 3 stress incontinence.[31] In the elderly, it generally results from repeated operative trauma or diabetes, but occasionally no precipitant is identified.

Outlet Obstruction. Outlet obstruction is the final lower urinary tract cause of incontinence and the second most common cause in older men.[43,53] If caused by neurologic disease, it is invariably associated with a spinal cord lesion. In this situation, pathways are interrupted to the pontine micturition center, where outlet relaxation is coordinated with bladder contraction. Then, rather than relaxing when the bladder contracts, the outlet contracts simultaneously, leading to severe outlet obstruction, a "Christmas tree bladder," hydronephrosis, and renal failure—a condition termed detrusor-sphincter dyssynergia. Alternatively, and much more commonly, obstruction results from prostatic enlargement, carcinoma, or urethral stricture in men; anatomic obstruction is uncommon in women in the absence of a large cystocele, which can prolapse and kink the urethra if the patient strains to void.

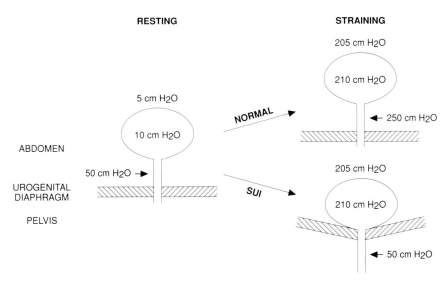

Figure 12–1. Pathophysiology of stress incontinence (SUI) due to urethral hypermobility. Normally, resting urethral pressure is greater than bladder pressure; with a stress maneuver (such as coughing, straining, laughing, or bending over) the increase in abdominal pressure is transmitted equally to the bladder and the outlet, and the individual remains dry. In women with urethral hypermobility, however, the proximal urethra "herniates" through the urogenital diaphragm (UGD) into the pelvis with a stress maneuver. Because abdominal pressure is no longer transmitted equally, instantaneous leakage occurs. (From Rowe and Besdine,[43a] p 251, with permission.)

Clinically, it is useful to rearrange these four basic pathophysiologic mechanisms into two categories: disorders of storage (detrusor overactivity or outlet incompetence), in which the bladder empties at inappropriate times; and disorders of evacuation (detrusor underactivity or outlet obstruction), in which the bladder empties incompletely, leading to progessive urine accumulation and overflow. In the first category, the bladder is normal in size; in the second, it is distended.

FUNCTIONAL INCONTINENCE

Of course, factors other than lower urinary tract dysfunction can contribute to established incontinence in the elderly, since continence is also affected by environmental demands, mentation, mobility, manual dexterity, and motivation. These factors are important to keep in mind because small improvements in each can result in marked amelioration of both incontinence and functional status. In fact, once one has excluded serious lesions of the urinary tract, attention to these factors will often obviate the need for further investigations.

THE DIAGNOSTIC APPROACH

The diagnostic approach has three purposes: to determine the cause of the incontinence; to detect related urinary tract pathology (Table 12–4); and to comprehensively evaluate the patient, the environment, and the available resources. The extent of the evaluation must be tailored to the individual and tempered by the realization that not all detected conditions can be cured (e.g., invasive bladder carcinoma), that optimal diagnostic and treatment strategies remain to be determined, that simple interventions may be effective even in the absence of a diagnosis,[44,57,64] and that for many elderly persons, diagnostic tests are themselves often interventions. Fortunately, however, the diagnostic approach outlined below is relatively noninvasive, accurate, easily

Table 12–4 SERIOUS CONDITIONS THAT MAY PRESENT AS INCONTINENCE

Lesions of the brain and spinal cord
Carcinoma of the bladder or prostate
Bladder stones
Hydronephrosis
Decreased bladder compliance
Detrusor-sphincter dyssynergia

Source: Adapted from Resnick.[44]

Table 12–5 CLINICAL EVALUATION OF THE INCONTINENT PATIENT

HISTORY
  Type (urge, reflex, stress, overflow, or mixed)
  Frequency, severity, duration
  Pattern (diurnal, nocturnal, or both; also, e.g., after taking medications)
  Associated symptoms (straining to void, incomplete emptying, dysuria, suprapubic discomfort)
  Alteration in bowel habit or sexual function
  Other relevant factors (cancer, diabetes, acute illness, neurologic disease, pelvic or lower urinary tract surgery)
  Medications, including nonprescription agents
  Functional assessment
PHYSICAL EXAMINATION
  Identify other medical conditions (e.g., congestive heart failure, peripheral edema)
  Test for stress-induced leakage when bladder is full
  Observe or listen to void
  Palpate for bladder distension after voiding
  Pelvic examination (atrophic vaginitis or urethritis; pelvic muscle laxity; pelvic mass)
  Rectal examination (resting tone and voluntary control of anal sphincter; prostate nodules; fecal impaction)
  Neurologic examination (mental status and elemental examination, including sacral reflexes and perineal sensation)
INITIAL INVESTIGATION
  Voiding-incontinence chart
  Metabolic survey (measurement of eletrolytes, calcium, glucose, and urea nitrogen)
  Measurement of postvoiding residual volume (PVR)
  Urinalysis and culture
  Renal ultrasound*
  Urine cytology*
  Uroflowmetry*
  Cystoscopy?*

*See text.
Source: Adapted from Resnick[44] and Resnick and Yalla.[47]

tolerated, and will detect most underlying pathology (Tables 12–4 and 12–5).

History

The first step is to characterize the voiding pattern and determine if symptoms of abnormal voiding are present, such as straining to void or a sense of incomplete emptying. One must be careful in eliciting these symptoms, however, because many patients strain at the end of voiding to empty the last few drops. On the other hand, many patients have been straining for so long that they fail to acknowledge it. Thus, additional observations by the physician and family members are extremely useful.

One then elicits a detailed description of the incontinence, focusing on its onset, frequency, severity, pattern, precipitants, palliating features, and associated symptoms and conditions. It is also helpful to know if the patient leaks at night. Generally, individuals with detrusor overactivity gush intermittently both day and night, while those with pure stress incontinence are usually dry at night because they are in the supine position and not straining. However, individuals with type 3 stress incontinence, especially those who also have a poorly compliant bladder, may leak only at night if they allow their bladder to fill to a volume greater than their weakened outlet can withstand. These individuals may admit to postural-related dribbling as well, leaking continually while sitting or standing.

Prostatism is another symptom complex worth additional comment. Regardless of whether the patient has "irritative" or "obstructive" symptoms, the physician can easily be misled. Several investigators have found that about one third of patients referred for prostatectomy are not obstructed.[3,16] Usually, the problem is an overactive detrusor, which, if unaccompanied by outlet obstruction, may be exacerbated by operative intervention.[1] Thus, symptoms are a clue to the diagnosis of obstruction, but are alone insufficiently specific to confirm it.

Voiding Record

One of the most helpful components of the history is the voiding record kept by the patient or caregiver. Recorded for a 48- to 72-hour period, these charts note the time of each void at 2-hour intervals. Many incontinence records have been proposed; a sample of ours is shown in Figure 12–2.

To record the volume voided at home, an individual can use a measuring cup, coffee can, pickle jar, or other large container. Information regarding the volume voided provides an index of functional bladder capacity and, together with the pattern of voiding and leakage, can be quite helpful in pointing to the cause of the leakage. For example, incontinence that occurs only between 8 A.M. and noon may be caused by a morning diuretic. If a chairfast man with congestive heart failure wets himself frequently at night but remains dry during a 4-hour daytime nap in his wheelchair, the problem is probably not prostatic enlargement but rather the postural diuresis associated with heart failure.[42] A patient may also void frequently because of polyuria due to a metabolic abnormality. One woman's chart showed a single episode of leakage each day, always at 1 A.M. Closer questioning revealed her regular use of a "nightcap" to induce sleep!

The information gathered from the history and voiding record permits symptomatic characterization of the incontinence as *urge*, in which precipitant leakage of a large volume is preceded by a brief warning of seconds to minutes; *reflex*, in which precipitant leakage is not preceded by a warning; *stress*, in which leakage occurs coincident with, and only in association with, increases in abdominal pressure; *overflow*, in which continual dribbling occurs; and *mixed*, which is usually a combination of urge and stress.[23] Each of these types correlates fairly well with the pathophysiologic mechanisms already mentioned: urge and reflex with detrusor overactivity; stress with an in-

Time	Wet/Dry	How wet? (mild, moderate, severe)	Volume voided	Comments
8:00	W	Severe	1 oz	On way to bathroom
10:00	D	——	4 oz	Voided before going out
12:00	D	——	——	
2:00	W	Moderate	5 oz	Abrupt urge—couldn't get to bathroom in time

Figure 12–2. Sample voiding/incontinence record. The chart is completed for 24 to 72 hours, with information recorded every 2 hours. Voiding habits should not be changed (i.e., the patient should not be told to void every 2 hours while obtaining this baseline data.) The physician should review the record with the patient as part of the clinical evaluation (see text). (Adapted from Resnick,[42] p 286.)

competent outlet; overflow with outlet obstruction or detrusor underactivity; and mixed with both an overactive detrusor and an incompetent outlet.

Targeted Physical Examination

The examination should check for signs of neurologic disease—such as delirium, dementia, stroke, PD, cord compression, and neuropathy (autonomic or peripheral)—as well as for functional impairment and general medical illnesses, such as heart failure and peripheral edema. Additionally, one should check for spinal column deformities or dimples suggestive of dysraphism, for bladder distention (pointing to an evacuation disorder), and stress leakage. Stress incontinence is assessed by asking the patient, whose bladder should be full, to assume a position as close to upright as possible, to relax, spread her legs, and cough. The diagnosis of stress incontinence can be missed if any of these maneuvers is omitted. If leakage occurs, it is also important to note whether it occurs coincident with the stress maneuver or is delayed for more than 5 to 10 seconds. If delayed, such leakage suggests detrusor overactivity (triggered by coughing) rather than outlet incompetence.

The rectal examination checks for fecal impaction and masses. The size of the prostate is less important to assess because, as determined by palpation, it correlates poorly with the presence or absence of outlet obstruction.[34,42] The remainder of the rectal examination is actually a detailed neurourologic examination since the same sacral roots (S-2 to S-4) innervate both the external urethral and the anal sphincters. With the finger in the rectum, one assesses motor innervation by asking the patient to volitionally contract and relax the anal sphincter. Since abdominal straining may mimic sphincter contraction, it is useful to place one's other hand on the patient's abdomen to check for this. Many neurologically unimpaired elderly patients are unable to volitionally contract their sphincter, but if they can it is strong evidence against a cord lesion. One can assess motor innervation further by testing the anal wink (S - 4 to S - 5) and bulbocavernosus reflexes (S - 2 to S - 4). In an older person, however, the absence of these reflexes is not necessarily pathologic, nor does their presence exclude an underactive detrusor (caused by a diabetic neuropathy, for example). Finally, afferent supply is assessed by testing perineal sensation.

In women, one should check for pelvic muscle laxity (cystocele, rectocele, enterocele, uterine prolapse). It is important to realize, however, that the presence or absence of pelvic floor laxity reveals little about the cause of an individual's leakage. Detrusor overactivity may exist in addition to a cystocele, and stress incontinence may exist in the absence of a cystocele. Thus, knowledge of pelvic muscle strength is useful primarily in informing the surgeon's choice of operation. The one exception to this statement occurs in the woman with a large cystocele: descent of the cystocele may kink the urethra and cause obstruction.

Atrophic vaginitis must also be sought. It is characterized by mucosal friability, petechiae, telangiectasia, and vaginal erosions[55]; loss of rugal folds and the presence of a thin, shiny-appearing mucosa are signs of vaginal atrophy rather than atrophic vaginitis. The bimanual examination excludes pelvic masses.

A final caveat: One should not check for stress leakage when the patient has a strong urge to void since the urge may be due to an uninhibited contraction. If the contraction is accompanied by physiologic sphincter relaxation and if the patient then coughs, she will leak instantaneously, prompting the physician to misdiagnose a detrusor abnormality as outlet incompetence. Finally, if stress testing provokes delayed leakage of a large amount, suggestive of detrusor overactivity, the patient should be asked to interrupt the stream. If she is able to do so, this probably augurs well for bladder retraining.

The examination concludes when the patient voids and is catheterized for a postvoiding residual volume (PVR). Adding the PVR to the voided volume provides an estimate of total bladder capacity and a crude assessment of bladder proprioception. A PVR above 50 to 100 mL suggests either bladder weakness or outlet obstruction, but smaller values do not exclude either diagnosis, especially if the patient strained to void. Thus, it is important to observe or listen to the voided stream. If straining is observed, one must ask the patient whether this is typical and take it into account when interpreting the PVR. Of note, relying on the ease of catheterization to establish the presence of obstruction can be misleading, since difficult catheter passage can be caused by urethral tortuosity, a "false passage," or catheter-induced spasm of the distal sphincter, while easy passage can be seen even in severely obstructed patients.[28]

Laboratory Investigation[44]

In addition to a urinalysis, urine culture, and PVR determination, one should measure the blood-urea-nitrogen (BUN) and serum creatinine. If the voiding record suggests polyuria, serum concentrations of glucose and calcium should be measured as well. In a man whose PVR exceeds 150 to 200 mL, renal sonography should be performed to exclude hydronephrosis. In any patient with suprapubic discomfort or sterile hematuria, or in a patient at high risk for bladder carcinoma (e.g., a male smoker), a urine cytology should be obtained. If positive, or if suprapubic discomfort is present, cystoscopy is warranted. In the remaining majority of patients, however, the role of cystoscopy remains to be determined; the roles of uroflowmetry and radiography are discussed later.

Although the literature is replete with statements and uncontrolled studies asserting that "the bladder is an unreliable witness" and that the clinical evaluation is an unreliable guide to the cause of incontinence, our experience differs. In a prospective and blinded study, we found that the clinical evaluation correctly predicted the urodynamically determined cause of leakage in over 90% of cases.[50] The discrepancy between our experience and that of others may arise because we do not rely on any single symptom or sign. Rather, we dissect each symptom for its full diagnostic significance, and we integrate information from the history with that from the voiding record, physical examination, observed void, and PVR determination. Furthermore, even in nursing home patients, an algorithmic approach—relying only on information obtainable at the bedside by a nurse—has yielded the correct diagnosis in 83% of cases and correctly guided treatment in 93%.[54] Therefore, although the specificity of a given symptom may be low, we believe that an informed, carefully performed, and comprehensive clinical evaluation can determine the cause of incontinence most of the time.

Urodynamic Testing

If the cause of the patient's incontinence still cannot be determined, urodynamic evaluation is the next step to consider. Although "bedside testing" has long been advocated,[38,61,63] its marginal utility is unknown for the 10% to 20% of patients whose diagnosis eludes clinical evaluation. Urodynamic testing is probably warranted when diagnostic uncertainty may affect therapy, when empiric therapy has failed and other approaches would be tried, when surgical intervention is planned, and to exclude obstruction that would be corrected in the patient with overflow incontinence.[47,53]

"Urodynamics" consists of a battery of tests. Generally, the evaluation includes the simultaneous measurement of bladder, urethral, and rectal pressures during the filling and emptying phases of the micturition cycle. Optimally, the study is fluoroscopically monitored, and periurethral electromyography may occasionally be required. Some of the more commonly used tests will be described.

CYSTOMETRY

Cystometry (CMG) evaluates bladder proprioception, compliance, capacity, and stability (regarding detrusor overactivity). It assesses only the bladder—not the outlet—and only during filling, not voiding. Therefore it yields only one fourth of the information needed to establish a diagnosis. It is performed by inserting a catheter into the bladder, filling it with gas or fluid, and plotting the bladder's pressure response to increasing volume. Artifacts are common, especially when investigating the elderly, but they can be minimized by having the test performed by a knowledgeable physician (not a technician), by infusing fluid rather than gas, by using moderate infusion rates rather than rapid ones (<100 mL/min), by using fluoroscopy, and by measuring abdominal and bladder pressures simultaneously to differentiate rises in bladder pressure from rises in abdominal pressure.

Uninhibited contractions are phasic bladder contractions and are usually seen easily. They may be missed, however, especially in patients in whom detrusor hyperactivity coexists with detrusor weakness (DHIC).[49] DHIC can be distinguished from obstruction by the use of pressure-flow studies and micturitional urethral profilometry (MUPP), as described later. If these tools are unavailable, however, the distinction can be quite difficult. We are currently devising ways to simplify the diagnosis of DHIC, examining the importance of the distinction, and exploring whether DHIC will exacerbate or simplify our ability to treat detrusor hyperreflexia.

URETHRAL PROFILOMETRY
(DURING FILLING AND VOIDING)

There are two types of profilometry, depending on whether urethral presure is measured during bladder filling or contraction. The first is urethral closure pressure profilometry (UCPP) and the second is MUPP. UCPP is performed by inserting a catheter into the bladder, slowly withdrawing it through the urethra, and plotting urethral pressure at each point.[56] Although there is a correlation between the presence of stress incontinence and both the strength of the sphincter and the length of the urethra, the values overlap considerably, reducing the utility of these parameters for the individual patient. Similarly, values obtained for prostatic length and area are of limited value. Nonetheless, UCPP is occasionally useful to test the bulbocavernosus reflex, and for fluid bridge testing; the latter is an extremely sensitive test for stress incontinence.[62,72]

Urethral profilometry is also used to exclude detrusor-sphincter dyssynergia. Generally, only the distal urethral sphincter is evaluated; normally it should relax just prior to, or coincident with, detrusor contraction. The response of the smooth muscle sphincter is more complex, and is reviewed elsewhere.[51]

The MUPP is quite useful for evaluating men,[71] especially those with PD, since bladder dysfunction in PD can closely mimic obstruction. The MUPP is performed by simultaneously measuring pressure in the bladder and along the urethra as the patient voids. In the setting of a urethral obstruction, the pressure distal to the obstruction will be lower than bladder pressure. If an obstruction is detected, fluoroscopy will usually localize the site. MUPP is more accurate than cystoscopy for determining the presence of an obstruction and judging its severity.

UROFLOWMETRY

Uroflowmetry is often used in men to screen for obstruction. However, although its sensitivity may increase with age, its specificity almost certainly declines. The flow rate depends not only on the presence of an outlet obstruction, but also on the strength of detrusor contraction. Although age-related norms have been devised to facilitate interpretation of the test, the studies on which they are based are flawed and included few patients over age 70.[43] Thus, the utility of isolated uroflowmetry in elderly men remains undefined. One can, however, derive some information from it. In the older man with symptoms of prostatism, a normal flow rate and a low PVR probably exclude clinically significant obstruction. On the other hand, when performed in conjunction with a full urodynamic evaluation, uroflowmetry is quite helpful in assessing detrusor contractility and detecting obstruction.

Electromyography[5]

Electromyography (EMG) evaluates the distal urethral sphincter by determining the integrity of its innervation, testing its response to reflex stimuli (such as bladder filling [guarding reflex] and bulbocavernosus stimulation); and characterizing its behavior during voiding. A variety of techniques are available for EMG, depending on whether one employs surface or needle electrodes, records the response of single or multiple nerve fibers, and evaluates the nerve supply to the urethral sphincter or the pelvic floor musculature (through vaginal, anal, or perineal probes). The most accurate technique is to insert a needle electrode directly into the distal urethral sphincter. Although most elderly patients can tolerate this, the results can be difficult to interpret (e.g., are a few polyphasic potentials in a 90-year-old really abnormal?), the equipment is expensive, and, if urodynamic testing is performed as already detailed, EMG adds little. If fluoroscopically monitored multichannel urodynamic capability is not available, however, EMG is useful. Unfortunately, in these situations only surface or anal EMG is usually performed. Since these techniques are fraught with artifact,

they should be interpreted with caution.

Radiographic Evaluation

Optimally, the radiographic and urodynamic evaluations are performed simultaneously, allowing correlation of visual and manometric information. If this is not feasible, substantial information can still be gleaned from cystography. A full evaluation includes posterior-anterior and oblique (or lateral) views of the bladder, at rest and during straining and voiding. These films check for bladder trabeculation, diverticula, masses, bladder neck competence, and ureteral reflux. Although the urethrovesical angle and axis are also generally measured, their reliability and relevance are controversial.[17] The voiding films allow one to check for outlet obstruction. Postvoiding residual volume can also be assessed radiographically, but there are pitfalls. Elderly patients are frequently rushed through busy radiography departments and may feel too inhibited to void to completion; the radiologist, who may have been absent during the examination may then erroneously conclude that the residual volume is elevated. Conversely, a low volume does not exclude a weak bladder if the patient augmented voiding by straining. Therefore, the radiographer should be viewed as a partner in the evaluation rather than being asked to read films blindly after the examination is completed.

The precise role of urodynamic testing in the evaluation of the incontinent elderly individual remains to be determined. Although it pinpoints pathologic abnormalities, unless it is performed by a trained urodynamicist and incorporated into the overall clinical evaluation, it may not identify which of the abnormalities actually causes the patient's incontinence.[53]

Whatever its role, however, urodynamic evaluation of elderly patients is reproducible, safe, and feasible to perform, even in frail and debilitated individuals. In our series of over 100 consecutively evaluated nursing home patients, whose mean age was 89 and all of whom received prophylactic antibiotics, we induced only three cases of asymptomatic bacteriuria; no cases of urosepsis, pyelonephritis, endocarditis, or cardiac ischemia were observed. All but two patients were able to complete the examination at one sitting, and the original diagnosis was confirmed in all 30 cases in which the examination was repeated. It must be emphasized, however, that an extra person was employed whose sole job was to explain the procedure and comfort the patient during the test. Several modifications in the urodynamic suite were made as well.[52]

THERAPY

Like the diagnostic approach, treatment must be individualized because factors outside the lower urinary tract are also important (Table 12–6). For instance, although both may have detrusor overactivity that can be managed successfully, a severely demented and bedfast patient will be treated differently from one who is ambulatory and cognitively intact. Thus, this section will suggest several treatments for each condition and try to provide some guidance for their use. It assumes that serious underlying conditions and transient causes of incontinence have already been excluded.

Detrusor Overactivity

Detrusor overactivity or hyperactivity is the generic term for uninhibited contractions. If they occur in the setting of an upper motor neuron lesion, the condition is termed detrusor hyperreflexia; in the absence of such a lesion the condition is termed detrusor instability. Regardless, detrusor overactivity is characterized by frequent but periodic voiding; the patient is generally dry in between. Leakage is moderate to large in volume, nocturnal frequency and incontinence are common, sacral sensation and reflexes are preserved, voluntary control of the anal sphincter is intact, and the postvoiding residual volume is generally low. A residual volume in excess of 50 mL in a patient with detrusor overactivity suggests outlet obstruction (although the residual may be nil in early obstruction), DHIC, or pooling of urine in a cystocele. It is also found in patients with PD or spinal cord injury.[49]

Initial management involves identification and treatment of reversible causes. Suspicion of a spinal cord disorder (an appropriate history and/or the finding of a dermatomal sensory "level") warrants a complete neurourologic evaluation. Sterile hematuria, if present, must be evaluated to exclude a bladder stone, carcinoma in situ, or carcinoma. Uroflowmetry, if available, can exclude important outlet obstruction, as described above.

It cannot be overemphasized that obstruction and stress incontinence may cause *secondary* detrusor overactivity that will remit with correction of the outlet abnormality.[2,32] Failure to evaluate the outlet may not only cause the patient harm (e.g., prescribing an anticholinergic agent to an obstructed patient) but will also lead to overlooking easily correctable incontinence. Obstruction and stress incontinence are common in the elderly, even frail and cognitively impaired individuals.[53] With recent medical and surgical advances, treatment of outlet abnormalities is now feasible even for these patients.[43,53] Thus evaluation of the outlet is critically important.

Unfortunately, however, many of the causes of detrusor overactivity are not amenable to specific therapy, or a cause may not be found. Treatment must then be symptomatic. Simple measures such as providing a bedside commode or urinal are often successful. Toileting regimens, based on analysis of the voiding record, are also beneficial, even in patients with advanced cognitive impairment.[10,22] For the demented patient,

Table 12–6 TREATMENT

Condition	Clinical Type of Incontinence	Treatment*
Detrusor hyperactivity with normal contractility (DH)	Urge	1. Bladder retraining or prompted voiding regimens 2. ± Bladder relaxant medication (anticholinergic, smooth muscle relaxant, calcium channel blocker), if not contraindicated 3. In selected cases, induce urinary retention pharmacologically and add intermittent or indwelling catheterization
Detrusor hyperactivity with impaired contractility (DHIC)	Urge§	1. If bladder empties adequately with straining, behavioral methods (as above) ± bladder relaxant medication (low doses) 2. If residual urine high (e.g., >150 mL), augmented voiding techniques† or intermittent catheterization ± bladder relaxant medication. If either is not feasible, undergarment or indwelling catheter may be used. UTI prophylaxis can be used for recurrent symptomatic UTIs if catheter is not indwelling.
Stress incontinence	Stress	1. Conservative methods (weight loss if obese; treatment of cough or atrophic vaginitis; and rarely, use of pessary/tampon) 2. Pelvic muscle exercises ± biofeedback 3. Imipramine (or doxeipn) or α-adrenergic agonists, if not contraindicated 4. Surgery
Urethral obstruction	Urge-overflow‡	1. Conservative methods (including adjustment of fluid intake, bladder retraining/prompted voiding ± bladder relaxants), if hydronephrosis, elevated residual urine, recurrent symptomatic UTI, and gross hematuria have been excluded 2. Bladder suppressants if DH coexists, PVR volume is small, and surgery is not desired or feasible 3. α-Adrenergic antagonists, if not contraindicated and if the patient prefers them or is not a surgical candidate 4. Surgery
Underactive detrusor	Overflow	1. If duration is unknown, decompress for several weeks and perform a voiding trial 2. If fails, or retention is chronic, try augmented voiding techniques ± α-adrenergic antagonist if any voiding possible 3. If fails, intermittent or indwelling catheterization 4. Bethanechol rarely if ever useful

*All patients should have adequate toilet access, contributing conditions treated (e.g., atrophic vaginitis, heart failure), and unnecessary medications stopped. For additional recommendations, details, and drug doses, see text.

†Augmented voiding techniques include Crede and Valsalva maneuvers and "double" voiding.

‡Also can cause postvoid "dribbling" alone, which is treated conservatively (e.g., sit to void and allow more time, "double void," gently "milk" the penile urethra after voiding).

§Also may mimic stress or overflow incontinence

the technique known as prompted voiding is used. One uses the voiding record to predict when leakage is likely to occur, and escorts the patient to the bathroom in advance. Positive reinforcement is employed, while negative reinforcement is avoided. A blinded controlled study conducted in two nursing homes found nearly a 50% decrease in incontinence within the first day of using the technique in this manner, a decrease that persisted as long as it was utilized.[57] In nondemented patients, techniques such as behavior modification permit the voiding interval to be progressively lengthened. For instance, if the incontinence chart reveals that the patient is wet every 3 hours, one asks the patient to void every 2 hours. Once the patient remains dry for 3 consecutive days using this regimen, the interval is lengthened by ½ hour, and the process is repeated. One need not ask patients to void at night; once they are dry during the day, they are generally dry at night as well. Biofeedback may be added to this regimen, but its marginal benefit is unclear.

The voiding record can be helpful in another way. For instance, as noted above, patterns of fluid excretion alter with age. If incontinence is worse at night and the chart discloses a nocturnal diuresis, incontinence can be ameliorated by altering the pattern of fluid intake or judiciously prescribing an evening diuretic; nocturnal use of an antidiuretic agent has proved less effective.[41,43] If noctural diuresis is due to peripheral edema in the absence of heart failure, a pressure-gradient stocking may avert fluid accumulation and the resultant nocturnal leakage. Another example is the patient with DHIC whose voiding record and PVR reveal that uninhibited contractions are provoked only at high volumes. By voiding every few hours during the day she may remain dry, but nocturnal leakage will persist, since functional bladder capacity is low. However, catheterization just before bedtime will remove the residual urine, and thereby increase bladder capacity and restore both continence and sleep. Significantly, in each of these cases pharmacologic suppression of detrusor contractions can be avoided.

Pharmacologic intervention can be added, but there is a dearth of data regarding efficacy and toxicity in this population, and comparative or controlled trials are rare.[43] Smooth muscle relaxants, such as flavoxate (300 to 800 mg/d) and calcium channel blockers have been used, as have anticholinergic agents such as propantheline (15 to 120 mg/d). Oxybutynin (5 to 20 mg/d), combining both smooth muscle relaxant and anticholinergic properties, and imipramine (25 to 100 mg/d), whose mechanism of action is more complex, are also frequently successful. So, too, is terodiline, a drug soon to be released in America, but extensively tested in Europe.[63a] All these drugs are given in divided doses. The decision regarding which drug to employ is often based on factors unrelated to bladder function.[43,47] In the incontinent patient with dementia or the patient taking other anticholinergic agents, propantheline is best avoided. In the patient with associated hypertension, angina pectoris, or abnormalities of cardiac diastolic relaxation, a calcium channel blocking agent may be preferred. Orthostatic hypotension often precludes the use of imipramine and nifedipine and should be watched for if these agents are used. Occasionally, combining low doses of two agents with complementary actions, such as oxybutynin and imipramine, will maximize benefit and minimize side effects. Medications with a rapid onset of action, such as oxybutynin, can be employed prophylactically if incontinence occurs at predictable times. But regardless of which medication is used, since urinary retention may develop, the PVR and common indexes of renal function (BUN, serum creatinine, and urine output) should be monitored, especially in DHIC where the detrusor is already weak. On the other hand, inducing urinary retention and using intermittent catheterization may be a viable approach for patients whose incontinence defies other remedies (such as those with DHIC) and for whom intermittent catheterization is feasible. Other remedies for urge incontinence, including electrical stimulation, bladder distension, and selective nerve blocks, are less widely used, although some are successful in selected situations.

Adjunctive measures, such as pads and special undergarments, are invaluable if incontinence proves refractory, and a wide variety of these are now available, allowing the recommendation to be tailored to the individual's problem. For instance, for bedridden individuals a launderable bedpad may be preferable,[8] while for those with a stroke, a diaper or pant that can be opened using the good hand may be preferred. For ambulatory patients with large gushes of incontinence, a wood-pulp-containing product is generally preferable to those containing a polymer gel, since the polymer gel generally cannot absorb the large amount and rapid flow these individuals produce, while the wood-pulp product can easily be doubled up if necessary. Optimal products for men and women also differ because of the location of the "target zone." Finally, one must know whether the patient has fecal incontinence as well, in order to choose the most appropriate product.[8,70]

Condom catheters are helpful for men, although they are associated with skin breakdown and, often, a decreased motivation to become dry. A satisfactory external collecting device has not yet been devised for women, especially for elderly women in whom the problem is further complicated by the high prevalence of atrophic vaginitis and vaginal stenosis. Indwelling urethral catheters are not recommended for this condition because they usually exacerbate detrusor overactivity. If they must be used (e.g., to allow healing of a pressure sore in a patient with refractory detrusor overactivity), a small catheter with a small balloon is preferable to minimize irritability and consequent "leakage around the catheter." Such leakage almost invariably results from bladder "spasm," not a catheter that is too small. Increasing the size of the catheter and balloon only aggravates the problem and, over time, may result in progressive urethral erosion and sphincter incompetence. If "bladder spasm" persists, agents such as oxybutynin can be employed. Especially in the elderly, alternative agents with more potent anticholinergic side effects (e.g., belladonna suppositories) should be avoided.

Stress Incontinence

Involuntary leakage that occurs only during stress is common in elderly women, but uncommon in men unless the sphincter has been damaged by surgery. The definition excludes overflow incontinence, which, although exacerbated by stress, occurs at other times as well and is associated with bladder distention. Typical stress incontinence is characterized by daytime loss of small to moderate amounts of urine, infrequent nocturnal incontinence, and a low postvoiding residual volume in the absence of urine pooling in a large cystocele. The sine qua non of the diagnosis is leakage that, in the absence of bladder distension, occurs coincident with the stress maneuver. The usual cause is "urethral hypermobility" due to pelvic floor laxity (Fig. 12–1), but other conditions must be considered. These include intrinsic "sphincter incompetence" (type 3 stress incontinence), stress-induced detrusor overactivity, and urethral instability.[6,30–32]

Sphincter incompetence (type 3 stress incontinence) was described earlier. One should realize that the term is actually a misnomer because if the weight of urine in the bladder exceeds the ability of the weakened sphincter to retain it, leakage can occur even when the patient sits quietly, a helpful diagnostic point.

Stress-induced detrusor instability is merely an uninhibited bladder contraction triggered by stress maneuvers. These uninhibited contractions usually occur at other times as well, giving rise to urgency, frequency, nocturia, urge incontinence, and nocturnal incontinence. The key point is to assess the integrity of the outlet as described earlier. If it is competent, then the problem is detrusor-mediated and should be treated as detrusor overactivity. If the outlet is incompetent, then the patient has either stress incontinence or mixed incontinence (discussed later) and should be treated as such.

Urethral instability occurs when the sphincter abruptly and paradoxically relaxes in the absence of a detrusor contraction. In our experience this condition is rare in the elderly. In fact, it may be less common than believed in younger individuals as well, since most investigators have failed to use fluoroscopic monitoring. This omission may lead one to miss an uninhibited contraction (DHIC) and mistakenly identify the accompanying physiologic sphincter relaxation as a pathologic sphincter abnormality.[49,53]

The most common cause of stress incontinence, however, is urethral hypermobility, which is improved by weight loss if the patient is obese, by therapy of precipitating conditions such as coughing or atrophic vaginitis, and occasionally by insertion of a pessary.[4] Pelvic floor muscle exercises are time-honored and frequently effective.[22,43,68] The patient is instructed to sit on the toilet and begin voiding. Once voiding has started, she is asked to interrupt the stream by contracting the sphincter for as long as possible. Initially, most elderly women are able to do so for no more than a second or two, but after a few weeks, many can prolong the duration of the contraction. Once she recognizes which muscle to contract, she can do the exercises at any time and during any activity. The optimal regimen remains to be determined. We advise patients to increase the duration of muscle contraction to about 10 seconds, to contract the muscle as many as 15 times per set, and to complete three to four sets per day. When the patient is able to comply, the exercises are extremely efficacious. However, many older women are unable or unmotivated to follow this regimen. If so, we contact them more frequently or add biofeedback, if available. If not contraindicated by other medical conditions, treatment with an α-adrenergic agonist such as phenylpropanolamine (50 to 100 mg/d in divided doses) may be added and is often beneficial for women, especially when administered with estrogen. In fact, these two agents work for women with sphincter incompetence as well. Phenylpropanolamine is inexpensive, available without a prescription, and contained in many "diet pills." However, the physician should prescribe the dose and guide the choice of preparation, since some capsules contain additional agents such as chlorpheniramine in doses that can be troublesome for elderly patients. Imipramine, with beneficial effects on the bladder and the outlet, is a reasonable alternative for patients with evidence of both stress and urge incontinence if postural hypotension has been excluded.

If these methods fail, further evaluation of the lower urinary tract may be warranted. If urethral hypermobility is confirmed, surgical correction may be performed and is successful in the majority of selected elderly patients.[43] If sphincter incompetence is diagnosed instead, it too can be corrected, but a different surgical approach is often required, morbidity is higher, and precipitation of chronic urinary retention is more likely than with correction of urethral hypermobility.[6,43] Other treatments for sphincter incompetence include periurethral injection of Teflon or collagen and insertion of an artificial sphincter, all of which are effective in selected cases.[43]

If all other interventions fail, prostheses such as condom catheters or penile clamps may be useful for men, but most such prostheses require substantial cognitive capacity and manual dexterity, and are often poorly tolerated. An alternative product for men is a penile sheath, such as the McGuire prosthesis (similar to an athletic supporter) or the self-adhesive sheath produced by several manufacturers, especially if it is lined with a polymer gel or cellulose. Unfortunately, no similar satisfactory prostheses are available for elderly women. As discussed above, pads and undergarments are employed as adjunctive measures, but in these cases, thin, superabsorbent polymer gel pads are frequently successful because the gel can more readily absorb the smaller amount of leakage. Some products (e.g., Tranquility) consist of pads that can actually be flushed down the toilet, which is quite convenient for ambulatory women. Electrical stimulation is promising, whether applied rectally or vaginally, but is still investigational.[43]

OUTLET OBSTRUCTION

Outlet obstruction is the cause of incontinence in up to 5% of elderly women.[43,53] As noted earlier, the etiology is usually a large cystocele that distorts or kinks the urethra during voiding.[43] Other causes of obstruction include bladder stones and bladder neck obstruction, which are rare, and distal urethral stenosis, which may afflict as many as 2% to 3% of incontinent women.[53] If a large cystocele is the problem, surgical correction is usually required and should include an outlet suspension if urethral hypermobility is also present. Prior urodynamic evaluation is helpful as well: If bladder neck incompetence or low urethral closure pressure ($<20\,cmH_2O$) is observed, a different surgical approach may be required to avoid converting incontinence due to obstruction into incontinence due to sphincteric incompetence. Bladder neck obstruction is also corrected easily, using local anesthesia, and is thus feasible for even the frailest elderly patient. Distal urethral stenosis can be dilated and treated with estrogen. If meatal stenosis is present, more extensive intervention may be necessary; alternatively, dilation can be repeated at fairly frequent intervals. It should be noted that many women who undergo dilation do not have urethral stenosis but rather an underactive detrusor; for these women, dilation is usually unhelpful and may be harmful.

In men, the cause of obstruction is usually a stricture, carcinoma, or prostatic enlargement. As noted above, neither the size of the prostate nor a past history of prostatectomy correlates well with obstruction since estimates of prostatic size are unreliable[34] and following a prostatectomy the patient may have a bladder neck contracture or stricture. Although transurethral resection prostatectomy (TURP), or even suprapubic or retropubic prostatectomy, is optimal and feasible for the elderly,[33] newer approaches (e.g., bladder neck incision with bilateral prostatotomy)[35,43] have made surgical decompression feasible for even the frailest individuals. These procedures, as well as a TURP in some instances,[60] can be done with local anesthesia and can be completed in less than 30 minutes of operating time. Unlike the TURP and open resections, these newer procedures do not fully resolve the problem, but in frail elderly individuals recrudescence of obstruction 2 to 3 years later may not be an issue.

Another new approach to the obstructed individual involves administration of α-adrenergic antagonists, such as prazosin or phenoxybenzamine. Numerous double-blind placebo-controlled trials have documented the symptomatic efficacy of these agents, and in some trials postvoiding residual volume, outlet resistance, and urinary flow rate have improved as well.[11] Phenoxybenzamine in adequate doses (5 to 20 mg/d) is probably superior to prazosin (1 to 2 mg two to four times a day), but concern about its carcinogenic potential in mice has mitigated against its use. Neither agent is a panacea for outlet obstruction. Rather, each allows the physician to treat the problem symptomatically until more definitive therapy is necessary and feasible.

UNDERACTIVE DETRUSOR

Incontinence due to an underactive detrusor is associated with a large PVR and overflow incontinence. Leakage of small amounts of urine occurs frequently throughout the day and night. The patient may also notice hesitancy, diminished and interrupted flow, a need to strain to void, and a sense of incomplete emptying. If the problem is neurologically mediated, perineal sensation, sacral reflexes, and control of the anal sphincter are frequently impaired. Before this entity can be diagnosed, one must first exclude outlet obstruction.

Management of detrusor underactivity is directed at reducing the residual volume, eliminating hydronephrosis (if present), and preventing urosepsis. The first step is to use indwelling or intermittent catheterization to decompress the bladder for up to 1 month (at least 7 to 14 days), while reversing potential contributors to impaired detrusor function (fecal impaction and medications). If this does not restore bladder function, once obstruction has been excluded, augmented voiding techniques (such as double voiding and implementation of the Crede or Valsalva maneuver) may help if the patient is able to initiate a detrusor contraction. An alpha blocker such as prazosin may further facilitate emptying by reducing outlet resistance. Bethanechol (40 to 200 mg/d in divided doses) is occasionally useful in a patient whose bladder contracts poorly because of treatment with anticholinergic agents that cannot be discontinued (e.g., neuroleptic agents). In other patients, bethanechol may decrease the PVR if sphincter function and local innervation are normal, but evidence for its efficacy is equivocal[15,18] and residual volume should be monitored to assess its effect.

On the other hand, if after decompression the detrusor is acontractile, these interventions are apt to be fruitless, and the patients should be started on intermittent catheterization or an indwelling urethral catheter. Intermittent self-catheterization is preferable and requires only clean, rather than sterile, catheter insertion. The individual can purchase two or three of these catheters inexpensively. One or two are used during the day and another is kept at home. Men can carry their catheter in a coat pocket, and woman can carry theirs in a purse (the catheter used for females is only a few inches long). The catheters are cleaned daily, allowed to air dry at night, sterilized periodically, and may be reused repeatedly. Prophylaxis against urinary tract infection is probably warranted if the individual gets more than an occasional infection or has an abnormal heart valve. Intermittent catheterization is painless, safe, inexpensive, and effective, and allows individuals to carry on with their usual daily activities.

Unfortunately, despite the benefits and proven feasibility of intermittent catheterization, most elderly individuals choose indwelling catheterization instead. Complications of chronic indwelling catheterization include bladder and urethral erosions, bladder stones, and bladder cancer, as well as urosepsis. There is still no consensus regarding the optimal composition of the catheter or the best time to change it, but several points should be mentioned. First, asymptomatic bacteriuria is ubiquitous in the chronically catheterized individual.[66,67] It is pointless to treat these asymptomatic infections, since all one does is replace one organism with a more virulent one; symptomatic infections, on the other hand, should be treated. Second, recent studies have revealed that organisms colonizing catheter encrustations may be unrelated to the organism causing a given bladder infection.[21] For this reason, before treating a symptomatic infection, one should pull the old catheter and obtain a culture from a newly inserted one. Third, the use of mandelamine for the chronically catheterized patient is useless, both theoretically and in practice. Mandelamine is inert unless activated, a process that takes at least 60 to 90 minutes in acidic urine. Because urine in the catheterized patient remains in the bladder for only a few minutes, mandelamine will do nothing to sterilize it.

When indicated, indwelling catheters can be extremely effective, but their use should be restricted. They are indicated in the acutely ill patient to monitor fluid balance, in the patient with a nonhealing pressure sore, and in the patient with overflow incontinence refractory to other measures. Even in long-term care facilities, they probably should not be used in more than 1% or 2% of patients.[43]

MIXED INCONTINENCE

Especially in the elderly, more than one type of incontinence may be present. For example, urge incontinence may develop in a woman with a history of stress incontinence. Such mixed incontinence differs from stress-induced detrusor overactivity; in the latter only detrusor overactivity is present, whereas in the former both detrusor overactivity and impaired outlet integrity are present. Urodynamic evaluation is frequently helpful in such cases because it can help the physician decide which is the predominant lesion and target therapy more effectively.

CONCLUSION

Incontinence is a common, morbid, and costly condition that has been neglected too long. While the approach to it can be time consuming, it can also challenge one's diagnostic and therapeutic skills, and its successful treatment can be tremendously gratifying to patient, caregiver, and clinician alike.

The approach to the incontinent elderly patient should be stepped. Transient causes and serious underlying pathology should be excluded, and contributing factors identified and pursued. If incontinence persists, the clinician must weigh the risks and benefits of empiric therapy against those of further investigation. While urodynamic investigation will probably be necessary in only the minority of cases, when it is indicated it can be done safely, and it can be extremely helpful if conducted by an experienced urodynamicist. In sum, if the clinician is prepared to devote patience, skill, and compassion to the problem, most incontinent patients can be helped.

REFERENCES

1. Abrams, PH: Prostatism and prostatectomy: The role of urine flow rate measurement in the preoperative assessment for operation. J Urol 117:70–71, 1977.
2. Abrams, PH: Detrusor instability and bladder outlet obstruction. Neurourol Urodynam 4:317–328, 1985.
3. Abrams, PH and Feneley, RCL: The significance of the symptoms associated with bladder outflow obstruction. Urol Int 33:171–174, 1978.
4. Bhatia, NN, Bergman, A, and Gunning, JE: Urodynamic effects of a vaginal pessary in women with stress urinary incontinence. Am J Obstet Gynecol 147:876–844, 1983.
5. Blaivas, JG: Sphincter electromyography. Neurourol Urodynam 2:269–288, 1983.
6. Blaivas, JG, and Olsson, CA: Stress incontinence: Classification and surgical approach. J Urol 139:727–731, 1988.
7. Boscia, JA, Kobasa, WD, Abrutyn, E, Levinson, ME, Kaplan, AM, and Kaye, D: Lack of association between bacteriuria and symptoms in the elderly. Am J Med 81:979–982, 1986.
7a. Brandeis, GH, Baumann, MM, Yalla, SV, Resnick, NM: Detrusor hyperactivity with impaired contractility: The great mimic. J Urology 143:223A, 1990.
8. Brink, CA and Wells, TJ: Environmental support for incontinence: Toilets, toilet supplements, and external equipment. Clin Geriatr Med 2:829–840, 1986.
9. Brocklehurst, JC, Andrews, K, Richards B, and Laycock, PJ: Incidence and correlates of incontinence in stroke patients. J Am Geriatr Soc 33:540–542, 1985.
10. Burgio, KL and Burgio, LD: Behavior therapies for urinary incontinence in the elderly. Clin Geriatr Med 2:809–827, 1986.

11. Caine, M: The present role of alpha-adrenergic blockers in the treatment of benign prostatic hypertrophy. J Urol 136:1–4, 1986.

12. Castleden, CM, Duffin, HM, Asher, MJ, and Yeomanson, CW: Factors influencing outcome in elderly patients with urinary incontinence and detrusor instability. Age Ageing 14:303–307, 1985.

13. Chetkowski, RJ, Meldrum, DR, Steingold, KA, Randle, D, Lu, JK, Eggena, P, Hershman, JM, Alkjaersig, NK, Fletcher, AP, and Judd, HL: Biologic effects of transdermal estradiol. N Engl J Med 314:1615–1620, 1986.

14. Diokno, AC, Brown, MB, Brock, BM, Herzog, AR, and Normolle, DP: Clinical and cystometric characteristics of continent and incontinent noninstitutionalized elderly. J Urol 140:567–571, 1988.

15. Downie, JW: Bethanechol chloride in urology—A discussion of issues. Neurourol Urodynam 3:211–222, 1984.

16. Eastwood, HDH: Urodynamic studies in the management of urinary incontinence in the elderly. Age Ageing 8:41–48, 1979.

17. Fantl, JA, Beachley, MC, Bosch, HA, Konerding, KF, and Smith, PJ: Bead-chain cytourethrogram: An evaluation. Obstet Gynecol 58:237–240, 1981.

18. Finkbeiner, A: Is bethanechol chloride clinically effective in promoting bladder emptying? A literature review. J Urol 134:443–449, 1985.

19. Fossberg, E, Sander, S, and Beisland, HO: Urinary incontinence in the elderly: A pilot study. Scand J Urol Nephrol (Suppl)60:51–53, 1981.

20. Goldsmith, MF: Research on aging burgeons as more Americans grow older. JAMA 253:1369–1405, 1985.

21. Grahn, D, Norman, DC, White, ML, Cantrell, M, and Yoshikawa, T: Validity of urinary catheter specimen for diagnosis of urinary tract infection in the elderly. Arch Int Med 145:1858–1860, 1985.

22. Hadley, E: Bladder training and related therapies for urinary incontinence in elderly people. JAMA 256:372–379, 1986.

23. Hald, T, Bates, P, and Bradley, WE: The Standardisation of Terminology of Lower Urinary Tract Function. Glasgow: International Continence Society, 1984, pp 1–34.

24. Hellstrom, PM and Sjoqvist, A: Involvement of opioid and nicotinic receptors in rectal and anal reflex inhibition of urinary bladder motility in cats. Acta Physiol Scand 133:559–562, 1988.

25. Herzog, AR, Diokno, AC, and Fultz, NH: Urinary incontinence: Medical and psychosocial aspects. Annu Rev Geriatr Gerontol 9:74–119, 1989.

26. Hu, T: The economic impact of urinary incontinence. Clin Geriatr Med 2(4):673–687, 1986.

27. Jensen, J, Riis, BJ, Strom, V, Nilas, L, and Christiansen, C: Long-term effects of percutaneous estrogens and oral progesterone on serum lipoproteins in postmenopausal women. Am J Obstet Gynecol 156:66–71, 1987.

28. Klarskov, P, Andersen, JT, and Asmussen, CF: Symptoms and signs predictive of the voiding pattern after acute urinary retention in men. Scand J Urol Nephrol 21:23–28, 1987.

29. Matthew, TH, McEwen, J, and Rohan, A: Urinary incontinence secondary to prazosin. Med J Aust 148:305–306, 1988.

30. McGuire, EJ: Reflex urethral instability. Br J Urol 50:200–204, 1978.

31. McGuire, EJ, Lytton, B, Pepe, V, and Kohorn, EI: Stress urinary incontinence. Obstet Gynecol 47:255–264, 1976.

32. McGuire, EJ and Savastano, JA: Stress incontinence and detrusor instability/urge incontinence. Neurourol Urodynam 4:313–316, 1985.

33. Mebust, WK, Holtgrewe, HL, Cockett, ATK, Peters, PC, and Writing Committee: Transurethral prostatectomy: Immediate and postoperative complications: A cooperative study of 13 participating institutions evaluating 3,885 patients. J Urol 141:243–247, 1989.

34. Meyhoff, HH, Ingemann, L, Nordling, J, and Hald, T: Accuracy in preoperative estimation of prostatic size. Scand J Urol Nephrol 15:45–51, 1981.

35. Orandi, A: Transurethral incision of prostate (TUIP): 646 cases in 15 years—A chronological appraisal. Br J Urol 57:703–707, 1985.

36. Ory, MG, Wyman, JF, and Yu, L: Psychosocial factors in urinary incontinence. Clin Geriatr Med 2:657–671, 1986.

37. Ouslander, JG, Kane, RL, and Abrass, IB: Urinary incontinence in elderly nursing home patients. JAMA 248:1194–1198, 1982.

38. Ouslander, JG, Leach, G, Abelson, S, Staskin, D, Blaustein, J, and Raz, S: Simple versus multichannel cystometry in the evaluation of bladder function in an incontinent geriatric population. J Urol 140:1482–1486, 1988.

39. Overstall, PW, Rounce, K, and Palmer, JH: Experience with an incontinence clinic. J Am Geriatr Soc 28:535–538, 1980.

40. Pannill, FC, III, WIlliams, TF, and David, R: Evaluation and treatment of urinary incontinence in long-term care. J Am Geriatr Soc 36:902–910, 1988.

41. Pedersen, PA and Johansen, PB: Prophylatic treatment of adult nocturia with bumetanide. Br J Urol 62:145–147, 1988.

42. Resnick, NM: Urinary incontinence in the elderly. Med Grand Rounds 3:281–290, 1984.

43. Resnick, NM: Voiding Dysfunction in the Elderly. In Yalla, SV, McGuire, EJ, Elbadawi, A, and Blaivas, JG (eds): Neurourology and Urodynamics: Principles and Practice. Macmillan, New York, 1988, pp 303–330.

43a. Resnick, NM: Urinary Incontinence— A Treatable Disorder. In Rowe, JW and Besdine, RW (eds): Geriatric Medicine, ed 2. Little, Brown, and Co, Boston, 1988, pp 246–265.

44. Resnick, NM: The initial evaluation of the incontinent patient. J Am Geriatr Soc 38:311–316, 1990.

45. Resnick, NM and Paillard, M: Natural History of Nosocomial Incontinence: Proceedings of the 14th Annual Meeting, International Continence Society, Innsbruck, 1984, pp 471–472.

46. Resnick, NM, Wetle, TT, Scherr, P, Branch, L, and Taylor, J: Urinary Incontinence in Community-Dwelling Elderly: Prevalence and Correlates: Proceedings of the 16th Annual Meeting, International Continence Society, Boston, 1986, pp 76–78.

47. Resnick, NM and Yalla, SV: Management of urinary incontinence in the elderly. N Engl J Med 313:800–805, 1985.

48. Resnick, NM and Yalla, SV: Aging and its effect on the bladder. Semin Urol 5:82–86, 1987.

49. Resnick, NM and Yalla, SV: Detrusor hyperactivity with impaired contractile function: An unrecognized but common cause of incontinence in elderly patients. JAMA 257:3076–3081, 1987.

50. Resnick, NM and Yalla, SV: The bladder is a "reliable witness": A prospective, blinded study (abst). J Urol 141(412): 575A, 1989.

51. Resnick, NM and Yalla, SV: Initiation of voiding in human subjects: The temporal relationship and nature of urethral sphincter responses, submitted.

52. Resnick, NM, Yalla, SV, and Laurino, E: Feasibility, safety, and reproducibility of urodynamics in the elderly. J Urol 137(4/2):189A, 1987.

53. Resnick, NM, Yalla, SV, and Laurino, E: The pathophysiology and clinical correlates of established urinary incontinence in frail elderly. N Engl J Med 320:1–7, 1989.

54. Resnick, NM, Yalla, SV, Laurino, E, and Prout, V: Evaluation of a clinical algorithm to identify the cause of incontinence in the elderly. J Urol 135:168A, 1986.

55. Robinson, JM: Evaluation of Methods for Assessment of Bladder and Urethral Function: In Brocklehurst, JC (ed): Urology in the Elderly. Churchill Livingstone, New York, 1984, pp 19–54.

56. Schmidt, RR, Witherow, R, and Tanagho, E: Recording urethral pressure profile: Comparison of methods and clinical implications. Urology 10:390–397, 1977.

57. Schnelle, JF, Traughber, B, Morgan, DB, Embry, JE, Binion, AF, and Coleman, A: Management of geriatric incontinence in nursing homes. J Appl Behav Anal 16:235–241, 1983.

58. Semmens, JP, Tsai, CC, Semmens, EC, and Loadholt, CB: Effects of estrogen therapy on vaginal physiology during menopause. Obstet Gynecol 66:15–18, 1985.

59. Sier, H, Ouslander, J, and Orzeck, S: Urinary incontinence among geriatric patients in an acute-care hospital. JAMA 257:1767–1771, 1987.

60. Sinha, B, Haikelm, G, Langem, PH, Moonm, TD, and Narayan, P: Transurethral resection of the prostate with local anesthesia in 100 patients. J Urol 135:719–721, 1986.

61. Stamey, TA: Endoscopic suspension of the vesical neck for urinary incontinence in females. Ann Surg 192:465–471, 1980.

62. Sutherst, JR and Brown, MC: Detection of urethral incompetence in women using the fluid bridge test. Br J Urol 52:138–142, 1980.

63. Sutherst, JR and Brown, MC: Comparison of single and multichannel cystometry in diagnosing bladder instability. Br Med J 288:1720–1722, 1984.

63a. Tapp, A, Fall, M, Norgaard, J, Massey, A, Choa, R, Carr, T, Korhonen, M and Abrams, P: Terodiline: A dose-titrated, multicenter study of the treatment of idiopathic detrusor instability in women. J Urol 142:1027–1031, 1989.

64. Tobin, GW and Brocklehurst, JC: The management of urinary incontinence in local authority residential homes for the elderly. Age Ageing 15:292–298, 1986.

65. Torrens, M and Morrison, JFB (eds): The Physiology of the Lower Urinary Tract. Springer-Verlag, New York, 1987.

66. Warren, JW: Urine collection devices for use in adults with urinary incontinence. J Am Geriatr Soc, 38:364–367, 1990.

67. Warren, JW, Muncie, HL, Bergquist, EJ, and Hoopes, JM: Sequelae and management of urinary infection in the patient requiring chronic catheterization. J Urol 125:1–8, 1981.

68. Wells, TJ: Pelvic (floor) muscle exercises. J Am Geriatr Soc 38:333–337, 1989.

69. Wheeler, JS, Siroky, MB, Bell, R, and Babayan, RK: Vincristine-induced bladder neuropathy. J Urol 130:342–343, 1983.

70. Willington, FL: Problems in urinary incontinence in the aged. Gerontol Clin 11:330–365, 1969.

71. Yalla, SV and Resnick, NM: Vesicourethral static pressure profile during voiding: Methodology and clinical utility. World J Urol 1984; 2:196–202.

72. Yalla, SV, Finn, D, and DeFelippo, N: Fluid bridge test in the evaluation of male urinary continence. J Urol 128:1241–1245, 1982.

73. Yarnell, JWG and St Leger, AS: The prevalence, severity, and factors associated with urinary incontinence in a random sample of the elderly. Age Ageing 8:81–85, 1979.

Chapter 13

THE NEUROLOGIC CONSULTATION AT AGE 80. II: SOME SPECIFIC DISORDERS OBSERVED IN THE ELDERLY

Leslie Wolfson, M.D., and Robert Katzman, M.D.

In this third section of our book, we have considered a number of special issues in geriatric neurology. Separate chapters have been devoted to Alzheimer disease (AD), the diagnosis and management of dementia, delirium, syncope, gait disturbances, and incontinence. Neuropathies of aging are considered in regard to the gait disturbances produced. In this chapter, several disorders not covered in prior chapters, but frequently observed in the neurologic consultation of the 80-year-old, are discussed.

STROKE AND AGING

Stroke is a major cause of disability and death among the elderly. The death rate, incidence, and prevalence of stroke all rise exponentially with age. Thus, stroke is an age-dependent disorder according to the strict definition described in Chapter 1.

In the US Vital Statistics tables of age-specific mortality, data by 5-year age groups are available for all cerebral vascular disease and for four subheadings: hemorrhage, thrombosis, embolism, and "other or late consequences of stroke." The death rate for cerebral thrombosis is a sharply rising semilogarithmic function of age (Fig. 13–1). The death rate data for cerebral hemorrhage, however, are not a simple exponential function of age; rather it rises steeply to about age 45, then continues on a gentler slope. The rapid rise at younger age groups primarily reflects the deaths due to subarachnoid hemorrhage, the latter slope primarily intracerebral hemorrhage. As a consequence, at age 50, the death rate due to cerebral hemorrhage is four times that

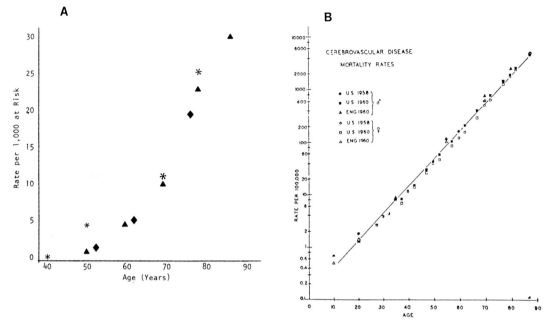

Figure 13–1. *A*, Stroke as a function of age. The symbols represent data from three studies. *B*, Semilog plot of mortality rates from stroke. (From Katzman, R and Terry, R [eds]: The Neurology of Aging, FA Davis, Philadelphia, 1985, p 9, with permission; and Kurtzke,[47] p 156, with permission.)

of cerebral thrombosis; at age 85, the death rate due to cerebral hemorrhage is one third that of cerebral thrombosis.

During the past 20 years there has been a remarkable decrease in the death rate due to strokes. Thus, the US death rate per 100,000 population for all types of cerebrovascular disorders has fallen from 101.9 in 1970 to 62.1 in 1986. The figure is more dramatic if the US Vital Statistics age-adjusted mortality figure is used; this figure recalculates the death rate based on the age distribution of the US population in 1940. These age-adjusted figures have fallen from 76.3 (per 100,000 total population) in 1963 to 66.3 in 1970 to 31.0 in 1986. The most dramatic decrease has been in the death rate from intracerebral hemorrhage, which has fallen 60% since 1970 and 89% since 1950. The cerebral thrombosis death rate actually rose from 1950 to 1970 but has since fallen to one third of the 1970 rate, one half of the 1950 rate.

Presumably, this reduction in the death rate has been in large part due to the improvement in the treatment of

hypertension, one of the major risk factors for stroke. The stroke rate is particularly high in countries such as Japan and Finland and in the United States among blacks. All three populations have excess hypertension; all three are noted for increased salt consumption. In the Framingham Study, stroke was related primarily to systolic hypertension. Other major risk factors for stroke include age, diabetes, transient ischemic attack (TIA), and prior stroke. Stroke is 30% more common in men than in women at younger ages, but the gender difference narrows at advanced ages. Auricular fibrillation, smoking, hypercholesterolemia, and elevated hematocrit are other important risk factors that have been found in epidemiologic studies.

It is not clear, however, whether these risk factors retain their importance in those who have survived without stroke to age 80. Thus, a history of hypertension only modestly elevated stroke rates in the Bronx Aging Study[43] subjects, whereas diabetes was a much more significant risk factor. Further data in regard to risk factors at advanced ages are urgently needed.

It has been surprising therefore that recent reports from the Framingham and other studies indicate that the incidence of new cases of stroke has not changed significantly over the past 20 years. Indeed, in our own experience the incidence of 2.0% per year in an 80-year-old cohort in the Bronx is not dissimilar from the 80-year-old incidence rates published during prior decades.[47] In part this discrepancy has occurred during a period in which no effective treatment for stroke per se had been developed and may reflect three factors: (1) improved survival due to improved treatment of coincident complications such as pneumonia and arrhythmias; (2) a decrease in the number of large life-threatening strokes and an increase in lacunes among hypertensive individuals whose life has been prolonged by treatment of the hypertension; (3) and the improved ability to diagnose small strokes such as lacunes based on improved clinical criteria and the use of high-resolution computed tomography (CT) imaging or magnetic resonance imaging (MRI). The National Institutes of Health (NIH) stroke data bank suggests that lacunes are now more common than large-vessel strokes. Lacunar strokes and their relationship to Binswanger disease and vascular dementia have been discussed in Chapter 8 and their relationship to gait disturbances has been discussed in Chapter 10.

An additional factor that must be considered in regard to the reduction in life-threatening strokes during the past 15 years is the possibility that the development of comparatively safe carotid endarterectomies in patients with TIAs has played a role; the number of such endarterectomies in the United States each year is sufficient to have had an impact on stroke mortality, although there is still controversy as to the value of this procedure in averting thrombotic strokes. It should be noted that the rate of carotid endarterectomies began to decline in 1986 and is now at the lowest rate since 1981. Meanwhile, as noted earlier, stroke incidence has been reported to be increasing in 1988.

Although the treatment of predisposing conditions has had a major impact on the occurrence of major stroke and stroke death, the treatment of stroke, once the pathologic process has begun, has been frustrating. Attempts to abort developing thrombotic strokes by administration of heparin to prevent further clot formation have been largely fruitless. Treatment of the edema that occurs in some very large strokes by use of hyperosmotic agents or steroids has not had the success accorded treatment of edema secondary to tumors.[44] It has only been with the recent introduction of tissue plasminogen activator (TPA), the recombinant form of the natural factor that dissolves thrombin clots, that there has been the possibility of an effective treatment. If administered within the first few hours, TPA has the ability to dissolve the clot rapidly in both animals and humans, thereby permitting re-establishment of perfusion. In experimental models, hemorrhage has not been an important complication. The clinical efficacy and safety of TPA in the treatment of stroke is now in clinical trial. In addition, other experimental drugs including calcium channel blockers and N-methyl-D-aspartate (NMDA) receptor antagonists have proved to be effective in limiting brain damage in animal models of experimental stroke. Calcium channel blockers have already been used in clinical trials, but the data are inconclusive. If safety problems can be overcome, NMDA receptor antagonists will enter clinical trials in patients; the latter could represent the first set of drugs that can alter the evolution of a stroke and the size of the subsequent infarct.

In this regard, the pathogenesis of the evolution of a thrombotic stroke needs to be reviewed. Thirty years ago one assumed that, if a region of the brain were totally deprived of oxygen and glucose supply, the region would die (become infarcted) within a few minutes. During the 1960s and 1970s, experimental and clinical data altered this concept. Biochemical and electron microscopic studies of evolving experimental strokes demonstrated the long delay before one could demonstrate changes in structural elements after ischemia. In total brain ischemia experiments, it was found that part of the damage occurred on reperfusion, and if this were limited, the animal brain was partially functional after 30 to 60 minutes of total ischemia. Swelling of the brain after experimental occlusion of the middle cerebral artery was found to begin intracellularly after several hours and then be followed after many hours by extracellular edema. This was paralleled by observations on radioisotope brain scans and CT scans in which it was found that infarcts usually could not be detected for 12 or more hours, with the full extent of extracellular edema being expressed after several days. Regional xenon studies in patients demonstrated the rather considerable area of partial blood flow around a smaller core of absent blood flow following occlusion of large vessels. These latter data were presumably due to collateral blood flow. Altogether, the experimental and clinical findings suggested that it might be possible to institute treatment to limit brain damage. Attempts to use hypothermia or barbiturate anaesthesia during the first several days after stroke onset were disappointing. The rationale for the use of the NMDA receptor antagonists developed after it was found that certain neuronal toxic substances such as kainate and quisqualate acted on the glutamic acid receptor. The concept of excitotoxicity then arose and in turn led to experiments that demonstrate a protective effect during ischemia of NMDA receptor antagonists.

The basic mechanisms of stroke are the same in younger and older individuals. There are, however, some differences in clinical presentation, at least in regard to dominant-hemisphere strokes that produce aphasia. It has been consistently found that nonfluent aphasics, with lesions presumed to be in the Broca area within the frontal lobe, are younger than patients with fluent aphasias presumed to result from lesions of the Wernicke area on the posterior portion of the superior temporal gyrus.[8,24,58] The question then has arisen as to whether this results from a predisposition to posterior lesions in older patients, a difference in the size of lesions as a function of age, or to a difference in clinical expression of a language deficit as a function of age. Studies using CT measurements have demonstrated that this is not due to a more posterior location of lesions in older subjects, but rather due to the occurrence of fluent aphasia with anterior lesion in elderly patients[8,35]; for example, Basso and colleagues[8] found that, in aphasic patients with CT lesions confined to an anterior site, the average age of the nonfluent patients was 57.5 years, and the average age of the fluent aphasics, 75.8 years.

Increasing age also correlates negatively with recovery after strokes that involve the language area, but there are many exceptions. In a study by Pashek and Holland[61] of patients with severe aphasia at the onset of ischemic strokes, one third of those over 70 showed complete or partial recovery or evolution of aphasia (for example, evolving from a Wernicke aphasia to an anomic aphasia) after 1 year, whereas two thirds of those under 70 showed improvement or evolution. A further complication of dominant hemisphere stroke with aphasia in the elderly is the onset of dementia after stroke. In the Pashek and Holland study, one fourth of those over age 70 with global aphasia demonstrated symptoms the authors defined as dementia, including behavior and/or language inappropriate to context or evidence of overall cognitive decline. (See also Chap. 7 in regard to multiple infarct dementia.) Communication deficits masked dementia symptoms in the first month after onset. Yet, the aphasia evolved even in the face of dementia. In their study, no aphasic patient under the age of 70 developed dementia. A final complication of stroke in some elderly are postinfarction seizures, particularly common in subjects with cortical infarcts extending to subcortical structures.[34] Seizures in the elderly are discussed in greater detail later.

In regard to the management of stroke, the condition of the patient, particularly the presence of coexistent diseases, whether they be cardiac or neurologic disorders, rather than age should be the determinant of how aggressive treatment is. For example, AD patients at any age do not do well following neurosurgical or other interventional procedures. On the other hand, an 85-year-old without prior cognitive changes should be an excellent candidate for carotid endarterectomy and perhaps, in the future, the infusion of TPA. One exception is that hemodilution therapy, which is routinely used in stroke patients in Europe, should be used with great caution in the elderly, due to reduced homeostatic reserve.

SLEEP DISORDERS IN THE AGING

During aging, an alteration in daily sleep pattern characterized by more arousals during the night, early morning awakening, and shortened period of sleep together with recurring brief naps during the day is frequently noted.[72] Community surveys have shown that significant sleep complaints are present in 25% to 40% of the elderly.[72] Sleep studies in selected volunteers have shown that there is no consistent change in stage 2 sleep (spindle-K-complex stage) or rapid-eye-movement (REM) sleep. There is, however, a marked decrease in slow wave sleep, particularly stage 4 sleep, which declines by as much as 90%.[42] There is a small increase in the number of night time awakenings with aging but a marked increase in the length of each awakening.

Changes in sleep patterns with aging are not well understood, and although they may likely reflect aging changes in noradrenergic and serotonergic neuronal systems, the data in this regard are scanty. There are, however, several treatable conditions that the physician must consider initially in regard to sleep complaints. Sleep alterations are one of the major symptoms of depression.[1] The sleep disturbance in depression usually manifests itself by early morning awakenings or difficulty in falling asleep, but alternatively some depressed individuals have hypersomnia. If other symptoms of depression are also present, then a trial of a sedating antidepressant medication is worthwhile.

Two additional major causes of insomnia or daytime sleepiness are sleep apnea and periodic leg movements. Both lead to frequent arousals and hence daytime sleepiness.[46] Ancoli-Israel and colleagues[2] found that sleep apnea may be more frequent than previously anticipated; in a community study of randomly selected elderly, it occurred in about 25% of the subjects.[2]

Periodic leg movements or excessive nocturnal myoclonus is defined as more than 40 jerks per night. This also affects about 20% of the elderly in a community sample. In the short term it can be controlled by the use of benzodiazepines. It is interesting to note, however, that studies show a considerable variation in frequency of nocturnal myoclonus from night to night in the same subject.

Sleep fragmentation is particularly evident in patients in nursing homes. In a study of over 200 patients in a skilled nursing facility, subjects averaged only 39.5 minutes of sleep per hour in any hour of the night and 50% woke up at least two or three times per hour.[3] The presence of sleep apnea was not correlated with the occurrence of dementia. There was, however, a strong association of mortality and measures of sleep apnea, especially in the women in this series.

A major problem facing the clinician is that of treatment of insomnia, whether it be due to delayed sleep onset or to frequent awakenings, or early morning awakening. If depression is present, sedative tricyclics and other antidepressant medications can be very effective and may be used safely for a period of months. Many of the antidepressant medications act on the serotonin system, particularly by blocking serotonin reuptake; because the precursor amino acid tryptophan is often limited in normal dietary sources, tryptophan has been suggested as a "natural" hypnotic; however, very high doses, in the gram range, must be taken for tryptophan to be effective. Moreover, tryptophan in high doses is toxic or causes allergic reactions in many individuals.

Nonmedication techniques to improve sleeping that are currently fashionable include increasing daily exposure to sunlight and increasing or instituting a program of daily exercise; such techniques have been reported to improve sleep, but available studies have been on limited groups. Old standbys such as a high carbohydrate meal (presumably acting to improve tryptophan transport) or a glass of warm milk at bedtime will occasionally suffice. Self-hypnosis is occasionally useful. In practice, however, these alternative methods frequently do not work. Thus, the clinician is faced with the difficult choice of whether to prescribe hypnotic medication.

The most popular hypnotics today are the over-the-counter antihistaminics and the prescription short-half-life benzodiazepines such as triazolam. The former have daytime sedative side effects. The latter are very effective for short periods of treatment, and the hypnotic effect is often gone by the time of arising due to the rapid metabolism of this molecule. We have treated patients with sedative benzodiazepines successfully on an occasional or intermittent (two or three times a week) basis. Kripke[46] has pointed out, however, that, in clinical practice, sleeping medications are most often prescribed on a chronic basis and there is no evidence that the benzodiazepines are ef-

ficacious after the first month of usage; in fact, there is limited clinical data that suggest they do not improve sleep after weeks but that users remain on them because of withdrawal insomnia that can occur. This may be of concern; Kripke[46] cites epidemiologic data suggesting a 50% increase in mortality in chronic hypnotic medication users compared with nonusers, although confounding factors have not been ruled out. In view of the popularity of these medicines, further studies of their efficacy and safety in chronic users need to be carried out.

ACCIDENTAL HYPOTHERMIA

The elderly are at special risk for developing the potentially fatal syndrome of "accidental hypothermia."[10] Hypothermia is arbitrarily defined as a core (rectal, esophageal, urinary) body temperature less than 35°C (92.3°F). The diagnosis requires only awareness of the possibility of cold exposure and the availability of a low-temperature thermometer, now present in most large hospital emergency rooms. During 1976 to 1985, there were 7450 deaths caused by hypothermia in the United States, with persons over age 60 accounting for more than half of the deaths (according to the *Morbidity and Mortality Weekly Report*[55]). There are approximately 5.5 times as many persons treated in emergency rooms with hypothermia as there are deaths.[15] When core body temperatures were below 34°C and the full syndrome was present, there had been a 30% to 80% death rate,[64] although this has now fallen to about 20% because modern emergency room CPR techniques are used.[15] In the United States, deaths attributed to hypothermia averaged 300 to 400 per year in the early 1970s, but rose to 634 in 1977; the death rate in persons over age 75 was 17 per million in that year;[19] in 1985 the number of deaths were nearly 1000.[55] This rise is probably due in part to the energy crisis and to increased fuel costs, because there are older individuals who are unable to maintain body heat when the ambient temperature is below 60°F, and even some for whom 65°F is inadequate,[10] and in part due to the increase in the number of the homeless. Nevertheless, this number is much lower than the British experience; in 1975, 3.6% of all persons over age 65 admitted to the University College Hospital in London were hypothermic.[30] In view of the fact that the number of excess deaths in the United States in a typical winter is 20,000, some additional undiagnosed cases undoubtedly occur.

In the United States, accidental hypothermia is usually reported in the context of alcoholism, drug intoxication, sepsis, immersion, or exposure to severe cold,[15,41,64,71] but in Great Britain it is most often observed during winter months in elderly individuals living at home.

In the British experience, the typical patient with accidental hypothermia is elderly, lives alone, and is discovered by a visitor to be confused, stuporous, or comatose.[18,19,23,52,65] The most important presenting sign is an alteration in mental state. The skin is cold and pale and occasionally cyanotic. Reflexes are sluggish, with increases in both contraction and relaxation times of the Achilles reflex.[52] Muscles are stiff. There is a bradycardia, usually caused by a slow sinus rhythm, but atrial fibrillation may be present. In about one third of all patients, a pathognomic electrocardiographic sign, the J wave, a characteristic extra deflection at the junction of QRS and ST segments recorded over the left ventricle, may be observed.[23] Respiration may be slow and shallow, and bronchopneumonia is often present. Acute pancreatitis can occur in association with hypothermia without the presence of abdominal signs or symptoms.[63]

A variety of conditions predispose toward development of the malignant form of the accidental hypothermia syndrome: diabetic acidosis and hypothyroidism are the best documented.[18,29,52,65] Senile dementia may predispose toward development of the syndrome, as do stroke, sepsis, and drug intoxication.[18,64] In each of the latter situations, it may be assumed that the primary condition has interfered with the subject's ability to respond to the cold. Moreover, with intracranial disease, there may be hypothalamic involvement, interfering with central control of temperature regulation.[64]

However, there is a group of elderly persons with normal mental status who develop accidental hypothermia. MacMillan and associates[53] were able to study eight such individuals after recovery from their bout of hypothermia and found several common characteristics in these patients. All had lower than normal body temperatures. During bouts of hypothermia, their core body temperatures ranged from 27.5° to 33.5°C. When fully recovered, their core body temperatures ranged from 34.8° to 36.5°C, clearly below temperatures of most individuals of the same age. Six of eight did not shiver when exposed to cold sufficient to reduce their skin temperatures to 21°C. They also had less vasoconstriction of peripheral arteries when exposed to cold.

In a multicenter study of hypothermia in emergency rooms in the United States, a total of 428 patients were treated by 13 emergency departments during a 2-year study. The core temperatures in the subjects ranged from 35° to 15.6°C, with 272 cases below 32.2°C. There were 73 fatalities (17.1%), 30 of which occurred in December and January; wet clothing was a contributing factor in 21 of these fatal cases; other predisposing conditions included infections, injury, immersion, frostbite, and overdose. In this study it was found that standard cardiopulmonary resuscitation techniques, including tracheal intubation particularly in those with temperatures below 32.2°C, contributed to survival, but it was not clear whether passive or active rewarming was preferable.[15]

A large-scale survey of body temperatures in community-residing elderly persons (over age 65) was carried out in Great Britain using urinary temperature as a measure of core body temperature. Ten percent of the sample had urinary temperatures lower than 35.5°C.[28] A subsample of these individuals was studied intensively and found to have low resting peripheral blood flow with failure to develop vasoconstriction in response to cold.[13] These persons also showed a higher than usual incidence of orthostatic hypotension. These findings demonstrate the presence of autonomic dysfunction in 10% of the "normal" elderly. The coexistence of orthostatic hypotension, abnormalities in vasoconstriction, and low resting body temperature suggests (but does not prove) that an autonomic neuropathy may be present that predisposes toward the development of hypothermia in some elderly persons in moderately cool environments well tolerated by others.

HEAT STROKE

Heat stroke also takes its toll among the elderly.[21,49,67] In general, the number of deaths from heat stroke today is less than in the past owing to the availability of air conditioning. Compare, for example, 765 deaths due to heat stroke that occurred in a 10-day heat wave in 1896 in New York City with less than 30 deaths during the 1973 New York City heat wave of similar degree and duration.[21,22] Today, the elderly at special risk are those who reside in a nursing home designed for air conditioning, rather than natural ventilation, in which the air conditioning breaks down.

A detailed study of such a catastrophe has been reported.[70] Twenty-one of 90 nursing home residents developed hyperpyrexia, and 5 died because of a 5-day failure of the air conditioning unit. It is significant that the survivors' mean temperature rose to 101.5°F by the last day of the heat wave. In general, excess mortality during heat waves—in persons over age 65, it may actually triple—is due to cardiovascular or cerebrovascular events. But these in turn reflect the inability of the body to cope with a rising body temperature.

The difficulty experienced by the elderly in maintaining core temperature in hot and humid environments results from diminished sweating.[18,21] The sweating threshold, which reflects temperature perception, hypothalamic regulation, and the integrity of the autonomic nervous system, is impaired in the elderly. Thus, in one study, almost half of the subjects over age 70 had a sweating threshold in excess of that of the younger controls; that is, sweating did not begin in the old subjects until body core temperature had been raised above 37.4°C (ambient temperature being 30°C). Presumably, the hyperpyrexia sometimes associated with neuroleptic medication may result from the effect of this medication on hypothalamic temperature regulations. In addition, the rate of sweating in the elderly subjects was half that of young controls, apparently owing to loss of the eccrine gland, since injection of a cholinergic agonist failed to restore full sweating.[27] Depending on its severity, hyperpyrexia may require urgent medical intervention with fluids and cooling.

SEIZURES IN THE ELDERLY

Hauser and Kurland[39] report that the incidence of epilepsy is stable through adult life at about 15 new cases per 100,000 per year, starting to rise at 50 years of age, reaching 50 new cases per 100,000 per year at age 60, rising to 75 per 100,000 per year by age 75. An even higher incidence was noted by Luhdorf and colleagues[50,51] who, in a prospective series of subjects over the age of 60 from an urban area in Denmark, found that new cases of seizures reached a peak of 130 per 100,000 per year in those aged 70 to 74.

Seizures in the elderly often occur as a result of stroke. Thus, in the Luhdorf series, 32% of those with a first seizure in later life had a prior history of stroke and 14% had a brain tumor. In a series of 102 patients with occlusive vascular disease, approximately 12% of the patients developed recurrent seizures during a 4- to 22-month follow-up.[62] In a retrospective study of 90 patients with postinfarction seizures, Gupta and colleagues[34] found that one third occurred within 2 weeks of the stroke, 73% in the first year, with 22% becoming recurrent seizures. In this regard it is interesting that in one series of seizures beginning in the elderly,[39] the largest group were those with focal onset, whereas in another series[50] the majority had grand mal seizures without focal onset. A small but significant number of patients develop seizures during the course of AD. Although Hauser and Kurland[39] were unable to demonstrate a reason for the increase in seizures in elderly patients, it seems likely that the increase is related to the high incidence of occlusive vascular disease and AD in these individuals. Luhdorf and colleagues[50] do not comment on it, but in their series of 151 patients over the age of 60 with a first seizure, 66 had dementia, and an identical number had focal neurologic findings. The authors did not report what proportion of the demented subjects had vascular dementia, or what proportion had AD. Seizures also occur in older patients as a result of tumors, chronic subdural hematomas, infections, and alcoholism.

Commonly used anticonvulsant medications are tolerated well by elderly subjects. Hydantoin is generally initiated at levels of 200 to 300 mg/d, while carbamazepine should be initiated slowly (initially 100 mg twice daily) because surprisingly small doses of carbamazepine are frequently effective. The primary measure of therapeutic efficacy is control of seizures or the occurrence of symptoms indicative of toxicity. Blood levels are useful to monitor compliance or unusual metabolism. The optimum therapeutic levels as measured in plasma are the same as in younger subjects and provide a convenient goal in establishing the proper dose of medication. If multiple seizures occur in a short time span, initial oral or parenteral loading (depending on the urgency) should be undertaken to rapidly reach a therapeutic level.

In most instances, seizures should be evaluated with an imaging procedure, an EEG, and the appropriate blood chemistries. Although neurologists tend to avoid treating single seizures in younger patients, this must be individualized to a particular older patient. There have not been adequate studies in the elderly that would provide firm guidelines in regard to a decision to treat after a single seizure; certainly, recurrent seizures must be treated. The decision then is based on clinical experience. In our experience, an elderly patient with a 3-month-old middle cerebral artery infarct who has a focal seizure with secondary generalization should probably be treated after the initial ictus (the seizure will likely recur), while in a healthy older person without a focal abnormality, this may be unnecessary. Patients with dementia who develop a single seizure, usually generalized, are also at high risk for recurrent seizures and should be treated if there are no contraindications. Since these patients have difficulty reporting symptoms of toxicity, regular monitoring of blood levels is necessary.

DIZZINESS AND VERTIGO IN THE ELDERLY

Dizziness, one of the most common complaints of adults of any age visiting a physician's office, always presents a diagnostic challenge because of the multiplicity of disorders that may produce this symptom.[4,17] However, persistent dizziness in the elderly is more likely to be associated with specific disorders, particularly of the peripheral vestibular system, than in younger patients. Thus, Baloh and colleagues[5] found that they were able to make a specific diagnosis in about 85% of a series of patients over the age of 70 who presented with persistent dizziness. Peripheral vestibular problems presented in about 50% of the patients, and cerebrovascular disease presented in 22%. This experience contrasts with their findings in a group of younger patients in whom psychophysiologic dizziness was the most common diagnosis with peripheral vestibular disorders accounting for only 21% of the cases. In the Drachman and Hart[17] series, 38% had peripheral vestibular disorders.

Drachman and Hart[17] classified the symptoms of their "dizzy" patients as (1) definite rotational sensation, (2) sensation of impending faint, (3) dysequilibrium or loss of balance without head sensation, and (4) ill-defined light-headedness. Patients with orthostatic hypotension have a sensation of impending faint or ill-defined light-headedness. Demonstrating orthostatic changes may require multiple determinations of lying and standing blood pressure. Ill-defined light-headedness is otherwise a difficult symptom from which to establish a diagnosis and for which to devise an effective treatment.

Positional vertigo is often the result of labyrinthian disorders.[66] Such disorders may occur in greater frequency in the elderly because of calcifications that affect the vestibular organ in an asymmetric fashion. The most common form of peripheral vestibular disorder in the elderly is benign positional vertigo. In this condition, frequent but brief episodes, usually lasting less than 30 seconds, occur, often induced by a change in position. The diagnosis is readily made using the Nylen-Barany maneuver: With eyes open, the patient is moved abruptly from a seated to a prone position with the head hanging 45° below horizon and rotated 45° to side; the patient is observed for nystagmus and vertigo. In patients with benign positional vertigo, nystagmus is induced. This phenomenon is fatigable and Baloh recommends positional exercises, in which the patient carries out this maneuver on his or her own; in his

experience remissions often occur after a series of such exercises. Baloh also recommends such exercises rather than antivertigo drugs in patients with vestibular neuronitis. Even though there may be greater discomfort for a few days, the length of the period of disability is foreshortened. The success of such exercises argues for the ability of the brain, even in the elderly, to learn to compensate for asymmetric vestibular excitation.

Vertigo may occur as a result of cerebrovascular disorders, almost always of the posterior fossa, although rarely temporal lobe lesions also give rise to this symptom. Typically, episodes of vertigo due to vascular disease are longer than those due to benign positional nystagmus and last minutes. Specific diagnosis depends on the presence of accompanying localizing signs. These authors ascribe the vertigo in such patients to ischemia of the superior vestibular labyrinth due to involvement of the anterior vestibular artery, which is supplied by the vertebrobasilar system. According to Grad and Baloh,[32] isolated episodes of vertigo may precede other signs of vertebrobasilar insufficiency. In these instances diagnosis becomes increasingly urgent today. It is now often possible to visualize blood flow through the basilar artery on MRI so that a diagnosis can be confirmed with a noninvasive imaging procedure and therapy with anticoagulants or thrombolytic therapy instituted if indicated.

ORTHOSTATIC HYPOTENSION

Orthostatic hypotension accounts for a small but significant number of falls by elderly patients.[25,59,68] The falls are often related to postural changes, although they may be associated with standing for a while. Patients usually experience light headaches and a brief loss of consciousness. Focal neurologic signs do not occur in these circumstances. Orthostatic changes in blood pressure should be readily demonstrable on rapid arising (20 mm Hg drop in systolic pressure).

Orthostatic hypotension is common among the elderly. In a series of 494 elderly patients living at home, Caird and co-workers[11] reported falls in systolic blood pressure with a postural change of 20 mm Hg or more in 34% of the individuals studied. The occurrence of these orthostatic changes was significantly higher in patients aged 75 and older than in those between 65 and 74 years of age (30% vs 16%). However, other series have reported a somewhat lower incidence of orthostatic changes.[25]

Orthostatic hypotension may be related to dysfunction at several loci (e.g., hypothalamic, brainstem, spinal cord, nerve transmission, or effector), but is most often associated with an autonomic neuropathy seen in some elderly, or as part of the polyneuropathy of diabetes. The use of medication, including antihypertensives, L-dopa, phenothiazines, butyrophenones, and tricyclic antidepressants, can produce orthostatic hypotension. The condition often is the presenting symptom of the Shy-Drager syndrome,[6] and can frequently be seen in patients with idiopathic PD[33] as well. Finally, orthostatic hypotension can be related to a depletion of blood volume, which may be due to diabetes insipidus, adrenal insufficiency, or a salt-losing nephropathy. Patients may respond to the treatment with salt-retaining steroids, ergotamine, or mechanical methods to prevent blood pooling.[25]

TEMPORAL ARTERITIS

Temporal arteritis is an age-related systemic disease, occurring after age 50, that is frequently associated with the occurrence of headache and systemic symptoms. The arteritis involves primarily extracranial branches of the carotid artery and if untreated may lead to retinal or optic nerve infarction resulting in severe visual loss. With prompt diagnosis, treatment is effective.

Temporal arteritis has rarely been reported under age 50. The incidence increases more than 10-fold in the sixth through ninth decades with a 2:1 preponderance in women.[9] The primary symptom is boring or throbbing headache often centered over the temples but also involving the face, mouth, occiput, or neck. Approximately one half of patients demonstrate generalized scalp tenderness with localized tender nodular and pulseless superficial temporal arteries.[31] Jaw claudication, highly suggestive of temporal arteritis, occurs in more than one third of patients.[31] Constitutional signs and symptoms, which include diaphoresis, fever, anorexia, weight loss, and malaise, are common.[31] About half of patients complain of aching and stiffness involving primarily axial muscles without associated weakness (i.e., polymyalgia rheumatica[40,57]). When polymyalgia occurs without headache, it still suggests an underlying vasculitis requiring treatment.[38] Blindness is unusual as the initial manifestation of temporal arteritis (4%) and in recent years with prompt diagnosis and treatment, its occurrence has decreased to 10%. The most common neurologic abnormalities are diplopia, ophthalmoparesis, and ptosis.[26] This may be produced by cranial nerve ischemia[7,16] induced by arteritis of the meningohypophyseal trunk or recurrent collaterals of the ophthalmic arteries.[26,74] The clinical manifestations of temporal arteritis are almost always associated with a markedly elevated erythrocyte sedimentation rate.

The arteritis produces patchy involvement of the extracranial branches of the carotid artery, particularly the superficial temporal artery as well as the ophthalmic and ciliary arteries. Large arteries throughout the body are involved as well as occasionally the vertebral arteries, but only rarely are intracranial vessels affected. The arterial media is infiltrated by inflammatory cells and ultimately is destroyed, to be replaced by fibrous connective tissue. There is severe intimal proliferation leading to arterial narrowing or occlusion. The unique pathologic component is the presence of multinucleated giant cells at the intima-media border.[37] Diagnosis can be strongly suspected by the clinical manifestations and elevated sedimentation rate. It is confirmed by demonstrating the above pathologic changes in a specimen of biopsied superficial temporal artery. Because of the patchy nature of the disease, even a large biopsy specimen may not demonstrate the diagnostic pathologic changes. Therefore, therapeutic intervention based on the clinical diagnosis is often indicated, although histologic verification allows for more confidence in the long-term use of steroids.

Treatment with prednisone (40 to 60 mg/d) should be instituted as soon as possible (suspicion of diagnosis is sufficient) to prevent visual loss. The response is often rapid with decrease in headache and constitutional symptoms after hours. Long-term treatment with the lowest effective steroid dose minimizes complications.

COMPLICATIONS OF NEUROLEPTIC TREATMENT

Previous studies have reported tardive dyskinesia to be more common in older individuals[14] and those with preexisting brain damage.[20] The widespread use of neuroleptics as a sedative in the demented elderly, and occasionally as a sleeping medication, has produced an upsurge of this disorder. In our experience, relatively low doses over surprisingly brief periods may produce the typical buccolingual and masticatory movements. The movements often persist in these elderly patients long after the drug has been discontinued, although they rarely produce significant disability. Restricting the use of neuroleptics to instances of severe agitation that require pharmacologic treatment seems prudent. Agitated depression should be treated primarily with antidepressants. Frequent re-examination of the necessity of continuing such treatment is also advised.

A rare complication of neuroleptic treatment that we recently observed in an elderly patient is the neuroleptic malignant syndrome.[12,56] During neuroleptic treatment (haloperidol and fluphenazine are most often incriminated), patients develop stupor, muscular rigidity, and fever and appear catatonic. This idiosyncratic drug reaction, which may be lethal if untreated, responds to discontinuance of *neuroleptics* and use of *anticholinergics* such as trihexyphenidyl.

TUMORS IN THE ELDERLY

Although the incidence of nervous system tumors decreases after middle age, several tumors occur with some frequency in the seventh through ninth decades. The tumors with the highest incidence in this age group are glioblastoma, meningioma, neurolemmomas, and metastatic cancer.[75] These comprise 82% of the tumors encountered in these patients above 60.[76] The literature does not address differences in the biology or host interactions in brain tumors occurring in the elderly. It has been reported, however, that the median survival time after surgery in patients 60 or older is less than half that of patients younger than 50 (18 weeks versus 40 weeks),[45] suggesting a poorer prognosis in elderly patients.

The site of the tumor determines the clinical manifestations. Glioblastomas occur predominantly within the hemisphere and are therefore accompanied by signs and symptoms characteristic of hemispheric lesions (e.g., hemiparesis, parietal sensory loss, aphasia, and homonymous hemianopsia). Although metastatic lesions most often involve the hemisphere at multiple sites, the cerebellum and epidural space of the spinal canal are also frequently affected by tumor. Signs of cerebellar dysfunction (e.g., ataxia or incoordination) or back pain and myelopathy are produced by local compression. By contrast, neurolemmomas develop from nerve root sheaths (spinal or cranial), thereby initially producing manifestations of nerve dysfunction (e.g., radicular pain, motor-sensory loss, tinnitus, and hearing loss) before compressing adjacent structures (e.g., spinal cord, other cranial nerves, and brainstem). Meningiomas arise from the dura and thereby involve the hemisphere(s), brainstem, cranial nerves, and spine, producing numerous syndromes by compressing local structures.

The history and examination will usually establish the site of the tumor and provide some insight into differential diagnosis. Most often, the etiology can be confirmed with CT or MRI.

In younger patients, slowly growing, benign, extra-axial tumors are effectively treated surgically, most often resulting in positive outcomes. Common sense suggests that in elderly patients surgery should be considered in individuals who are either symptomatic or at risk for imminent major complication (e.g., compression of the brainstem or spinal cord). The older and frailer and/or the more difficult the resection, the more compelling the indications must be. In younger individuals, establishing a tissue diagnosis of glioblastoma and partial removal at surgery provides a beneficial first step often followed by radiotherapy and chemotherapy. In frail elderly, the practitioner may be faced with the necessity of omitting the first step and relying on radiotherapy. The treatment of old and young with malignant tumors is comparable, although chemotherapy is used rarely in elderly patients. Glioblastoma and metastatic cancer respond (often dramatically) in all age groups to treatment with steroids. After the initial success, steroids should be

tapered or discontinued as elderly are even more susceptible to the complications of long-term treatment than younger patients. In both glioblastoma and metastatic cancer, the goal is to maximize function over a significant time span. Treatment as outlined here sometimes achieves these goals.

DISORDERS OF THE SPINAL CANAL

The spinal canal consists of a series of vertebrae separated by flexible fibrocartilagenous material (disks) anteriorly. The bone arches around the spinal cord and posteriorly forms a series of small apophyseal joints with adjacent vertebrae. The cervical spine is the most flexible portion of the canal with a large range of motion (ROM) for both flexion-extension (ROM, 100°) and rotational movement (ROM, 180°). The lumbar spine has, by comparison, limited ROM but structurally supports the upper body and head, resulting in weight-bearing stresses. While the water content of the disks decreases during aging and they lose their flexibility, it is bony overgrowth of osteophytes reminiscent of osteoarthritis that compromises the canal and roots. The osteophytes form long bars on the posterior aspect of the vertebral bodies adjacent to the disk space that compress the contents of the spinal canal. In addition, there are osteophytes that project from the apophyseal joints in a manner similar to the bony overgrowth seen in osteoarthritis involving other joints. The osteophytes project laterally into the neuroforamina, compressing nerve roots in the lateral recesses of the canal. Individuals with congenitally narrow spinal canals are at greater risk from these processes. The flexion-extension movements of the neck further narrow the canal and may propel the osteophytic bars against the spinal cord. Significant osteophytic narrowing of the spinal canal occurs in 75% of individuals over 50 and is almost universal after 70.[60] Compression of neural elements occurs in only a fraction of those at risk.

Cervical spondylosis may manifest itself as pain radiating from the neck into the upper extremities in a nerve root (dermatomal) distribution. It is often accompanied by loss of reflexes, atrophy, weakness, and sensory loss in one or more nerve roots. Spinal cord compression by osteophytic bars usually occurs in men 65 or more years of age. The progression is usually slow, often extending over 1 to 2 years. Pain is not prominent (unless there is a coincident radiculopathy), and the usual presentation is that of gait impairment due to a spastic paraparesis (rarely quadriparesis). Often there is an associated sensory loss (usually dorsal column). Urinary dysfunction is unusual. MRI and CT scan allow for noninvasive delineation of bony and soft tissue compression of neural elements. ALS may be difficult to distinguish from the above, although sensory abnormalities and electrophysiologic techniques demonstrating denervation in other areas may be useful.

Lumbar spondylosis may narrow the spinal canal with anterior spondylotic bars, apophyseal overgrowth, or herniated disk material. When there is compression of neural elements in the lateral recess or in the neural foramina, most often root symptoms occur. The dysfunction engendered produces radicular pain in the lower extremities but may also be accompanied by appropriate weakness and sensory loss. The pain engendered by lumbosacral root compression is quite common and is a major cause of "sciatica" in elderly patients. Narrowing of the spinal canal produces compression of the cauda equina most often at the L-4 (23%) and L-5 (71%) levels.[54]

The primary symptom is severe pain in one or both legs, which occurs during walking and is relieved by flexing forward (sitting or standing) or squatting. The onset is slow (4 years). The examination is often normal, although mild motor and sensory signs occasionally

accompanied by urinary dysfunction may be present. Treatment of radicular symptoms, either lumbar or cervical, is directed toward control of pain. The use of nonsteroidal anti-inflammatory agents and analgesics may provide some relief. Traction and a soft collar for control of movement may aid in control of cervical pain. A hard bed, bed rest, and local heat to decrease muscle spasm may be useful for both cervical and lumbar root symptoms. Often the pain remits and only occasionally is more aggressive therapy warranted.

Lumbar stenosis may seriously impair the mobility and quality of life. Rarely do the symptoms remit. Medication, bed rest, and a lumbar surgical corset help only marginally. In healthy vigorous elderly, with stenosis at a single level, surgery may yield a vast improvement in the quality of life.

A soft collar that limits neck movement should be used in spondylosis of the cervical canal resulting in myelopathy. Conservative therapy results in a significant improvement in one third[48] to a little less that one half[73] of patients, so this appears a reasonable first course of action, especially in frail patients. Although the progression is usually slow, rapid deterioration might influence a decision in favor of surgery. In several series, a significant improvement following surgery is reported in the majority (60%) of patients.

REFERENCES

1. American Psychiatric Association Task Force on Nomenclature and Statistics: Diagnostic and Statistical Manual of Mental Disorders (DSM-III), ed 3. American Psychiatric Association, Washington, DC, 1980.
2. Ancoli-Israel, S, Kripke, DF, and Mason, W: Characteristics of obstructive and central sleep apnea in the elderly: An interim report. Biol Psychiatry 22:741–750, 1987.
3. Ancoli-Israel, S, Parker, L, Sinaee, R,

Fell, RL, and Kripke, DF: Sleep fragmentation in patients from a nursing home. J Gerontol 44:M18–M21, 1989.

4. Baloh, RW: Dizziness, Hearing Loss, and Tinnitus: The Essentials of Neurology. FA Davis, Philadelphia, 1984.

5. Baloh, RW, Honrubin, U, and Jacobson, K: Benign positional vertigo: Clinical and oculographic features in 240 cases. Neurology 37:371–378, 1987.

6. Bannister, R: Degeneration of the autonomic nervous system. Lancet 2:175–179, 1971.

7. Barricks, ME, Traviesa, DB, Glaser, JS, and Levy, IS: Ophthalmoplegia in cranial arteritis. Brain 100:209–221, 1977.

8. Basso, A, Bracchi, M, Capitani, E, Laiacona, M, and Zanobio, ME: Age and evolution of language area functions: A study on adult stroke patients. Cortex 23:475–483, 1987.

9. Bengtsson, BA and Malmvall, BE: The epidemiology of giant cell arteritis including temporal arteritis and polymyalgia rheumatica. Arthritis Rheum 24:899–904, 1981.

10. Besdine, RW: Accidental hypothermia: The body's energy crisis. Geriatrics 34:51–59, 1979.

11. Caird, FI, Andrews, GR, and Kennedy, RD: Effect of posture on blood pressure in the elderly. Br Heart J 35:527–530, 1973.

12. Caroff, SN: The neuroleptic malignant syndrome. J Clin Psychiatry 41:79–82, 1980.

13. Collins, KJ, Dore, C, Exton-Smith, AN, Fox, RH, MacDonald, IC, and Woodward, PM: Accidental hypothermia and impaired temperature homeostasis in the elderly. Br Med J 1:353–356, 1977.

14. Crane, G: Persistent dyskinesia. Br J Psychiatry 122:395–405, 1973.

15. Danzl, DF, Pozos, RS, Auerbach, PS, Glazer, S, Goetz, W, Johnson, E, Juli, J, Lilja, P, Marx, JA, and Miller, J: Multicenter hypothermia survey. Ann Emerg Med 16:1042–1055, 1987.

16. Dimant, J, Grob, D, and Brunner, NG: Ophthalmoplegia, ptosis, and myosis in temporal arteritis. Neurology 30:1054–1058, 1980.

17. Drachman, DA and Hart, CW: An approach to the dizzy patient. Neurology 22:323–334, 1972.

18. Duguid, H and Simpson, RG: Accidental hypothermia. Lancet 2:1213–1219, 1961.

19. Editorial: Action needed to prevent deaths from hypothermia in the elderly. JAMA 243:407–408, 1980.

20. Edwards, H: The significance of brain damage in persistent oral dyskinesia. Br J Psychiatry 116:271–275, 1970.

21. Ellis, FP; Mortality from heat illness and heat-aggravated illness in the United States. Environ Res 5:1–58, 1972.

22. Ellis, FP, Nelson, F, and Pincus, L: Mortality during heat waves in New York City, July, 1972, August and September, 1973. Environ Res 10:1–13, 1975.

23. Emslie-Smith, D: Accidental hypothermia: A common condition with a pathognomonic electrocardiogram. Lancet 2:492–495, 1958.

24. Eslinger, PJ and Damasio, AR: Age and type of aphasia in patients with stroke. J Neurol Neurosurg Psychiatry 44:377–381, 1981.

25. Exton-Smith, AN: Disturbances of autonomic regulation. In Isaacs, B (ed): Recent Advances in Geriatric Medicine. Churchill Livingstone, New York, 1978, p 4.

26. Fisher, CM: Ocular palsy in temporal arteritis. Minn Med 42:1258–1268, 1959.

27. Foster, KG, Ellis, FP, Dore, C, et al: Sweat responses in the aged. Age Ageing 5:91, 1976.

28. Fox, RH, Woodward, PM, Exton-Smith, AN, Green, MF, Donnison, DV, and Wicks, MH: Body temperatures in the elderly: A national study of physiological, social and environmental conditions. Br Med J 1:200–206, 1973.

29. Gale, EAM and Tattersall, RB: Hypothermia: A complication of diabetic

ketoacidosis. Br Med J 2:1387–1389, 1978.

30. Goldman, A, Exton-Smith, AN, Francis, G, and O'Brien, A: A pilot study of low body temperatures in old people admitted to hospital. J R Coll Phys Lond 11:291–306, 1977.

31. Goodman, BW: Temporal arteritis. Am J Med 67:839–852, 1979.

32. Grad, A and Baloh, RW: Vertigo of vascular origin: Clinical and electronystagmographic features in 84 cases. Arch Neurol 46:281–284, 1989.

33. Gross, M, Bannister, R, and Godwin-Austen, R: Orthostatic hypotension in Parkinson's disease. Lancet 2:174, 1972.

34. Gupta, SR, Naheedy, MH, Elias, D, and Rubino, FA: Postinfarction seizures: A clinical study. Stroke 19:1477–1481, 1988.

35. Habib, M, Ali-Cherif, A, Poncet, M, and Salaman, G, Age-related changes in aphasia type and stroke. Brain Lang 31:245–251, 1987.

36. Hagnell, O, Lanke, J, Rorsman, B, and Ojesjo, L: Does the incidence of age psychosis decrease? Neuropsychobiology 7:201–211, 1981.

37. Hamilton, CR, Shelley, WM, and Tumulty, PA: Giant cell arteritis: Including temporal arteritis and polymyalgia rheumatica. Medicine 50:1–27, 1971.

38. Hamrin, B: Polymyalgia arteritica. Acta Med Scand 533(Suppl):1–164, 1972.

39. Hauser, WA and Kurland, LT: The epidemiology of epilepsy in Rochester, Minnesota, 1935 through 1967. Epilepsia 16:1–66, 1975.

40. Healey, LA and Wilske, KR: Manifestation of giant cell arteritis. Med Clin North Am 61:261–270, 1977.

41. Hudson, LD and Conn, RD: Accidental hypothermia: Associated diagnoses and prognosis in a common problem. JAMA 227:37–40, 1974.

42. Kales, A, Wilson, T, Kales, JD, Jacobson, A, Paulson, MJ, Kollar, E, and Walter, RD: Measurements of all-night sleep in normal elderly per-

sons: Effects of aging. J Am Geriatr Soc 15:405–414, 1967.

43. Katzman, R, Aronson, M, Fuld, PA, Kawas, C, Brown, T, Morgenstern, H, Frishman, W, Gidez, L, Eder, H, and Ooi, WL: Development of dementia in an 80-year-old volunteer cohort. Ann Neurol 25:317–324, 1989.

44. Katzman, R, Clasen, R, Klatzo, I, Meyer, JS, Pappius, HM, and Waltz, AG: Brain edema in stroke: Report of Joint Committee for Stroke Resources. Stroke 8:512–540, 1977.

45. Kornblith, PL, Wicker, MD, and Casady, JR: Neurologic Oncology. JB Lippincott, Philadelphia, 1987.

46. Kripke, DRF, Ancoli-Israel, S, and Okudaira, N: Sleep apnea and nocturnal myoclonus in the elderly. Neurobiol Aging 3:329–336, 1982.

47. Kurtzke, JF: Epidemiology of Cerebrovascular Disease. Springer-Verlag, Berlin, 1969.

48. Lees, F, and Turner, JWA: Natural history and prognosis of cervical spondylosis. Br Med J 2:1607–1610, 1963.

49. Levine, JA: Heat stroke in the aged. Am J Med 47:251–258, 1969.

50. Luhdorf, K, Jensen, LK, and Plesner, AM: 1. Etiology of seizures in the elderly. Epilepsia 27:135–141, 1986.

51. Luhdorf, K, Jensen, LK, and Plesner, AM: 2. Epilepsy in the elderly: Incidence, social function, and disability. Epilepsia 27:458–463, 1986.

52. Maclean, D, Taig, DR, and Emslie-Smith, D: Achilles tendon reflex in accidental hypothermia and hypothermic myxoedema. Br Med J 2:87–90, 1973.

53. MacMillan, AL, Corbett, JL, Johnson, RH, Smith, AC, Spalding, JMK, and Wollner, L: Temperature regulation in survivors of accidental hypothermia of the elderly. Lancet 2:165–169, 1967.

54. Micknael, MA, Ceric, I, Tarkington, J, and Vick, NA. Neuroradiologic

evaluation of the lateral recess syndrome. Radiology 140:97–1076, 1981.

55. Morbidity and Mortality Weekly Report. 37:780–782, 1988.

56. Morris, HH, McCormick, WF, and Reinarz, JA: Neuroleptic malignant syndrome. Arch Neurol 37:462–463, 1980.

57. Mowat, AC and Hazleman, BL: Polymyalgia rheumatica: A clinical study with particular reference to arterial disease. J Rheumatol 1:190–202, 1974.

58. Obler, LK, Albert, ML, Goodglass, H, and Benson, DF: Aphasia type and aging. Brain Lang 6:318–322, 1978.

59. Overstall, PW, Exton-Smith, AN, Imms, FJ and Johnson, AL: Falls in the elderly related to postural imbalance. Br Med J 1:261, 1977.

60. Pallis, C, Jones, AM, and Spillaine, JD: Cervical spondylosis: Incidence and implications. Brain 77:274–289, 1954.

61. Pashek, GV and Holland, AL: Evolution of aphasia in the first year postonset. Cortex 24:411–423, 1988.

62. Ramirez-Lassepas, M, Hauser, WA, Bundlie, SR, and Cleeremans, BB: Epileptiform Activity, Acute Seizures and Epilepsy with Acute Cerebral Vascular Disease (abstr). In Wade, JA and Penry, JK (eds): Advances in Epileptology. Xth Epilepsy International Symposium. Raven Press, New York, 1980, p 188.

63. Read, AE, Emslie-Smith, D, Gouch, KR, and Holmes, R: Pancreatitis and accidental hypothermia. Lancet 2:1219–1221, 1961.

64. Reuler, JB: Hypothermia; Pathophysiology, clinical settings management. Ann Intern Med 89:519–527, 1978.

65. Rosin, AJ and Exton-Smith, AN: Clinical features of accidental hypothermia, with some observations on thyroid function. Br Med J 1:16–19, 1964.

66. Rudge, P: Clinical Neuro-otology. Churchill Livingstone, New York, 1983.

67. Schuman, SH, Anderson, CP, and Oliver, JT: Epidemiology of successive heat waves in Michigan in 1962 and 1963. JAMA 189:733–738, 1964.

68. Sheldon, JH: On the natural history of falls in old age. Br Med J 2:1685, 1960.

69. Sluss, TK, Gruenberg, EM, and Kramer, M: The Use of Longitudinal Studies in the Investigation of Risk Factor for Senile Dementia-Alzheimer Type. In Mortimer, JA and Schuman, LM (eds): The Epidemiology of Dementia. Oxford University Press, London, 1981, p 132.

70. Sullivan-Bolyai, JZ, Lumish, RM, Smith, EWP, Howell, JT, Bregman, DJ, Lund, M, and Page, RC: Hyperpyrexia due to air-conditioning failure in a nursing home. Public Health Rep 94:466–470, 1979.

71. Tolman, KG and Cohen, A: Accidental hypothermia. Can Med Assoc J 103:1357–1361, 1970.

72. Weitzman, ED: Sleep and Aging. In Katzman, R and Terry, RD (eds): The Neurology of Aging. FA Davis, Philadelphia, 1983, p 167.

73. Wilkinson, M: Cervical Spondylosis. In Brain, L (ed): Recent Advances in Neuropsychiatry, ed 7. Churchill Livingstone, London, 1962.

74. Wilkinson, IMS and Russell, RWR: Arteries of the head and neck in giant cell arteritis: A pathological study to show the pattern of arterial involvement. Arch Neurol 27:378–391, 1972.

75. Youmans, JR: Neurologic Surgery, Vol III. WB Saunders, Philadelphia, 1973.

76. Zulch, KJ: Brain Tumors, Their Biology and Pathology. Springer-Verlag, Berlin, 1986.

Chapter 14

ETHICAL ISSUES IN THE MANAGEMENT OF THE ELDERLY

John W. Rowe, M.D.

THE SCOPE OF ETHICAL DECISIONS
AN APPROACH TO DECISION
  MAKING
ABUSE AND NEGLECT

The past decade has seen dramatic increases in concern regarding ethical issues in the management of elderly patients. This concern is fueled by increasing recognition of the rights of elderly people to participate in decisions regarding their care, concerns regarding the legal implications of physician's decisions to limit care, and growing interest in rationing health services to patients least likely to benefit from additional care. Discussions regarding decision making in geriatrics take on special focus in patients with neurologic disorders for several reasons. Patients with dementia are often considered unable to participate in decisions regarding their care. In addition to dementia, however, other neurologic diseases are important with regard to ethical issues. Many stroke patients are unable to communicate their wishes effectively despite the fact that they may be decision capable. The inevitability of the progressive decline in function seen in amyotrophic lateral sclerosis (ALS) has obvious implications. This chapter provides an overview of the principles emerging regarding decision making

for life-sustaining technologies in the elderly. The reader is referred to more extensive discussions for additional information.[3,13]

THE SCOPE OF ETHICAL DECISIONS

A broad scope of ethical issues impact on the care of elderly persons. These decisions go well beyond the traditional preoccupation with Do-Not-Resuscitate (DNR) orders and include considerations regarding decisions to hospitalize elderly, decisions to treat with antibiotics or other life-sustaining technologies such as dialysis and chronic ventilation, and questions as to whether or not to feed or provide intravenous or oral fluid replacement. Issues of feeding and fluid replacement seem to have a special significance since there is conflict regarding whether feeding and fluid replacement represent an extraordinary treatment, such as dialysis or ventilation, or whether they represent a more basic right of all patients. Regardless of the particular issue under consideration—resuscitation, dialysis, ventilation, or feeding—an emerging set of principles provide guidance for individuals who find themselves participating in the management of elderly individuals.[7]

356

AN APPROACH TO DECISION MAKING

There is general agreement on the right of an individual patient to participate in treatment decisions. This view is supported not only by a number of legal decisions, but also by the Older Americans Act,[8] the Federal Council on Aging Bicentennial Charter for Older Americans,[1] and the Nursing Home Patient's Bill of Rights.[6] Even individuals who may be marginally capable of making decisions should be involved, to whatever extent possible, in decision making regarding their own care. A physician who refuses to follow the wishes of a competent patient regarding life-sustaining technologies should withdraw from the case.

When an individual is judged not to be decision capable, alternative approaches to decision making are required. The *process* employed in decision making should be well documented and include the family and all relevant health care providers. Careful attention should be given to accumulating all appropriate data and to revisiting the decision over time. When such a process has been employed, if the ultimate decision is to withhold therapy, one's confidence in this decision is greatest and the distress such a decision causes for family members and health care providers is minimized.[4,14] Health care providers should be aware of the fact that a decision to withhold treatment can and should be revised on significant change in the patient's clinical status or the availability of additional information regarding the value history or previous intentions or expectations of the patient. These decisions are not and should not be written in stone, but rather should be open to constant reconsideration to assure the most open process and the greatest likelihood of consideration of all the appropriate data and involvement of all appropriate individuals.

In the absence of a decision-capable patient, *advance directives,* such as a living will or other clearly documented written evidence of a patient's intentions and preferences, are exceptionally helpful as a guide for decision making. In those cases in which a patient's underlying disease is likely to be untreatable and progressive such as Alzheimer disease or ALS, such advance directives should be developed early in the course of the illness and revisited at regular intervals to assure that they continue to accurately describe the patient's preferences and intentions. In the absence of advance directives, *substituted judgment* is generally applied whereby another individual, generally a member of the patient's family, is asked to provide the decision for the patient. While the family would seem to be the logical choice to play a major role in this decision making, a minority of states have formally provided the family with the legal authority to do so. However, in many states this right of the family seems to have evolved informally as a matter of common law. In substituted judgment, another individual is asked to make the decision that the patient would have made. In this regard, a conflict often arises around the choice of a decision that one believes the patient would have made versus a decision one believes to be in the best interest of the patient. This conflict is clearly demonstrated in the study of Warren and co-workers[16] regarding the recruitment of demented individuals to participate in a research project. In this study, nearly one third of the individuals making decisions for the patient agreed to participation of the patient in the research study, because they viewed it as in the patient's best interest, despite their view that the patient, were he or she making decisions, probably would not agree to participate in the study.

Abdication of the responsibility by family members or health providers to make decisions regarding withholding care for patients deemed not decision-capable is far too common and can have serious deleterious effects. Reliance on the court system, which is slow, not designed to participate in these decisions, and, in many cases, not inclined to do so, can substantially impair the decision by removing it from the clinical setting and placing it in the hands of individuals who do not have experience either with these decisions or with the individual patient under consideration. Similarly, there seems to be little need or room for federal legislation concerning the initiation, withholding, or withdrawal of specific life-sustaining technologies.

The most straightforward approach to rationing health care for the elderly is to use a patient's *age* as an absolute criterion for withholding care. In such cases, individuals over a given age are deemed ineligible for care, independent of their individual clinical status. This pernicious and discriminatory approach neglects the remarkable heterogeneity of the elderly population. Age, by itself, is clearly an inadequate criterion on which to make decisions regarding withholding care.[7]

Diagnosis, while often considered to be a reasonable criterion, is also grossly inadequate. For instance, one could describe a patient as a 75-year-old man with diabetes, hypertension, and a history of myocardial infarction (MI). Such an age- and diagnosis-specific description does not provide information that would be useful in making a decision regarding withholding care. Indeed, such a 75-year-old hypertensive, diabetic man with a history of MI could be irreversibly, irretrievably ill in a long-term care facility or fully functional and sitting on the Supreme Court!

In addition to the remarkable variability *between* elderly patients even within diagnostic categories, there is substantial variability *within* patients on a day-to-day or week-to-week basis. Determinations as to whether a patient is decision-capable must take into account the fluctuating functional level of many elderly individuals and whenever possible should include serial prospective observations over time. It is not uncommon for individuals who appear to be decision-incapable at one time to recover their apparent capacity to make decisions at another point in time. This

is particularly common in patients with mild to moderate dementia, which is often complicated by intermittent reversible episodes of delirium associated with intercurrent illness or medication use. In addition, it should go without saying that patients should not be assumed to have an irreversible or untreatable form of dementia until treatable causes such as subdural hematoma, uremia, medication effects, and so forth, have been excluded.

The adverse consequences of decisions to withhold therapy cannot be overlooked.[2] For instance, a decision not to resuscitate a patient in the event of a cardiopulmonary arrest may very significantly adversely influence the quality and quantity of the care provided to the patient. Scrupulous attention is needed by the entire health care team to provide the finest, most humane care available at all times for those categories of care, that is, antibiotics, general care, and so forth, for which a decision has been made to continue care. The health care team must be made aware of the distinction between decisions to withhold certain types of care and decisions not to resuscitate. Too often, a DNR order is meant to translate into an *ignore* order for the markedly impaired, irreversibly ill, irretrievable, elderly patient.

ABUSE AND NEGLECT

One area of geriatrics laden with ethical considerations is the detection, management, and prevention of elder abuse and neglect. Several years ago a wave of reports of physical abuse of frail elderly triggered the passage of numerous state laws regarding reporting and punishing abuse. A productive byproduct of this increased interest in elder abuse was substantial research in this area. Recently, a number of research findings have emerged that broaden our understanding of this important problem.

The domains of elderly abuse and neglect should be viewed as subsets of a broader area of inadequate care of the elderly. Although many definitions have been offered, those of O'Malley and Fulmer[11] have practical utility. They define *abuse* as "active intervention by a caretaker such that unmet needs are created or sustained with resultant physical, psychological, or financial injury." As pointed out by this definition, it is important to recognize that abuse extends far beyond physical factors to include psychologic and financial abuse. They define neglect as "failure of a caretaker to intervene to resolve an important care need despite awareness of available resources." Clearly, taking this broad definition, neglect represents a failure of the informal support system of an individual.

The responsibility of the physician and other health providers is to detect cases of abuse and neglect as early as possible. In cases of neglect we must move to repair the deficit in the informal support system. In cases of abuse we must move to modify behavior or, in extreme cases, to remove the patients from the abusive environment and/or family member. Management of cases of abuse and neglect rarely includes legal efforts aimed at an abusive caregiver but more commonly includes clarification of the unmet needs and marshalling together the resources that are required to bolster the informal support system with formal supports.

Detection of cases of elderly abuse and neglect is of critical importance. Most cases present nonspecifically, and a physician must have a keen awareness of the patients who are at greatest risk. Most of the signs of physical abuse tend to be nonspecific and can be associated with worsening of common geriatric problems in the absence of abuse and neglect. Such symptoms include poor hygiene, poor nutrition including volume depletion, trauma, decubitus ulcer, or evidence of overmedication or undermedication.[9]

An important consideration in dealing with cases of elder abuse, which distinguishes it from child abuse, is that the competent elderly individual has control over the assessment and the intervention. It is common for elderly individuals to refuse evaluation or intervention in cases of abuse and neglect, often because of their fear of reprisals, feelings of hopelessness, or lack of confidence in the medical system.

With regard to detection, O'Malley and co-workers[10] identify seven characteristics of patients who are at risk for elderly abuse and neglect (Table 14–1). Assessment should include not only the possibility of the presence of abuse and neglect, but a careful evaluation of the risk of severe harm and how imminent that harm is likely to be. Through a comprehensive assessment, one can determine by the severity and likelihood of imminent harm whether an individual should be removed from the environment, or whether more paced approaches might be reasonable. In many cases, the goal is not to eliminate abuse and neglect, but rather to limit it to the point where it is tolerable for the patient and the risk is markedly diminished. Recalling that a competent elderly individual has control over the assessment and the intervention, one needs to take into account the needs of the patient for interaction with the family and other members of the informal support system. One should also

Table 14–1 ELDERLY PERSONS AT RISK FOR ABUSE AND NEGLECT

1. Those with accelerating care needs because of progressive or unstable conditions such as Alzheimer disease, parkinsonism, or severe strokes that exceed or will soon exceed their caretaker's ability to meet them.
2. Those with family members having a history of criminal or violent behavior.
3. Those with a family history of child or spouse abuse.
4. Those whose caretakers manifest signs of stress such as depression, anxiety, or "burnout."
5. Those who abuse drugs or alcohol or who live with family members who do.
6. Those whose caretakers are under sudden increased stress, for example, due to loss of job, health, or spouse.
7. Those who reside in an institution with the reputation of providing inadequate care.

Source: Adapted from President's Commission for the Study of Ethical Problems in Medicine and Biomedical and Behavioral Research.[13]

take into account that overzealous management of a problem, including premature removal of a patient from a neglectful or potentially abusive environment, generally will result in admission of the patient to a long-term care facility. Many older patients would prefer to be in a neglectful or even slightly abusive environment than to be institutionalized.[5,12,15,17]

REFERENCES

1. Administration on Aging. Federal Council on Aging Bicentennial Charter. Department of Health and Human Services, Washington, DC, 1976.
2. Bedell, SE, Pelle, D, Maher, PL, and Cleary, PD: Do not resuscitate orders for critically ill patients in the hospital: How are they used and what is their impact. JAMA 256:233–237, 1986.
3. Cassel, CK, Feier, DE, and Traines, ML: Selected bibliography of recent articles in ethics and geriatrics. J Am Geriatr Soc 34:399–409, 1986.
4. Dubler, NN: Some Legal and Moral Issues Surrounding Informed Consent for Treatment and Research Involving the Cognitively Impaired Elderly. In Karp, MB, Pies, HE, and Douders, AE (eds): Legal and Ethical Aspects of Health Care for the Elderly. Health Administration Press, Ann Arbor, 1985.
5. Fulmer, T and O'Malley, TA: Inadequate Care of the Elderly: A Health Care Perspective on Abuse and Neglect. Springer, New York, 1987.
6. Nursing Home Patient's Bill of Rights. See Code of Federal Regulations, 20 CFR 405.1121 (K) and 45 CFR 249.12(a)(1)b, 1974.
7. Office of Technology Assessment. Life-Sustaining Technologies and the Elderly. OTA—BA-306. US Government Printing Office, Washington, DC, 1987.
8. Older Americans Act, public Law 89-73, July 14, 1965 and as amended, Public Law 95-65, July 11, 1977.
9. O'Malley, HC, Segars, H, Perez, R, Mitchell, Z, and Knuetel, GM: Elder Abuse in Massachusetts: A Survey of Professionals and Paraprofessionals; Legal Research and Services for the Elderly. Boston, MA, 1979.
10. O'Malley, TA and Fulmer, T: In Rowe, RW and Besdine, RW (eds): Abuse, Neglect and Inadequate Care. In Geriatric Medicine, ed 2. Little, Brown & Co, Boston, MA, 1988, pp 89–98.
11. O'Malley, TA, Everitt, DE, O'Malley, HC, and Campion, EW: Identifying and preventing family mediated abuse and neglect of elderly persons. Ann Intern Med 98:998–1005, 1983.
12. Pillemer, CN and Wolf, R (eds): Elder Abuse: Conflict in the Family. Auburn House, Dover, MA, 1986.
13. President's Commission for the Study of Ethical Problems in Medicine and Biomedical and Behavioral Research: Deciding to Forego Life-Sustaining Treatment. US Government Printing Office, Washington, DC, 1983.
14. President's Commission for the Study of Ethical Problems in Medicine and Biomedical and Behavioral Research: Making Health Care Decisions, Vol I. US Government Printing Office, Washington DC, 1983.
15. US Department of Health and Human Services. Family Violence: Intervention Strategies. DHHS Pub. No. (OHDS) 80-30258. US Government Printing Office, Washington, DC, 1980.
16. Warren, JW, Sobal, J, Tenney, JH, Hoopes, JM, Damron, D, Levenson, S, DeForge, BR, and Muncie, HL: Informed consent by proxy. N Engl J Med 315:1124–1128, 1986.
17. Wolf, RS, Godkin, MA, and Pillemer, KA: Elder Abuse and Neglect: Final Report from Three Model Projects. University Center on Aging, Worcester, MA, 1984.

Index

An "f" following a page number indicates a figure; a "t" following a page number indicates a table.